A Collection of Classics in
Psychiatric Nursing Literature

A Collection of Classics in Psychiatric Nursing Literature

Editors:
Shirley A. Smoyak, RN, PhD
Sheila Rouslin, RN, MS

Library of Congress Catalog Number: 82-061592
ISBN: 0-913590-96-7
Printed in the United States of America by:
Charles B. Slack, Inc.
6900 Grove Road
Thorofare, NJ 08086

For Neil and Aaron

Contents

Introduction

Although psychiatric nursing has a hundred-year history of education and practice in the United States, it does not have a hundred-year history of specialty publication. However, publication was not far behind the 1882 date of the establishment of the first formally organized program for nurses in a psychiatric hospital. Indeed, it was in 1891 that Annie Payson Call, a nurse of "nervous patients," wrote what might be called the first book by a nurse on a psychological philosophy of treatment entitled *Power Through Repose.* Between that date and the publication of the first textbook on psychiatric nursing itself, written by Harriet Bailey in 1920, there were three possible outlets for the written word on psychiatric nursing. One was through the convention proceedings of organizations that were to become the National League for Nursing and the American Nurses' Association; another through *Trained Nurse and Hospital Review*, established in 1882; and another through the *American Journal of Nursing*, established in 1900.

It was to be sixty-three years into the century before the publication of specialty journals in psychiatric nursing in 1963: *The Journal of Psychiatric Nursing* (now *Journal of Psychosocial Nursing and Mental Health Services*) and *Perspectives in Psychiatric Care.* In the interim, psychiatric nurses published their works in *Nursing World* (established in 1950, formerly titled *Trained Nurse and Hospital Review*), in the *American Journal of Nursing*, in *Nursing Research* (established in 1951) and in *Nursing Outlook* (established in 1952). In addition, while some nurses published their writing in specialty journals of other psychiatric disciplines, others published through the National League for Nursing's *League Exchange Series.*

The League Exchange, Series No. 26, Aspects of Psychiatric Nursing, made available materials on psychiatric nursing that were not published elsewhere. Recognizing the lack of suitable publication media, the National League for Nursing urged members to write reports and submit them for consideration for publication. *Aspects of Psychiatric Nursing* was but one of forty-four nursing publications of the League Exchange. It was published in 1957, assisted through grants from the National Institute of Mental Health. Published papers were gathered from five regional conferences and one national conference on psychiatric nursing education in which nurses, psychiatrists and social scientists were asked to participate. This Series was divided into four sections: A. Concepts of Nursing Care; B. Therapeutic Concepts; C. Administration; and D. Education.

In a way, this Series was a prelude to the psychiatric nursing specialty journals, its contents providing a framework of basic components involved in the education for and practice of psychiatric nursing. Further, it was oriented in a cognitive direction, setting a tone of inquiry and suggesting theory-based therapeutic practice.

Psychiatric nursing had three staunch supporters who substantially aided the causes of including psychiatric nursing concepts into the whole of nursing and in promoting publication of psychiatric nursing papers. Julia Miller and Helen Nahm, who were in executive positions at the National League for Nursing, and Jeanette White, a psychiatric nurse who was an editor at the American Journal of Nursing, are to be recognized for their important roles in the development of the specialty.

Beginning in 1943, when the term "clinical specialist in psychiatric nursing" first appeared in the catalogue of program offerings in nursing education at The Catholic University of America, there arose many psychiatric nurses who became leaders overnight, particularly in graduate education, but also in consultation and practice. The list of these psychiatric nursing leaders enlarged when, in 1946, funds for graduate study in psychiatric nursing became available under the Mental Health Act. These leaders and their students were among the early contributors to the literature in psychiatric nursing:

Madge Bauman
Barbara Bernard
Kathleen Black
Annie Laurie Crawford
Nora Cline
Laura Fitzsimmons*
Lavonne Fry
Lee Fuller
Esther A. Garrison
Winifred Gibson
Ruth Gilbert*
Rose Godbout
Mildred Gottdank
Dorothy Gregg
Anne Hargreaves
Marion E. Kalkman
Cecile Lediger
Eleanor Lewis
Garland Lewis
Marguerite Manfreda
Ruth Matheney*
Anne K. McGibbon*
Dorothy Mereness
Agnes B. Middleton
Tirzah Morgan*
Theresa G. Muller*
Hildegard E. Peplau
Mary Redmond*
Alice Robinson
Mary M. Schmitt
Katherine Steele*
Dorris Stewart
Frances Theilbar*
Mary Topalis
Ruth von Bergen
Jeanette White*

*Deceased

However, while *Aspects of Psychiatric Nursing* provided material for a sound working basis for clinical practice, administration, and education, it tended to reach the educator audience and clinicians in academia more than it did the practicing clinical and administrative audiences.

All publishing patterns, however, had limitations. Since the nonspecialty nursing journals published articles in all areas of nursing, the number of psychiatric nursing specialty articles submitted for publication far exceeded the number that could be accepted. Furthermore, the first responsibility of specialty journals in other disciplines and professions was to publish their own members' work, not that of psychiatric nurses. Thus, for the first sixty-two years of this century, publication through a professional association and through professional periodicals was, at best, severely limited for psychiatric nurses, and, at worst, through omission or unavailability, not encouraged.

Interestingly, limited space and limited numbers of professional association contributors *did not* deter writing efforts. In fact, it was during this era that psychiatric nurses turned to writing books.

From 1952 onward, psychiatric nursing textbooks took a decided turn toward educated scrutiny of clinical work. With the publication of Peplau's book, *Interpersonal Relations in Nursing,* no subsequent psychiatric nursing text could ignore the influence of some notion of the "nurse-patient relationship," the "therapeutic interview," or the "participant observer" role of the psychiatric nurse. The nurse was now to be seen as an active, knowledgeable, knowledge-seeking therapeutic agent in work with patients. In one way or another, the impact of Peplau's introduction of an interpersonal concept of psychiatric nursing was reflected in books in the 1950's and 1960's such as the following: Kalkman's *Introduction to Psychiatric Nursing,* Mereness and Karnosh's *Psychiatry for Nurses,* Burton's *Personal, Impersonal and Interpersonal Relations,* Schwartz and Schokley's *The Nurse and the Mental Patient,* Muller's *The Nature and Direction of Psychiatric Nursing,* Hofling and Leininger's *Basic Psychiatric Concepts in Nursing,* Orlando's *The Dynamic Nurse-Patient Relationship,* Armstrong and Rouslin's *Group Psychotherapy in Nursing Practice,* Burd and Marshall's *Some Clinical Approaches in Psychiatric Nursing,* Hays and Larsen's *Interacting with Patients,* Bermosk and Mordan's *Interviewing in Nursing,* Manaser and Werner's *Instruments for the Study of the Nurse-Patient Relationship,* and Ujhely's *Determinants of the Nurse-Patient Relationship.*

The publication of books, nevertheless, brought with it several problems. First, these books tended to reach a growing but limited audience; educators and their students had the time and inclination to make their way through entire books, but the more pragmatic clinicians, pressed with the urgency of patient demands, could not afford such time and energy. As time progressed, books began to address the needs of the practicing clinician.

A second problem was that theory and practice presented in book form could not be critically examined and appraised in the process of its development the way it could be if it were to appear in smaller units, more quickly, through periodical literature. For theory to influence clinical practice, and vice versa, both writer and reader must have a vehicle for ongoing exchange; books inhibit rather than facilitate such an exchange process. And a third problem was that books tended to be written by nursing leaders or those to become leaders, especially in education. While that in itself was not a problem, the fact was that many competent clinicians who might not have had the inclination to write books, but could have contributed to specialty periodical literature, did not become authors. Had journals been in existence, they would have been a resource for clinician-writers. In the 1960's, the Burd and Marshall book served as the only available collection of previously unpublished papers, but these were limited to papers that had emerged from the Rutgers program in advanced psychiatric nursing.

In 1958, an historic film, Psychiatric Nursing: Nurse-Patient Relationships, was produced by the American Nurses' Association, the National League for Nursing, and Smith Kline & French Company. The free film, made widely available by Smith Kline & French Company, won several awards and stimulated publications related to clinical interactions of nurses with psychiatric patients. In general, however, 16mm films, like books, had response-time features inhibiting communication. But with the 1960's came video cassettes. They were welcomed for their live recording, easy interruption-for-discussion, and easy access capabilities. The video cassette and its counterpart, the cassette tape recorder, replacing the unwieldy reel-to-reel, brought psychiatric nursing concepts within reach and facilitated the immediate response of most psychiatric nurses.

When psychiatric nursing specialty journals became a reality in 1963, psychiatric nurses had the opportunity to communicate and critique the published theory, clinical practice, and educational and administrative practices of their colleagues in writing and with greater frequency than in past years. From that point on, as became so clear at a conference on "The State of the Art of Psychiatric Nursing" sponsored by the National Institute of Mental Health and Rutgers University, the periodical literature in psychiatric nursing proliferated. At that conference in 1974, a crucial, critical assessment of psychiatric nursing's components, as expressed through much of the literature from 1946 onward, was conscientiously presented in the papers constituting the proceedings.

It is now eight years since the "State of the Art" Conference. Obviously it is impractical to reproduce in one volume all significant books, articles, and reviews published since psychiatric nurses began to publish their ideas and observations. The books and periodical literature are readily available from most university libraries.

What *is* feasible is to provide the reader with some sense of the history and focus of psychiatric nursing through the written word prior to 1963. By doing so, today's psychiatric nurse can be exposed to the profession's roots, roots that otherwise would be lost, remaining only in the memory of the early leaders and their students and on the pages of certain documents currently uncirculated or out of print. With this in mind, the effort in this book is toward presenting psychiatric nursing "classics." For this purpose, a classic is defined as: 1. an important, early, unpublished work; 2. a selected publication that has significantly contributed to the field but is not readily available or was not widely disseminated when originally published; or 3. a selected article originally published in non-psychiatric nursing journals before psychiatric nurses had their own journals. All "classics" were written before 1963. Surely the names of early, significant contributors to psychiatric nursing literature have been inadvertently omitted. In the event that errors of omission are found by the reader, the editors welcome the information so that corrections can be made.

It should be noted that the decision to include these materials does not represent endorsement of either the ideas presented or their authors by the editors or by the *Journal of Psychosocial Nursing and Mental Health Services.* Additionally, these are not the only significant pieces of nursing literature from the time period covered. Rather, the material included represents selections of those psychiatric nurses who, within the constraints of severe time limitations, selected and retrieved significant portions of psychiatric nursing writings. A national advisory panel was constituted in January, 1982 in order to assure as thorough a search process as possible. For their work on the advisory panel, thanks are due to: Nancy Burke, Ann Cain, William Field, Doris Greiner, Carol Hartman, and Holly Wilson. In addition, the work of some twenty-six psychiatric nurses who assisted the advisory panel is greatly appreciated. In responding to the call for selections, they submitted substantial lists of suggestions.

The editors extend appreciation to those psychiatric nurses who helped bring psychiatric nursing into its historical perspective.

SHIRLEY SMOYAK
SHEILA ROUSLIN
May, 1982

A Collection of Classics in Psychiatric Nursing Literature

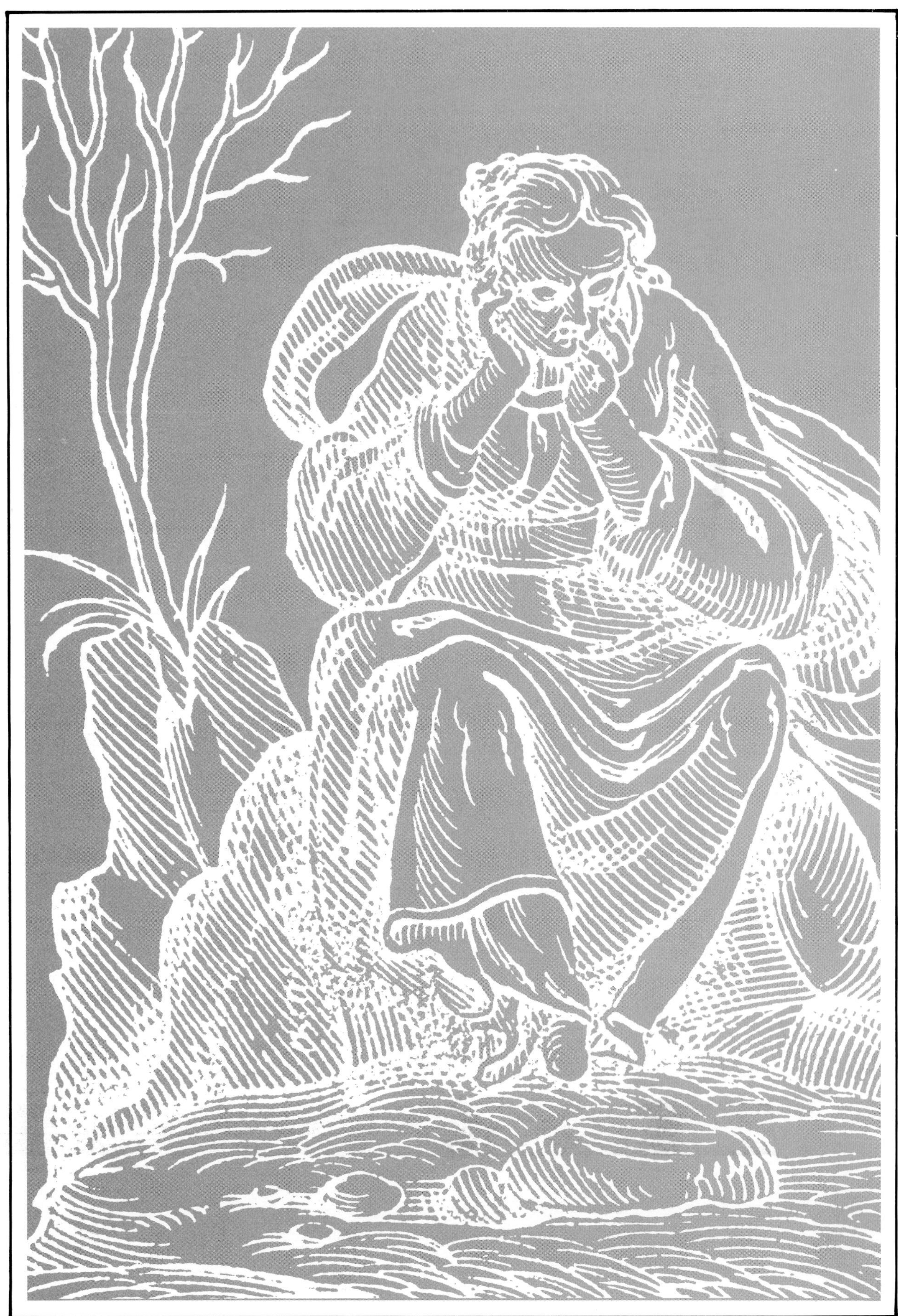

Important, Early, Unpublished Papers

Introduction

This section is composed of previously unpublished papers. Some, such as the Crawford papers and an accompanying "letter of rejection," have been virtually unshared with the psychiatric nursing community. Others, such as the Peplau paper on the workrole of the clinical specialist and the Peplau paper known unofficially by many as the "Williamsburg Report," are familiar to those educators and students of the late 1950's and early 1960's, but represent an unknown piece of history to today's psychiatric nurses and students. The content of some papers, such as the Norris paper on the teacher's use of self and Rector's work on hallucinations, has become so absorbed into the fabric of psychiatric nursing's education and practice that their origin has been forgotten. Each of these papers has had considerable impact on the field and is an integral part of psychiatric nursing's history.

Psychiatry: A Nursing Essential

Annie Laurie Crawford, R.N., B.S.

This paper was read at the South Carolina State Nurses' Association Annual Convention, October 6, 1934.

From Out of the Shadows

In the light of our modern understanding of mental and nervous disorders, it is not surprising to find that psychiatric nursing was recognized many thousands of years ago. In tracing its history we find that as civilization has risen and fallen, so has this important field of nursing. While the term "psychiatric nurse" is a fairly recent one, we find recorded evidences of a high type of specialized mental care in Egypt three thousand years before the time of Christ.

In the Greek temples, during the period of Aesculapius, the sick were treated. From far and near they came. The technique then used is interesting in its similarity to methods valuable even today. The patient was not treated at once upon admission, but placed in an Inn outside the temple, and made to observe certain rules of purification before he would be seen by the gods. He must not drink wine, must rest and diet, and bathe in cold salt water. Although the patient did not know this, it was indeed the first steps of his treatment, and this practice alone was often responsible for his betterment. Each day the patients were assembled and heard read the list of those cured by the gods, and thus gained confidence. The names of those who died probably did not appear. We also surmise that those cured seemingly by miracles were the auto-toxic, hysteric, or of "upset nerves." Much of the treatment was in no way beneficial, except as it enhanced the patient's confidence and contributed the assurance that he would be well. So sleep would come, as the gods had said, and their suggestions, combined with the simple hygienic living, practiced in preparation for the visit of the gods, added to the helpful planned attentions, proving definitely curative.

From Greek Mythology, we turn momentarily to the Bible, and quote three verses from the sixteenth chapter of First Samuel, relating a very beautiful example of psychiatric nursing: "And Saul's servant said unto him, Behold now, an evil spirit from God troubleth thee. Let the Lord now command thy servants, which are before thee, to seek out a man who is a cunning player on an harp: and it shall come to pass, when the evil spirit from God is upon thee, that he shall play with his hand, and thou shalt be well. And it came to pass, when the evil spirit from God was upon Saul, that David took an harp, and played with his hand: so Saul was refreshed and was well, and the evil spirit departed from him."

In the fifth century before Christ, a man was born who was to be not only the Father of Medicine, but the Father of Modern Psychiatry as well. For a hundred centuries man had struggled against disease, but always with his attention fixed on the invasion of the mind and body by spirits or demons as the cause of the malady. Hipprocrates, born on the Island of Cos, about 460 B.C., a member of the Guild of Aesculapidiae, all of whom claimed to be direct descendants of Aesculapius, taught that disease was to be found in nature, in the workings of the body, in the earthly surroundings of man. Quoting from his writings we are struck with the similarity of his theories to those of the psychiatrists of today who are bio-chemists: "As long as the brain is at rest, the man enjoys his reason, but the deprivement of the brain arises from phlegm and bile. Those who are mad from phlegm are quiet and do not cry and make a noise, but those from bile are vociferous malignant, and will not be quiet, but are always doing something improper. It is the brain which interprets the understanding...and therefore an extremely attenuated diet must be used....Melancholic diseases are most particularly exaggerated by beef....The physician must not only be prepared to do what is right himself, but also to make his patients, the attendants and externals cooperate." We recognize the external soundness of many of the ideas set forth in these writings.

From Hippocrates' time all medicine suffered a decline, and the humane care and treatment of the insane, the understanding care which would stimulate recovery or better adjustments in this unfortunate group, retreated into the murk of the "Dark Ages." As late as the middle of the seventeenth century it was commonplace for the curious to look upon the mentally ill, confined in filthy dungeons, by the payment of a fee collected and kept by the "keeper" for personal use, Middle Age "slumming" so to speak. Segregation was in no way a step to benefit the patient, but done merely as a protective measure to the community. Like wild beasts, inherently malicious, the mentally ill were brought under control by force.

The middle of the nineteenth century was to see the dawn of a new era in psychiatry, the beginning of sane care of the insane, the Humanitarian Movement. Phillippe Pinel, a prison physician in France, though timid and frail, sought, and by perseverance, secured from the Commune permission to remove the manacles and chains from the insane under his care, assured, we may be certain, that the responsibility must be his entirely, should harm come to him at the hands of his patients. The experiment proved successful, and gradually there spread among the physicians of Europe a conviction that Pinel's theory that insanity was an *illness* was correct, and here and there a hospital utilizing humane treatment was opened.

To an American woman, however, we owe the conception of a new ideal, sympathy for the mentally ill. Miss Dorothea Linde Dix, a Boston school teacher, spent more than forty years during the last half of the nineteenth century inspecting and describing conditions in prisons, almshouses, and the hospitals of this country, to the end that more than thirty state hospitals for the care and treatment of the insane were built, a direct result of her influence. Truly Dr. Charles N. Nichols of Bloomingdale Hospital could write after Miss Dix's death, "Thus has died and been laid to rest in the most quiet, unostentatious way, the most useful and distinguished woman America has yet produced."

So from out of the shadows we come to consider:

Psychiatric Nursing of Today

The past thirty years has seen more growth in this field than in any other branch of nursing.

Today the theory and practice of psychiatry includes all helpful familiarity with personality development and personality problems. Florence Nightingale once said, "A conscientious nurse is not necessarily an observing nurse, and life or death may lie with the good observer." With what emphasis we teach this principle to the psychiatric nurse! She must be trained to the keenest observation of her patient, to recognize in the depressed patient the symptoms which all too often, unnoticed, may precede suicide.

To see the underlying cause of the baffling retreat from reality of the neurotic individual, consider the following facts. A so-called "nervous" wife is probably unprepared to meet the demands which society makes upon the family of an aggressive, ambitious, and more than ordinarily successful business or professional man. Unconsciously desiring to avoid those situations in which she feels insecure or inferior, she finds an acceptable excuse in physical "ailments." The term ailments we use advisedly because what word can better describe the variety of symptoms presented by this group? The intelligent psychiatric nurse is promptly cognizant of the true difficulty, and brings to her patient not physical comfort alone, but institutes a program of reeducation. This, intelligently carried out, returns the patient to her home, and to the formerly distressing situation, fortified primarily by insight into her problem, and with determination to master it. This is only one example among hundreds of the broad training, deep insight, intelligence and social consciousness necessary for successful psychiatric nursing, the demands strikingly, often strangely, diverse from general hospital training.

With over 50% of all hospital beds in the United States already utilized for mental and nervous patients, the number who either consult the psychiatrist, visit mental hygiene clinics, or become hospitalized for periods of varying lengths is increasing annually. Does it not then become imperative that the nursing profession meet this need squarely and intelligently with an adequately trained personnel, trained especially in view of the modern program of re-education directed toward the ultimate goal which every psychiatrist desires for his patient, the assimilation of his illness. No longer do we cloak with evasions a frank discussion with the patient of the nature and significance of his mental disturbance. Understanding this, the pattern for living wisely will, in so far as is possible, avert subsequent attacks. Much of the attainment of this goal is in the hands of the nurse. She shall be blessed with those rare qualities so necessary in the nurse specializing in mental and nervous disorders. First, an ability to look upon her patient as ill and needing help, rather than as possessed with some terrible affliction which is to be tolerated, but not discussed. Second, the patience and the ability to convince the ill person of this fact. And above all, that God-given blessing, common sense. Given these qualities, she is indeed a psychiatric nurse of the highest type.

Let us, for a moment, discuss the qualities listed above in their relative importance with reference to general nursing. Patience, that virtue extolled by poets, husbands and wives alike through countless ages, plays a vital part in the improvement or recovery of any illness, but in diseases of the mind and nervous system, recovery is usually more deliberate than in the average physical illness. Hence a program of activity which will fill the long days of waiting till the depression lifts, or the confusion gives way to clear thinking and constructive self-planning, is most essential. Our nervous systems, unlike the average gastro-intestinal tract which rids itself of the unwelcome, pronto, often suffers long in silence or with only unheeded warnings until much damage has been done.

Then, months of careful treatment are required to bring it back to normal. Remember, skin, bone and muscle tissue, damaged, tend to rapid healing. Nerve and brain tissue, misused, recover sluggishly. During this time it is the nurse who listens sympathetically to the expressions of hopelessness; it is she who directs the limping mind to productive interests and activities in keeping with the ill one's reduced capacity. Again, when the patient emerges from the depths she will probably rebound to abnormal emotional heights, and it is the intelligent nurse who will conserve these activities from the otherwise most certain wastage. This all, every hour, exacts trained patience. Much of the time the patient can offer no whole-hearted cooperation in assisting to her own recovery. Complaining resistance to the best that the nurse is giving may be expected. Thus, patience and perseverance, even in the face of little evidence of accomplishment, must be the fortress of the psychiatric nurse.

These qualities, while recognized as important, are rarely stressed as first essentials in the nurse training for general nursing. Mechanical perfection, clock-like administration of those aids to normal recovery from various physical ills, are generally taught first, and rightly so. But what of the combination; is it not toward that Mecca we journey?

The patient is indeed rare who, suffering from any illness, does not need sympathetic understanding, and today we dare call no understanding sympathetic which is not intelligent, and modern psychiatric nursing must above all be intelligent.

With this standard in mind let us for a moment go beyond today, and think briefly on:

The Ideal of Psychiatric Nursing

This, like all branches of nursing, accepts prevention as the ideal. The machine age has practically hurled us forward into such complex living as our forefathers could not even visualize, and it is due to the resultant emotional strain that the large increase in the maladjusted,the borderline, and the frankly psychotic is credited. Most of the functional nervous disorders are emotional rather than intellectual. Mental hygiene clinics, with well-trained personnel, are gradually being established, and the theme of their work is prevention. We think of prevention as the preparation to meet change. We must develop the fearless courage to try what is new, while holding fast our faith in the proven good of the old. The challenge toward a world of less maladjustment and more integrated completeness and satisfaction in life is like the lamp of our Mother of Modern Nursing, ever a-glow.

Previously in our discussion we have given much thought to the justification of our title, and now it seems fitting to discuss it from a practical view point, hence the "headline" of the concluding paragraph.

Practically Speaking

At the risk of being misunderstood by the ninety percent of nurses who are general- rather than psychiatric-trained, we are going to tell you that the general hospital has all too often contributed toward providing the psychiatric hospital with patients. Please consider *with us* the situation for a moment, and you may agree that this is true, not through any failure of the general hospital nurse to care for her patient in a most acceptable manner, but by the failure, through lack of understanding and training, to sense the problem of the neurotic individual, and to treat him in a manner which discourages rather than enhances the neuroticism.

The neurotic patient, all too often, leaves the general hospital more fearful, more dependent, more truly invalidized than when he entered. The suggestible patient can seize upon any statement of the nurse to apply it unto himself, and quite adroitly encourage her to discuss symptoms, any symptom, with their relative danger to the individual. These patients are past masters in eliciting information concerning the other patients in the hospital; they are so interested and are such good listeners that the nurse, quite without realizing it, provides them with a list of suggestions which, upon returning home, and used as practice material on the family, sends the head of the house to a psychiatrist in consternation. More often than any one of them will tell you, the interview begins in this fashion, "Oh, Doctor, my wife is in a terrible fix; she had her appendix out three months ago and has never gotten well. She came from the hospital on the tenth day, but she just doesn't seem to get her strength back, and lately she complains of so many things." Thus we see the onset of the neurasthenic or hysteric illness. Under the care of the psychiatrist we find him and his specialized nurse painstakingly replacing the thought suggestions received in the general hospital. Let us hope they succeed in restoring this patient to usefulness, rescuing her from becoming a whining, sympathy-craving specimen of humanity.

This patient, and countless others, entered the general hospital conditioned for a neurotic reaction.

Her nervous system was not a sturdy one, and the natural shock of an operation, combined with the solicitous care of a nurse who spent hours concentrating on the physical comfort of the patient, serves to center her interest in her symptoms to the end that bigger and better ones are discovered. An interesting illustration of this is the case of the little girl who had her first illness at about the age of six. Her brothers and sisters gave her their choicest toys; the imported trained nurse planned comforts for her constantly, and aunts and uncles visited and inquired almost every day. Each morning when she was asked how she felt today, her reply was, "Just a little bit worster, this morning, thank you."

Today, wise nurses are recognizing this damaging possibility and more and more our accredited schools are adding courses in psychology, and are arranging affiliations with mental hospitals where the progressive nurse may learn the far-reaching necessity of caring for the patient as an individual, rather than as a case to be treated symptomatically.

Many a physician, crediting the nurse with intelligent observation, writes a p.r.n. order for sedative or narcotic drugs for his post-operative patient, and lives to regret his assumption that she would use this order judiciously. The danger to the weakling from drug addiction is ever-present. It is the intelligent and understanding nurse, trained to appreciate the usefulness of drugs which relieve intense suffering, and to abhor the damaging effect on the neurotic who becomes dependent thereon, who uses her ingenuity to make her patient comfortable. This nurse, when the period of acute suffering is reasonably over, assumes that a glass of hot milk, a tightening of the sheet, a warm bath for the patient's face, and careful adjustment of the light, will bring rest and comfort to her patient, and usually finds herself exactly right. The hypochondriac (one morbidly anxious about his physical health) we find in the general and psychiatric hospitals alike, presenting in the general hospital at first a most interesting list of unusual symptoms, intrigues the unsuspecting interns into all sorts of attention as they seek to discover an unusual disease. Truly, after weeks have passed, this patient becomes the despair, almost, of the nurse personnel in the average general hospital. Mrs. Jones eats well, sleeps well, and is bright and cheerful when her friends come, relating in the most minute detail her latest developments, assuring all that she just can't seem to get straightened out. "As soon as one part of me gets well, another shows up with a new disease," she says. Enjoying her poor health, a discerning nurse will soon observe.

Let us consider a middle aged woman of our acquaintance with many advantages of education and culture. It seemed regretfully necessary to her husband to consult a psychiatrist when, with other disturbing symptoms, she had had removed and replaced a bit of bridge work, consisting of one tooth, seventeen times. Could one wonder at the physician's first question, "Where is the dentist?" And yet the dentist had found himself rather helpless in the face of this situation. Mrs. Smith had been his patient for years, and he was reluctant to tell her husband that she was obviously "getting queer."

In order to be positively helpful to her patient, the nurse needs psychiatric training. All patients, no matter what the illness, are suggestible. The individual's ability to reason unemotionally, his self-confidence and cheerful outlook on life in general are naturally reduced by illness, while often the sense of inferiority is increased. The nurse, through her specialized training, acquires poise, knowing that tired irritability, emotional stress and tension are reflected in and exaggerated by a neurotic patient.

It is with this in mind that we would make a strong appeal to all nurses to develop a true sense of proportion. She must recognize the point of view of the patient, but maintain the logic of the situation in spite of the patient's whims. It is for the nurse to encourage independence in her patient, realizing that this becomes vital to perfect recovery. In regard to serenity and poise versus the Pollyanna attitude, probably the most apt comment in this connection is a quotation from a nervous, depressed patient who burst into the office of the Superintendent of Nurses in a psychiatric hospital and said, "If you don't move Miss Smith from the floor I am on, I shall lose my mind. She is forever and eternally smiling, a regular Pollyanna, and I can't stand it. Some mornings she comes on duty when I feel as if I cannot get through another day, bounces into my room with her cheerful, boisterous remarks and I want to scream. Why can't she realize that there is a time and place for all things, instead of eternally smiling when one doesn't even feel like seeing a smile?" In this case, the patient needed a smile, but a thoughtful one, one which bespoke a sympathetic understanding of the dark hours bound to come from time to time until the depression had definitely lifted, and not a grin reflecting the frothy optimism of a "shallow-pate." And this nurse had the best of intentions.

The physician is so obviously dependent on the report of the nurse in charge of his patient that it is of the utmost importance for her to be awake to the factors which influence the physical symptoms which her record discloses. It is known that anxiety will definitely alter the pulse rate, and that fear or worry in many cases retards recovery to a marked degree. Mood swings, surely, should always be reported together with the physical symptoms in any case of prolonged illness, that the physician may have these intelligent observations in planning his treatment.

We do not hesitate to emphasize the need of some psychiatric training in the life of every nurse who would represent her profession on the basis of modern standards. The psychiatrically trained nurse must remember, on the other hand, that all symptoms are not of mental origin. This fact has been long recognized so nurses trained in mental hospitals have wisely requested affiliation in general hospitals, thus avoiding the danger of overspecialization. Does it not seem rational, therefore, that the general hospital shall guarantee its nurse an equivalent knowledge of the workings of the patient's mind as the psychiatric nurse has of the workings of his body? Modern psychology reveals the close interrelation of the two; it recognizes the ceaseless interaction of one on the other. Should we not then more consistently work toward the ideal that every hospital shall graduate nurses trained in preventive and curative methods of caring for the inevitably associated physically and mentally ill?

The American
Journal of Nursing

1790 Broadway
New York, New York

Telephone
Circle 5-8000

March 31, 1942

Miss Annie Laurie Crawford
Box 390
Blackfoot, Idaho

Dear Miss Crawford:

I am so sorry that we are not "in the market" for an article on psychiatric nursing just now. The Journal carried a good deal on psychiatry in 1941, and we have at least one article on the subject in our files now, waiting till space is available. We have had so few articles from Idaho in the Journal that I am especially sorry to have to decline yours. Also, may I say that we rarely receive manuscripts with the bibliography and footnotes all in such good order.

We would so much like to know more about psychiatric nursing in Idaho especially at Blackfoot. Won't you let us know (for our information - not for publication) something about the hospital and the nursing program? Some of our questions are: Do you have affiliating or postgraduate students; where do you secure the graduate nurses for your staff; to what extent do schools of nursing in Idaho arrange for psychiatric nursing affiliations; and so on? I am also sending you one of our biographical data sheets which I hope you will be interested in filling out and returning to us. We are always eager to build up the Journal's files of biographical data.

I am returning your manuscript to you herewith with so much regret.

Sincerely yours,

Helen W. Munson

Mrs. Helen W. Munson, R.N.
Associate Editor

HWM:GH
ENC.

The Place of Mental Hygiene in a Health Program

Annie Laurie Crawford, R.N., B.S.

This paper was read at the annual meeting of the Idaho State Nurses' Association, September 6, 1940.

To place mental hygiene in a health program, let us consider briefly what mental hygiene implies. It is not difficult to stimulate a series of concrete mental pictures when we mention physical hygiene — sufficient warm clothing; adequate nourishing food; fresh air and sunshine; physical exercise; rest and sleep — these form the basic pattern of our response to any mention of physical hygiene. Such standards presume that, the individual being sound in organic and anatomic structure, he will enjoy good health. When we come to define mental hygiene, we are dealing with somewhat more abstract ideas. The New York State Health Commission defines mental hygiene as: "In its fullest meaning mental hygiene is directed to developing personality to its greatest possibilities, so that every individual gives his best to the world and knows the deep satisfaction of a life richly and fully lived."

Recently there has come to our attention a new term: psychosomatic medicine. Psychosomatic comes from a combining of two Greek words meaning mind and body. With this newer concept of the interrelation of physical and mental ills comes the awareness that any health program, to be effective, must correlate and integrate the factors which influence both mental and physical health. Perhaps a practical discussion of the opportunities presented various personnel for participation in a mental hygiene program will indicate what is meant by an integrated program.

The public health nurse makes her contact with the family as a unit. She is acquainted with all members of the family — adolescent boys and girls, the preschool child, and the infant. If she is socially conscious, discerning, and adequately trained, she can determine by observation and interested inquiry not only the physical health of the family, but something of the personal relationships which make up the life-pattern of each family. She will know whether the parents are in agreement on the set of moral and ethical values to be taught the children in order to make them happy and productive members of society; she will note indications that sixteen-year-old Mary is restless and moody, dissatisfied that she has plainer or fewer clothes than some of the other girls in her class; she will recognize the significance of the conspiracy among parents and brothers and sisters which protects from unpleasantness and coddles with sympathy six-year-old Johnny, only slightly crippled by poliomyelitis. She will be intelligently aware that adjustment and guidance in these problems is as necessary for adequate standards of health as is instruction in proper sterilization of the baby's bottles.

The public school teacher occupies a different, though no less important, place in the fostering and maintenance of mental health standards in a community. To her is given the opportunity, provided she is a well-integrated personality versed in the technique of human relationships as well as pedagogical methods, to direct activities in such a way that Samuel becomes more friendly and less shy; that Edith develops a sense of security in play instead of accepting her slight lameness as sufficient reason for isolation and self-pity; that John, outgoing and sure of himself, does not become more overbearing in his manner by monopolizing the class period or the playground; that Joan, sensitive to the bickerings of her parents at home, is stimulated by sympathetic understanding to give her attention to school work, instead of being punished for preoccupation and inattention. To meet satisfactorily these challenges for guidance is as essential in promotion of mental health as a hot lunch is in promoting physical health.

The part the social worker plays in our health program is a peculiarly important one. To her falls the task not only of determining the economic and social status of the family but of interpreting these in terms of community as well as individual welfare. She is frequently looked upon by the family as an interloper or meddler, prying into personal matters that do not concern her. She meets pride which refuses to accept charity; independence which manifests itself in an unwillingness to divulge even the most casual information concerning family matters; perhaps even a determination to continue standards of living and practices which are a detriment to community health and welfare. The social worker must come not as an investigator, but quite sincerely as a counselor and friend. She must develop a discrimination which expresses itself in an ability to offer moral support or sympathetic understanding, financial aid, or a positive, constructively critical attitude toward the potential or actual weakling.

Thus far I have spoken primarily in terms of ways

and means of insuring improved mental health through broader understanding of and directed attention toward the factors which enter into the making of mental health. Let us think briefly in terms of the usefulness and relationship of physical and mental hygiene in reducing the duration of illness and the probability of chronicity in the case of mental illness.

Most of you know that more than 50% of the hospital beds in the United States are occupied by patients suffering from various mental diseases. At least 15% of these illnesses are entirely preventable because 15% of all mental illness is caused by syphilis of the brain or central nervous system. Since a campaign to wipe out syphilis is being vigorously waged we can expect, by the end of the next quarter century, to see this 15% reduced to 1%.

In the mental hospitals we are concerned with two principles in treating mental diseases which directly concern the community. First of all is the absolute necessity for early diagnosis and treatment. Schizophrenia, or dementia praecox, is the most prevalent of all mental diseases. It occurs commonly in late adolescence or early adulthood and is characterized by emotional flatness and a gradual and progressive retreat from reality. Untreated patients often revert to a mere vegetative state. New developments in methods of treating this scourge of the young mind have, however, given us evidence that cases treated within the first six months of illness have up to 85% chance of recovery, while the case receiving initial treatment two years or more after the onset of illness has only a 10% to 15% chance of recovery and return to normal productive living. This statement alone should adequately emphasize our first principle.

Our second principle concerns the return of the patient to his normal place in the community when he has recovered from his illness. We do not regard with alarm the return from hospitalization of the person who has recovered from typhoid or pneumonia. Why then should we regard the person who has recovered from psychosis with suspicion and fear? Why should the recovered schizophrenic be stigmatized when the recovered typhoid patient is not? Typhoid is an entirely preventable disease. Moreover, it is a filth-borne disease; yet we do not lower our voices and glance significantly at the person who has spent two months in a hospital because he contracted typhoid. Frequently the attitude of a family or a community toward mental illness marks the difference between recovery and a progressive retreat to chronicity. Lack of the stamina necessary for the nervous system to withstand strain, or chemical and hormonal imbalance may precipitate a psychosis even in the presence of the best type of mental hygiene but, and this is important, that background of mental hygiene may be the factor which determines the insight and cooperation necessary for early and complete recovery. Therefore we would emphasize that it is not enough to insure early diagnosis and the most modern and scientific treatment. We must properly orient the patient's family and the community to the necessary environmental factors — the mental hygiene, if you please, which will contribute to the recovered patient's sense of security in the community. His readjustment to normal living and productivity will be in direct relationship to this sense of security.

When the Mental Hygiene Movement was instituted in 1908, the objectives as outlined by Clifford W. Beers and Dr. Adolph Meyer were: first, child guidance (and this was to include the guidance of normal healthy children as well as the maladjusted and handicapped); second, to aid in maintaining the normal individual at his highest functioning level; third, to prevent borderline conditions from developing into frank psychosis; fourth, to give skilled scientific care to the psychotic; and fifth, to aid in rehabilitation of the individual recovering from a psychosis.

In a practical approach to the place of mental hygiene in a health program, I have sought to indicate how these objectives may be met. I would also suggest for the individual worker a very real use of mental hygiene principles for himself — one cannot teach health standards effectively unless he practices them. For the group, I would suggest an integrated program planned so that each worker would function effectively in his own field with proper orientation to the part his co-workers will play in meeting the common goal. The theme of our convention, "Nursing for Better Health," is a timely one. A mentally and physically healthy society is a productive and contented society. We are faced today as never before in the history of our nation with the knowledge that the very foundation of our democracy rests upon our ability to function as productive society — as a mentally and physically healthy people.

Historical Development of Psychiatric Nursing: A Preliminary Statement of Some Facts and Trends

Hildegard E. Peplau, R.N., Ed.D.

A paper prepared for the Working Conference on Graduate Education in Psychiatric Nursing, held by the National League for Nursing at Williamsburg, Virginia, November 26-30, 1956, by Hildegard E. Peplau, R.N., Ed.D., Chairman, Psychiatric Nursing, College of Nursing, Rutgers, The State University, Newark, New Jersey.*

Here in Williamsburg, in 1773, the first psychiatric hospital in America was built. Now, in 1956, the National League for Nursing has brought together, in this historic city, a group of professional nurses who are specialists in graduate education in psychiatric nursing. This occasion provides an opportunity for nurses to confer with experts in allied disciplines about future directions of psychiatric nursing education and practice. These two facts mark the beginning and the end of a period of time in the history of America and of nursing, preceding this conference. In the course of the intervening 183 years, psychiatric nursing has been born and undergone many changes.

The Eastern Psychiatric Hospital, here in Williamsburg, was a going concern for 99 years, before training schools for nurses were formally established in 1872. It was not until 10 years later, in 1882, that "psychiatric nursing" actually got started with the opening of the training school for nurses at the McClean Hospital for the mentally ill, Waverly, Massachusetts. The workrole of the nurse in psychiatric facilities has had, therefore, a mere 74 years of historical development. In this paper, some of the facts and events related to this development are presented. A review of these materials may help serve the purpose of this conference, since guides for action in the future are also determinants, in some measure, of the continuing course of the history of psychiatric nursing. An examination of the turn of events, as they preceded this historic conference, can serve to pinpoint issues, illuminate trends, and can remind one of the long hard road that has been travelled in the establishment of psychiatric nursing, both as an aspect of all nursing and as a specialty in nursing.

In preparing this paper, the period in time, from 1773 to 1956, has arbitrarily been divided into five eras — each designated as a phase in the evolving history of psychiatric nursing. Each phase was determined and marked off, at its beginning and ending, by a specific event or occurrence which seemed to the author to have unusual significance, as if a greater step forward had thus been taken. Whether the phases stated are the best possible demarcation of dominant themes in the total history of psychiatric nursing to date can be left to more comprehensive study of the facts than was attempted for this paper. One day a competent historian will make this needed study available, taking into account the development of psychiatric nursing in the context of the evolution of total health services, and in the light of on-going changes in American society, and in relation to its contribution in the development of professional nursing.

The 183 years, from 1773-1956, can be divided into five phases, as follows:

I. 1773-1881 Background out of which emerged psychiatric nursing — 109 years

II. 1882-1914 Initial development of the work-role of nurse in psychiatric facilities —33 years

III. 1915-1935 Initial development of under-graduate psychiatric nursing education for all nurses — 21 years

IV. 1936-1945 Initial development of graduate education in psychiatric nursing — 10 years

V. 1946-1956 Widespread interest in psychiatric nursing education and initial development of consultation and research in psychiatric nursing practice — 10 years

Total — 183 years

What has been done in each phase has contributed something to the current status of psychiatric nursing. What has been accomplished has been due to the efforts of many nurses in many places, sometimes speaking as if in unison — sometimes expressing opposing views. As Roberts has pointed out: "Psychiatric nursing had no crusader to do for the schools what Dorothea Dix had done for the hospitals, although Linda Richards, Sara E. Parsons and Mary E. May struggled with the problem."[1]

*In the preparation of this work the assistance of the following persons is acknowledged: Margaret Larkin and Elizabeth Maloney, New Jersey State Hospital, Greystone Park, N.J.; Eleanor Franey, National League for Nursing Staff; and Mary M. Redmond: *Bibliography of Psychiatric Nursing References* (compiled from National League of Nursing Education Annual Reports — class material — The Catholic University of America, Washington, D.C.).

These nurses were among the many who served as leaders and spokesmen, keeping before the young and growing nursing profession the ever pressing problem of the care and understanding of persons in psychiatric facilities, and the preparation of nursing personnel for this work. But, most of all, Linda Richards — the first trained nurse in America — used every opportunity, direct and subtle, to keep before the nursing profession of her day the need for nurses not only in psychiatric facilities but also in tuberculosis hospitals. And so it is possible to say, from the dawn of nursing in America there has been a slowly evolving interest in psychiatric nursing as an important part of the care of all patients, and especially those in psychiatric facilities.

Phase I

Background Out of Which Emerged Psychiatric Nursing 1773-1881

In 1752, the first general hospital, Pennsylvania Hospital, admitted its first two patients. One was considered a "lunatic."[2,3] Even though the problem of care of the mentally ill thus presented itself at this very early point in the development of health services, it was too soon for public acceptance of the responsibility. By 1756, psychiatric patients at Pennsylvania Hospital were housed in the cellar. Attendants were called "cellkeepers" and their work consisted mainly of preventing escapes, securing conformity by physical punishment and mechanical restraints. These methods give a clue to the amount of anxiety that the observed behavior of psychiatric patients must have produced in the hospital workers. The public, however, had a responsibility to provide some form of care in the face of problems which the family and community, and even general hospital workers, could not handle with equanimity.

By 1773, a need was felt for specialized institutions of which the Eastern Lunatic Hospital, at Williamsburg, Virginia, was the first to be built. In 1765, just after Pennsylvania Hospital moved its psychiatric patients to the basement, and just before the Hospital here in Williamsburg had been built, the first medical school opened its doors. One hundred seven years would pass before a training school for nursing was started. The decision, therefore, about the form of institution and the pattern of care needed — for psychiatric patients at Pennsylvania Hospital — was made by laymen.

By 1783, Benjamin Rush had joined the staff of Pennsylvania Hospital and inaugurated the first course of study of mental illness. Meanwhile, in Philadelphia, the Friends encouraged the development of occupational means for effecting cures. Rush believed in the principle of education — the Friends believed in the principle of work; both combined to influence the emerging character of personnel and care programs.

The dominant emphasis in this era was on buildings, but there was interest also in the land, crops, and the task of feeding psychiatric patients. Two structural patterns emerged: the "Kirkbride plan" — which so long has dominated the architectural structure of psychiatric institutions — and the "cottage plan" which also can still be found in several states. These structures would ultimately influence the nursing program that could be designed by nurses for patients. By 1880 there were at least 30 hospitals built on the "Kirkbride plan," and also several on the "cottage" system.

As early as 1843, Dr. Thomas S. Kirkbride attempted to establish a training school for attendants at Pennsylvania Hospital — some 60 years after Dr. Rush began teaching about mental illness — some 13 years after "directions for attendants" were issued, in 1830, at both McClean and Worcester Hospitals. The time was not yet ripe for the development of a hospital worker to assist the physician in the care of mentally ill patients. Since the attendant "directions" predate nursing, Shyrock comments that "Hence the first interest in the training of nurses in these countries (England and America) may be claimed for the early asylum." However, in 1798 an organized course in nursing was being given at the New York Hospital, even though it was not until 1872 that training schools of nursing were established at the New England Hospital for Women and Children, and Woman's Hospital of Philadelphia. There apparently were no psychiatric services in either of these two hospitals at the time. In 1873, Linda Richards "graduated" as the first "trained nurse" in America and went to Bellevue as night superintendent — the first trained American woman to hold a hospital position.

The first phase — background out of which emerged psychiatric nursing — began with a need for personnel at Williamsburg, in 1773, a need that grew as more hospitals were built; the phase ended with the very early beginnings of what is now the profession of nursing. In this first phase psychiatric nursing was non-existent, although in 1878 Linda Richards collaborated with Dr. Edward Cowles in her organization of the training of the Boston City

Hospital. By 1879, "it was determined to establish a school for the training of attendants at McClean."[4] But, this interest in training personnel for psychiatric hospitals did not materialize in this era; only the need and the possibility of psychiatric nursing were there.

Phase II

Initial Development of the Workrole of Nurse in Psychiatric Facilities 1882-1914

In this second phase workers in psychiatric institutions were called "cellkeepers" at the outset, were then thought of as "custodial attendants," and slowly the concept of "nursing personnel" evolved.

In 1882, many persons were interested in the use of methods of "non-restraint" in the care of psychiatric patients — suggestion, persuasion and moral treatment were being discussed as more useful than former methods. Tucker, in a report to the government entitled "Lunacy in Many Lands," spoke firmly against the harsh measures still widely practiced.

> "Cages, iron chains, handcuffs, hobbles, straps, crib beds, and fixed chairs are common modes of restraint for patients, who being afforded no measure of occupation or diversion for mind or body, naturally become noisy and troublesome. The bath, either shower or immersion, is a favorite means of tranquilizing excited patients ...in some cases as punishment at the option of the attendants, without the sanction of a medical officer."[5]

Yet, Alabama, Columbus, and Norristown are reported as not using restraint in 1885. The plausible excuses given for using harsh means for controlling patients, seemed to be that hospital workers who cared for patients were unable to do otherwise, due to lack of education. It was now 39 years after Dr. Kirkbride's effort to start a training program for attendants, when, in 1882, such a program was started at McClean Hospital, Waverly, Massachusetts. This program soon became a training school for nurses, affiliated with a general hospital; it is still in operation today. It was the first formally organized school for nurses in a hospital for the mentally ill in the world.

By 1883, a similar school was established at Buffalo State Hospital — and soon there were many others. Even so, by 1891 there were only 35 schools of nursing and only 471 trained nurses.[6] And Harper Hospital had already adopted the eight-hour day.

Various explanations were given for this new development: Roberts states that "schools in Mental Hospitals developed because the Nightingale movement passed these institutions by." She comments that England had training standards for "mental nurses" before 1900, with emphasis on the administrative needs of the hospital rather than the education and professional growth of the nurse; in America, by 1906, the American Psychiatric Association had established standards here just as organized nursing was beginning its work to secure standards of nursing through state legislatures.

Bunker, quoting Zilboorg, states:

> "Since it enhanced the need for greater ingenuity in supervising and managing the mental patient, it naturally imposed the need for better training of supervisory personnel — the attendants and orderlies. This was the added circumstance which later created special training schools for psychiatric nurses."[7]

Malamud puts it this way:

> "The practice of good medical and surgical procedures made its way into some of the hospitals and had its effect not only upon the physicians but upon the rest of the personnel. One of the most important steps in the progress of psychiatric treatment was established in 1882 of the first nurses training school in a mental hospital at the McClean Hospital."[8]*

Meanwhile, the nursing profession was on the march: By 1893 the American Society of Superintendents of Training Schools (now the National League for Nursing) was formed. By 1897 the Nurses Associated Alumni of United States and Canada (now the American Nurses Association) was launched. By 1889 a toehold was gained in a university, when a course in hospital economics was offered for nurses under the auspices of Teachers College, Columbia University, and the International Council of Nurses was formed. And by 1900 there were 432 nursing schools in America.

Between these two events — the establishment of the McClean School and the establishment of an

*In Goodnow, Minnie, *Outlines of Nursing History*, Philadelphia, Saunders, 1935, p. 215, there appears a "composite picture of a fifteen-nurse class of 1886 at McClean Asylum, Waverly, Mass. (Century Magazine, November, 1887)." It prompts the question of why the faces of 15 nurses were submerged in the anonymous "composite picture" — one face.

organization of the members of the nursing profession — a "psychiatric nurse" made a very important contribution to the psychiatric literature of 1891. William James felt that the cause of "breakdowns" was related to "feelings of rush, hurry, tension, dissatisfaction, solicitude, and untoward anticipations." In this connection, James referred to the important work of Annie Payson Call, a nurse of nervous patients who worked out an unusually successful scheme of treatment and a philosophy of practice which is summed up in a remarkable book, *Power Through Repose.* Her methods were not purely physical as Weir Mitchell's were, at least theoretically. They involved relaxation exercises and mind training for rest, repose, and "power" for effective action. She believed that we have perverted nature's laws in our rush and strain of living. She advocated that one should learn to rest throughout the day by, for instance, relaxing while sitting in a train instead of trying to help it along, that one should learn to wait without tension and impatience, and that one should avoid rapid thought and misdirecting thought. She emphasized the effect of relaxed muscles in cultivating sleep. In her philosophy, Miss Call believed that body training was also mind training. To learn a new movement we must forget the old one and relax. She considered worry to be "brain tension" which leads to fatigue and illness. Along with her physical exercises and mind training, she utilized moral training in which she emphasized social relationships. As axioms, she used such thoughts as "One cannot be happy without considering others;" "One must develop tolerance;" "One must train oneself to yield as well as to direct."[9]

It is interesting that these techniques were extended and their significance supported by investigative evidence,[10] and were further developed in 1940,[11] yet no reference to their consideration or use by the nursing profession was found in the works consulted.

In 1894, Annual Reports of the American Society of Superintendents began to provide a vehicle for widespread dissemination of views of many nurses on their ideas and pressing problems. Maxwell[12] states that at the first convention "A gentleman made an appeal to our society, asking us to try to raise the standards of nursing in insane hospitals." The 1895 report indicates consideration of aspects of the psychiatric problem. Linda Richards, President, called for standards and uniformity of training of nurses in general, but commented specifically about "schools attached to special hospitals." Snively[13] stated that "schools attached to special hospitals... in the long run will benefit the nursing profession, and through them the general public. The effect will be to stimulate nurses to supplement the training they may have obtained...The aim is to make nurses all-around nurses, not those trained for specialties only." Drown,[14] in a paper given in 1895, said that "twenty years ago the hospitals for the insane in New England, in order to defend themselves from unworthy attendants who wandered from one asylum to another, contrived a plan by which all might be on their guard against such invaders." The plan is then described as an aid for general hospitals.

By 1896 the concerns were larger; the proceedings abound with discussion of "curriculum outlines," problems of the registries, and legal aspects of the nursing organization. But a list of "books on nursing" is recommended for use in the existing schools of nursing and C.K. Mill's text, *The Nervous and Insane,* is included.[15]

A year later, Mrs. Hunter (Isobel Hampton) Robb presented a provocative paper on "Nursing in the Smaller Hospitals and in those devoted to the care of Special Forms of Diseases." She made a plea for broader and more liberal education "of all who call themselves trained nurses." Reasons for the existence of these schools were cited. "If we think of the future of the women who enter these hospitals, it would seem that but little can be said in justification...free labor is more important to the hospitals...separate hospitals for the insane are necessities. It does not follow that they should organize a training school."[16] Five alternative courses of action which could be taken by such institutions were suggested:

1. Plan for nursing by graduates enrolled in post graduate programs;
2. Employ paid graduate nurse staffs;
3. Use attendants under the supervision of trained nurses;
4. Adopt a system of co-operative nursing; and
5. Offer nursing by members of religious orders who have had prior training.

Mrs. Robb continued: "Training schools in connection with hospitals for the insane are as yet few in number, but the tendency to increase them is growing and undoubtedly, in the care of this class of patients, there is room for much improvement. But can these hospitals, anymore than any special hospitals, offer sufficient variety in nursing to produce all-around trained nurses?"

From the references reviewed for this paper, admittedly an inexhaustive search, the first paper on the workrole of nurse in psychiatric facilities was given in 1899. The paper, by Mary E. May, was entitled "The Work of Nursing The Insane."[17] It consisted of a description of "State Care," the system adopted in New York in 1830, problems in control, a description of administration, and a statement of the "insanity law" passed in 1890. By law, there were 12 hospitals for the mentally ill in New York State, each with its own training school developed since 1896. A curriculum is outlined and the program offered to patients is presented. The textbook used by students in these "schools of nursing" was written by Dr. P.W. Wise, then President of the Commission on Lunacy. Miss May stated that:

> "The nurse...gains a very fair knowledge of the work required in caring for the different kinds of cases of insanity. Graduate nurses are in charge of all wards and of most of the industrial departments."

The word "treatment," used in a pragmatic sense, was defined as: "...all that works not only for the relief and cure, but for the general welfare of the patient. Great stress is laid on moral treatment of the insane, and a nurse may spend hours getting a patient to do what it would require a few minutes of the nurse's time to accomplish in the general hospital, simply for the good it will do the patient." She specified that one difference in the treatment of general and psychiatric patients was that in the latter the treatment took longer.

In this paper it is stated that the Rochester Training School started before the compulsory law, "in order to raise the standard of nursing in that hospital, and the attendants were trained with a view to retaining their services to the hospital after graduation." It can be speculated that graduated nurses were expected to have some mobility, being able to move from one psychiatric hospital to another or even to a general hospital, but that attendants were — hopefully — immobilized by training if it was completed.

Miss May's paper was followed by a discussion of the program at Kankakee by Miss McMillan.[18] This nurse apparently had been asked to appraise the Kankakee program but was not connected with that hospital. She reported "having carefully studied the plan of teaching...the impression vividly remains that the course is such as to produce nurses thoroughly instructed in the modern methods of care of the sick, and in addition, to send forth graduates who have been given every opportunity of absorbing tact and wisdom in dealing with the diseased mind...also the tendency is to aid the pupil toward attaining those rare and enviable attributes — leniency and patience toward human imperfections and tenderness towards their frailties."

A Miss Brown was then asked to describe the McClean program, which she did. A Miss McDonnel from Albany, New York commented that she "thought it necessary to have nurses trained to care for the insane, but if they were trained only in hospitals for the insane they were not fitted to do general nursing. There is little surgical or medical service and no obstetrics in a hospital for the insane."

Discussion of these presentations continued. An experimental exchange program whereby students from a general hospital and some from Utica State Hospital were "exchanged" — each having a chance to show how the training received worked in the other type hospital — was reported. The "experiment was not a success." The idea of conducting training schools in mental hospitals in order to get better care for patients was reiterated over and over throughout these papers.

Keating, near the close of the meeting, suggested that "if an arrangement could be made by which those nurses could receive general training and our nurses could have some experience with the nervous and insane, both would be benefitted." This suggestion gave rise to discussion of practical problems: the psychiatric institution provided no opportunity for practice among private patients; the experience of registries "is they (the nurses graduated from mental hospital schools) can work in hospitals for the insane but they cannot do general nursing without further training." One graduate of a state hospital school agreed with this opinion.

Mrs. Robb closed the meeting saying, "We, as nurses, have a distinct responsibility toward the insane. We cannot fairly criticize the methods of those endeavoring to meet their needs unless we have something to offer."[19]

By 1906, "Affiliation of Training Schools" became a topic for discussion.[20] This interest may have stemmed from the affiliation between Massachusetts General and McClean, and it may also have derived from the content of the 1899 convention. Papers given at the conventions were the one source of fresh thought in nursing; they were quoted in subsequent papers. For example, Lawler quotes a paper given at the "11th Annual Convention" entitled "Nursing in Psychotherapy."[21]

Lawler stated, "We should and must know the basic principles of mind action and be able to recognize even a slight deviation from normal." She felt that "a very great responsibility attached to the nursing of the mentally unsound, and a far-reaching opportunity always comes to the nurse...."[22] In this paper the form of treatment given is described; it included isolation, rest, proper diet, and psychic measures. Psychotherapy, in the form of suggestion and persuasion, were used "to cure by...utilization of the intellect and will of the patient as far as possible." She felt the nurses needed a "doctrine of optimism," that this work required "a special temperament."

In discussing Lawler's paper, Davis stated:

> "In insane work you will find the greatest difficulty is that nurses were taught in general schools to nurse and to study their case intelligently; they know in a general way what is going on, what to expect, what certain medicines must be given; they know what will probably be the outcome... recovery or death. In the case of the insane patient we lack that study....You cannot say that this is that or the other kind of insanity, because he had so many other symptoms that we cannot classify him, and we have to study, if we study blindly. That is very unsatisfactory to the nurses because they want to know in what class to put their patient and what to expect."

Kraepelin's system of classification of mental disorders, based though it was upon symptoms rather than causes, offered a system of classification and the hope that causes would follow description of the disease entity; by 1896 Kraepelin's system had been introduced by Meyer and adopted at Worcester. Miss Davis' comment seems to indicate that its use had not yet reached into nursing education.

A number of other events were occurring or had transpired in psychiatry at this time and would later influence psychiatric nursing.

In 1883, Adolph Meyer began his work at Kankakee, Illinois, moving in 1902 to the Pathological Institute of New York State Hospitals (now Psychiatric Institute). Meyer enlisted the help of social workers to study the environment and promoted the principle that the patient and not the disease was the object of treatment. In 1894, S. Weir Mitchell's now famous address led to reforms in the care of patients and gave rise to further interest in personnel. In 1895, Breur and Freud published "Studies in Hysteria" and in 1909 Freud was invited to come to America by G. Stanley Hall, a psychologist. Here Freud gave the lecture series at Clark University's 20th anniversary, thereby stimulating diversity of opinion which was later to encourage new thought among American psychiatrists. It was in 1903 that Clifford Beers was discharged, after three years spent as a patient in a mental hospital, and by 1909, the National Committee for Mental Hygiene was organized. By 1899, the various states began to require that the superintendent of psychiatric institutions be a licensed physician.

None of these ideas are included in Lawler's paper or its discussion in 1909. Instead, it is asserted that "it is very difficult to make (nurses) enthusiastic in the care of (insane) because in most instances the cases cannot be reasoned with and the outlook is hopeless...what was the use in trying to do more (than routine) for one who was surely going from bad to worse." That there was no private duty but only hospital work, in the care of the insane, seemed to be a much-discussed drawback.

Delano, however, commented, "To me, the important thought is the question of prevention," but Davis pointed out that the problem here was the "obscurity of early symptoms." Williard, however, felt that the problem was due to the fact that "nurses received their training in wards where there has not been sufficient time to consider patients as individuals, at least not to the extent necessary to fit them for this particular work." Nutting closed the session with a statement that "we should prepare to give to the insane the best nursing possible."

In 1909, The American Society of Superintendents appointed a "Sectional Committee of the Committee on Education" to study the care problem and to present recommendations. The committee was composed of Sara Parsons, Amy Hilliard, Linda Richards and Elizabeth May. In 1910 this subcommittee presented its report, which was based upon correspondence inasmuch as members could not get together in person.[23] The committee recommended that schools affiliate with psychiatric hospitals so as to give "optional or elective courses to students in the third year, if they have an inclination ....They would get a broader vision, would learn to know something of this sadly misunderstood phase of sickness." The members of the committee were, however, in disagreement as to how long the affiliation should be. Miss Richards proposed six months, another member nine months, one member wanted three months, and the fourth member felt it would "be out of the question to introduce it into the general curriculum." At this meeting, an outline of a post-graduate course was read, and books were recommended including Clara Barrus, M.D., *Nursing the Insane,* MacMillan; Wm. A. White, *Outline of Psychiatry;* and Burr, *Elementary Psychology of the Nursing of the Insane.* Discussion of the report brought the comment that "affiliations will soon be arranged to help the nurse in private and and hospital work." The committee apparently then disbanded as no further references are made to it in the 1911 or subsequent reports.

At the 1910 convention, there was also presented a "Report of Post Graduate Work."[24] The purpose of post-graduate courses is stated: (1) to supply the deficiency of the mother school — "this purpose we contend the post-graduate course should not be called upon to serve"; (2) to become acquainted with recent methods; (3) to offer opportunity for specialization. There were then in operation four post-graduate courses in this field; Adams Nervine Asylum, Massachusetts; Kings Park State Hospital, New York; Rochester State Hospital, New York; and Sheppard and Enoch Pratt, Maryland.

The question of specialization had already been raised in the profession of nursing. In 1900, De Witt said, "There is no need to urge nurses to take up specialties for there is no such demand for specialists in the nursing as in the medical profession, and there will always be enough who have marked ability in certain directions to fill the ranks."[25] But another nurse read something in the Boston Medical and Surgical Journal in August of 1900, and she was sufficiently stimulated to write about it for the November 1900 publication in the American Journal of Nursing.[26] The paper also quoted the "seven propositions" from the Boston Journal:

1) That some cases of illness are simply neuroses without appreciable pathological lesions;
2) That causes capable of producing such neuroses may act while disease is present and should be guarded against;
3) Purely psychic causes, as shock, grief, and the like, may pave the way for, if not directly cause, profound pathological disturbance;
4) Attention to the psychic is capable under some conditions of so turning the scale to health that it may arrest, even perhaps cure, otherwise fatal pathological conditions;
5) Attention to the psychic should be considered a routine measure in the treatment of delirium from toxic causes as alcohol, belladonna, ether, and the like;
6) Attention to the psychic should also be considered a routine measure in the treatment and in the prevention of delirium in febrile states, as of typhoid;
7) Nurses should be able to enter into psychic relations with their patients; otherwise the value of their services is much lessened and they may be harmful.

The early issues of the Journal presented several papers on psychiatric work: one in 1902 by Dr. Gulick[27] in which facts about treatment are presented; and two papers in 1901 by nurses.[28,29] Chapman pointed out the "ominous fact of increase in the number of insane patients and that serious consideration of the problem was needed in order to safeguard the progress of the nations." Laird presented a brief history of nursing of the insane, a description of what these patients were like, and forms of treatment used. This latter paper was discussed from the floor by a delegate from the "Asylum Workers Association," an association of superintendents of nurses in asylums, which had as its purpose "To bring about higher standards of attendants."

Moreover, in all of the earlier issues of the journal, there was a section entitled "Hospital and Training School Items" written by Linda Richards.[30] These were brief newsy notes about events within or related to nursing. In most of these notes Miss Richards referred to psychiatric nursing — either by a factual description of a hospital or of a program. For example, in 1900 she wrote a factual report on the Massachusetts law toward State Care of Insane; in other issues she described new institutions that had opened, or innovations in nursing programs by psychiatric facilities.

The interest in establishing affiliations between general hospital schools and psychiatric hospital services, for the purpose of enlarging the preparation of nurses, depended to a large extent on available descriptions of the nurse workrole in the treatment of "insane" patients and on the type of facilities that could be used for educational purposes. By 1906, the convention reports show interest in affiliations as previously stated in this paper. In this year, the American Psychiatric Association established a program for the purpose of effecting standardization of nursing schools in mental hospitals. Roberts[31] states that "there was no evidence of collaboration between the psychiatric association and existing nursing organizations until the early 30's." However, in 1914 the A.P.A. employed a nurse to assist when surveys of mental hospitals were made.[32] The full-scale development of the psychiatric aspect of undergraduate nursing education — for all nurses — could have been predicted from Taylor's paper given at the 1914 convention.[33] Taylor commented: "When the question (of affiliations) was closely studied it was felt that every nurse should at least have an opportunity of receiving instruction in this most important branch of the work, without which we now feel her training would be inadequate to meet the great demands made every day upon her in preventive work alone." The main issue in discussions to date seems to have been: Should the psychiatric affiliation be elective or should it be obligatory? There was also the question: How long should this period of instruction be? Miss Taylor commented, "Nothing less than six months was advised as satisfactory." At this convention, the program in undergraduate psychiatric nursing offered by Hopkins, at the Phipps Psychiatric Clinic, was outlined.

In this era the workrole of the nurse in psychiatric facilities seems to have been established. There were descriptions of the work available for other nurses to use in acquainting themselves with this work. There were even some efforts toward including preparation of all nurses for psychiatric aspects of nursing, in some schools. There are already many schools of nursing within mental hospitals. In all of the references consulted, no one seems to have questioned the lack of knowledge from which to develop the content of undergraduate curriculum in this area; it can be said that there were many varied efforts to bring about a solution to the psychiatric care problem. These efforts were in the direction of broad and general preparation of all nurses — or special preparation of nurses and attendants most particularly to meet the institutional needs of psychiatric hospitals. That the nursing profession supported the broader preparation as the one most likely to offer the greatest help in the long-run solution of the problem seems clear.

Phase III

Initial Development of Undergraduate Psychiatric Nursing Education for All Nurses 1915-1935

The twenty years in this era brought an awakening of interest in raising standards of care in psychiatric work, a growing realization of the role of nurses and the nursing profession in the needed improvements, and gradual inclusion in basic nursing curricula of the dominant psychiatric concepts available at this time.

In 1915, Tucker again brought before nurses the problem of "Nursing Care of the Insane in the United States."[34] She pointed out that 41 mental institutions were operating schools of nursing. (These developed in the 33 years since 1882.) These training programs were administered primarily by non-nurse superintendents, and not all of the products of such programs were eligible to take state board examinations. She gave these reasons for the nurses' seeming lack of interest: the hours of work were longer than hours expected of students in general hospitals, living conditions were poor, and standards of administration and education were lower than those in general hospitals. Her paper was clearly meant to stimulate awareness among nurses not only of the problem of care of the mentally ill, but of the role of nursing in the solution of the problem. She said: "Speaking generally, neither doctors, nurses nor the public have felt the need of nurses in this branch of medical work...nurses themselves should be educated to the needs of the mentally sick, for until nurses see their opportunity they can scarcely expect the doctors and the public to recognize it."

Miss Linda Richards, the first graduate nurse in the United States, organizer of several schools in general hospitals and in mental hospitals, remarked in 1915: "It stands to reason that the mentally sick should be at least as well cared for as the physically sick." She added that a course of study in a state hospital "often develops a pupil nurse in an astonishing manner. The average probationer does not possess a very large amount of patience or tact — two essential qualities in the making of a good nurse. In nursing the insane, these qualities must be cultivated."[35,36]

By 1915 the National Committee for Mental Hygiene and the American Nurses Association collaborated on a "Study of the Insane."

In this era not only journal articles (in the American Journal of Nursing) and convention proceedings (of the National League for Nursing Education) but also textbooks related to nursing, written by nurses, indicated a growing awareness of knowledge of psychiatric nursing practice. Sara E. Parsons published in 1916 her "Nursing Problems and Obligations,"[37] and in 1920, the first textbook of psychiatric nursing by Bailey appeared.[38,39]

By 1917, the nursing organization published its first "Standard Curriculum for Schools of Nursing."[40] In this work it is stated:

> "It is now recognized that if the sick patient is to have the most skillful and competent kind of nursing care, and if nurses are to keep pace with the advances of modern medicine, they must have something more than a mere deftness in precise manipulations and the scattered fragments of scientific knowledge which are all that can usually be given in the scant time allowed by most training schools. The development of more highly complicated procedures in diagnosis and

treatment, and the increased emphasis especially on dietetic, hygienic, occupational and mental factors, make it necessary that the nurse should assume an increasing measure of responsibility in the care and treatment of the patient. To safeguard her in those responsible duties, she must have a larger measure of scientific knowledge and she must be more highly trained both in observation and in judgment."

The nursing profession was already staking its claim that all "good nurses" attend to "mental factors."

In this curriculum, the therapeutic emphasis of the era is reflected; it is recommended that "special therapeutics" be included in the nursing education program in the form of such subjects as "hydrotherapy," "occupational therapy," and "serum therapy." A course in "Mental and Nervous Diseases" is specified. Twenty hours divided as follows are recommended: ten hours of lectures and clinics, preferably by a neurologist or psychiatrist; nine hours of class and demonstrations by a nurse with special training; and one hour of lecture on social aspects, by the head of a social service department or a specialist in mental hygiene. The objectives of this course were stated as:

1. To teach the student nurse the relationship between mental and physical illness and the application of general nursing principles to mental nursing.
2. To teach the underlying causes of mental disease with modern methods of treatment available both in the hospital and in the community, and to endeavor to overcome the stigma attached to mental illness or mental hospital care.
3. To train the nurse in observation of symptoms as expressed in earlier childhood and in later life through the behavior of patients, so that the early signs of mental illness may be understood and appreciated and so that nurses may give active and intelligent cooperation in movements for the prevention of mental illness.
4. To teach the importance of directed habits of thought, desirable associations and proper environmental conditions in early childhood and to show the relationship of make-up to mental disorders.
5. To assist in developing resourcefulness, versatility, adaptability and individuality in the nurse. To emphasize qualities essential to success in mental work and the importance of special training in this branch of nursing.[41]

All in twenty hours!

The importance of neuropsychiatric nursing in World War I was not thoroughly explored for this paper, due to lack of time. However, a few facts are available. World War I forced upon the medical and nursing profession the urgent need for mobilizing personnel for military service — of which neuropsychiatric nurses were at once new and necessary. The shortcomings "of undergraduate and graduate instruction in psychiatry and neurology" were soon evident. The separate existence of neuropsychiatry in the military was terminated in 1918, making it a subordinate branch of medicine. Many of "the precious few psychiatrically trained nurses were diverted to nonpsychiatric military nursing."[42] The lack of nurses required that enlisted men perform nursing functions. The total number of neuropsychiatric disabilities in World War I was 69,394.

By 1923, World War I being already a part of the past, many nurses were now speaking in many places for consideration of the new mental hygiene emphasis in nursing, and for some type of undergraduate experience in psychiatric work for all student nurses.

Sinclair,[43] in an honest discussion of "What Constitutes a Course in Psychiatric Nursing," in 1923, stated the purpose as: "To acquaint nurses with the problems of mental illness and psychiatric nursing, and to benefit the hospital by the students' period of service." Her conception of care of the insane is presented in this manner: "The treatment for the mentally ill patient is everything that is used as a means to help him return to his former self, and everything in the daily life of the patient can be used as a means toward this end, the technique of which is the nurse's mode of using this everyday living for her patient's welfare."

Williams, on those psychiatric situations where attendants should be replaced by psychiatric nurses, said "Only the highly trained psychiatric nurse (and she cannot be too highly educated for this work) should be assigned to (the care of acute mental cases) which can be supplemented by student nurses."[44]

In discussing this, Taylor said that "many of the mental hospitals should be, and could be nursed by students from affiliated schools, provided those students had had a sufficient amount of nursing experience previously."[45] She felt the students needed adequate teaching, supervision, and stabilization of services by employed graduates and attendants.

Roscoe[46] felt that every nurse should have psychiatric training in order to help people, to understand herself, and to prevent a "fall from the brink." She felt that psychiatric nursing was valuable only as placed in relation to the whole practice of nursing, commenting that many "physical ailments and difficulties of people are of purely mental origin, without physical basis." "We know that in the close relation of mind and body — one reacting upon the other — there are many physical illnesses so depleting and weakening that the various mental faculties weaken also." She felt that the nurse "trained to care for the purely physical diseases...is handicapped and limited very much in the development of many of her keener and finer faculties by the nature of the disease and by the short time patients can be kept in (the general) hospital; all of which keep up a certain excitement...of quick action, quick results and visible accomplishment...the nurse works mainly with the disease and misses the opportunity to work and study with the personality ...." She also commented that "...there are more mental patients in this country than all other patients put together...."

By 1924, the *Handbook of Attendants on the Insane* was published under the authority of the Medico-Psychological Association.*

Bowman felt that nurses were not interested in mental hospital work because the hours were too long, the wages poor, the living conditions were unsatisfactory, with some nurses even living on the wards with patients, and the location of the hospital being away from the city.[47] Misconceptions within the nursing profession about the nature of mental illness and mental hospitals, of the unsatisfactory nature of psychiatric work, and of the stigma attached to the disease and the worker also detracted nurses from this field of nursing practice. He felt that doctors needed to promote improvements and upgrade standards in order to promote training, which in psychiatric nursing is greater skill than in general nursing. He felt it was inconceivable to study and really become interested in psychiatric nursing and then to leave it.

In the 1927 Curriculum Guide, Nutting commented as follows:

> "Special hospitals present a peculiar problem. Many of them can contribute to the general scheme of training, and efforts should be made to utilize the special opportunities they provide. None of them are competent to conduct schools in which the main portion of the training given lies entirely outside the range of their activities or purposes. That they can cooperate largely, however, in educational work is clear, as more and more the special branches which they represent become incorporated into the regular accepted plan or scheme of training of nurses. Such subjects as obstetrics and children's diseases are now commonly required, and it seems probable that for public health work, training in contagious diseases, and possibly in mental and nervous disorders, may be called for."

These views are further developed in an essay with the title "Conditions Essential in Education of Nurses."[48]

The emphasis on orienting all nurses to psychiatric and mental hygiene concepts became widespread and seemingly overshadowed interest in preparing nurses for work in widespread facilities. The impact of the mental hygiene movement, growing lay interest, and recognition of the teaching and preventive possibilities inherent in the role of nurses in public health agencies all contributed to that emphasis. Nurse educators and leaders in general nursing and psychiatric nursing alike urged incorporation of psychiatric theory in the undergraduate curriculum. Suggestions included education about "normal living,"[49] psychiatric concepts useful in private practice and in nursing administration,[50] psychiatric concepts that would improve public health nursing,[51] assisting students to understand themselves and to recognize abnormal conditions in all patients,[52] and helping the student nurse to know, accept, and be herself, and to recognize internal conflicts.[53] One nurse commented vigorously in 1926, "There is no such thing as mental nursing apart from general nursing or general nursing apart from mental nursing"[54] and she recommended psychiatric training in the undergraduate curriculum in order to improve the nurse's function in prevention. And by 1926, there were 2,155 nursing schools.

The inclusion of psychiatric content in undergraduate curriculum was recommended by a curriculum committee in 1926.[55] The proposal was for thirty hours of lectures in psychology and thirty hours of lectures and clinics in psychiatry as well as two months of clinical experience. This proposal was an improvement over that recommended in 1917 (Standard Curriculum for Schools of Nursing), and it became a part of the established standard curriculum for nurses.[56] Actual clinical experience in a psychiatric hospital with patients was recommended and standardized in 1937.[57] The 1927 "Guide" had this to say:

**Handbook of Attendants on the Insane,* Chicago Medical Book Co., 1924.

"The importance of this phase (psychiatric) of nursing is being recognized more and more. It is now regarded as an essential part of the student nurse's basic experience. Though many general hospital patients have some psychiatric manifestations the best experience can be secured in the special hospital, where patients are recognized as mentally sick and a rational program of care can be carried out in an environment suited to their needs and where the various types of illnesses are separated and classified. The term should be divided in such a way that students will have an opportunity to participate in the care of patients suffering from milder types of mental disorders ranging up to a more serious disturbance including organic diseases. Time should be planned for experience in the hydrotherapy, physical training, and occupational therapy departments and in studying means for recreation and diversion. Experience should be given in planning work schedule and daily programs for patients. Time should be spent in the social service department or in the out-patient department in which early cases are usually seen and through which follow-up work and preventive measures are carried out. Opportunity should be afforded for the student to participate in the educational programs of patients and she should be a recognized factor in assisting them to make desirable readjustments.

"Where it is impossible to correlate the theory with practical experience in a special hospital, students should be assigned to the care of patients in the general wards who have mental disturbances in association with their physical illnesses, and the experience should be made as intense and varied as conditions will permit. Excursions and visits to state and mental hospitals, and child guidance and psychopathic clinics should be arranged and will provide at least a point of view. Special cases for study should be assigned and reports of findings compared and the student directed to an understanding of the patient as a whole. In order to accomplish results in the care and treatment of patients and in the training of nurses the careful and thoughtful assignment of cases is of the utmost importance. While bedside teaching is more difficult in the care of mentally sick patients it is not less important and must be accomplished in a tactful and unobtrusive way both for the safety and good of patients and for the teaching of the students."

It was further recommended that the teacher "should have special preparation in psychiatric work." Suggested "objects of the course" were:

1. To teach the student nurse that changes occur in the mental condition of physically ill patients and to explain the relation existing between physical and mental life and physical and mental illness.
2. To teach the student nurse the significance of looking upon behavior as a symptom and to observe and differentiate behavior in her patient as she is taught to observe and differentiate cardinal physical signs.
3. To teach underlying causes of mental disease in their physical, functional, and social relationships, with special emphasis on their prevention and to familiarize the student with the modern methods of nursing and medical, social, and educational treatment available both in the hospital and in the community.
4. To teach the importance of recognizing that the foundation for the majority of cases of nervous and mental disability is laid down during childhood and is not necessarily inherited; to illustrate the relationship between certain uncorrected, undesirable habits, tendencies and personalities during childhood and various forms of nervous and mental disorders in adult life.
5. To give the student nurse an elementary but authentic knowledge of the mental mechanisms which are known to motivate conduct; to direct attention towards a concept of mind expressed in individual behavior and adaptation to life experience, with a view to increasing the student's own mental stability and to develop a keener interest in and a more sympathetic understanding of human nature.

However, "compulsory inclusion of mental nursing and hygiene in the curricula of all schools for nurses," as well as post-graduate courses and the inclusion of psychiatric-mental hygiene content in the training for public health nursing, was suggested by "The International Committee" in 1929.[58]

McGibben,[59] however, suggested an "adaptation of the standard curriculum to meet the needs of a mental hospital." She felt that the three-year course could be given in a mental hospital providing there was an affiliation with a general hospital. She felt that the "30-hour course in psychiatric nursing should be enlarged and adjusted to provide a fuller program." Suggested theoretical content included medical psychology, psychiatry, mental nursing, hydrotherapy, and occupational therapy — "a total of 80 hours of such instruction is not too much; more would be valuable."

Ruggles,[60] urged nurses to seek "understanding and a well trained technique" and observed that the nurse "who cannot understand the patient's motivation is a liability and not an asset." He stated that nurses needed to have "understanding of the emotions as well as (of) the intellectual processes of herself." In the same year Pratt[61] suggested how to use nurses trained in psychiatric nursing to staff psychiatric departments in general hospitals and how such units could be used to train student nurses. The suggested program was to improve the generalized practice of nursing in the community.

In this era, the current workrole of nurse in psychiatric facilities was further refined and its traditional forerunners — its roots in the past — were reconsidered.

Hubbard[62] reminded nurses in 1927 that they were "in constant association — in closer touch with the patient. . .and that they often represent early figures to the patient." He suggested that the nurse ought to hear the patient out and help the patient to examine and check situations which cause distress. Russell[63] pointed out that psychiatric nursing required more "intelligence and broader capabilities," a statement which was in sharp contrast to the stereotyped view of psychiatric hospital worker.

In the 1929 issue of the Journal there appears a unique clinical paper written by a nurse.[64] This enterprising young woman asserted that ". . .doctors and nurses who have never made a special study of mental therapy are inclined to punish the mentally ill by withdrawing their interest." She felt that "case experience is absolutely necessary to make mental nursing piquant." In her paper there is indication of a spirit of inquiry used in nursing practice not easily duplicated in nursing literature of today. Miss Olsen stated: "For days, I forgot I was on duty. We played tennis, swam, and bathed, and then her neurosis would crop out with renewed strength." This patient's predicament forced this nurse to read, think and interest herself in what went on in the nursing situation. She seemed to overlap her role as socializing agent and as counselor with the patient, and attempted to present to her colleague an understanding of the dynamics of the situation, her technique, and her enthusiasm about this learning experience which was a mutual one for nurse and patient.

Richards,[65] whose assistance to nurses stands out in nursing literature, pointed out that "the nurse does not work for the doctor but with the doctor." She felt that "the nurse of the future will find herself poorly adapted to the job of institutional nursing, or private duty nursing, or public health nursing, unless she is able to practice nursing as an art, and nursing as an art inevitably involves educational training in a study of personal relationships." She felt that "nursing schools have the advantage over other educational institutions in being able to watch the student apply principles she has been taught over a long period of time. . .this advantage is not well utilized at the present."

Thus a nurse and a doctor sharply indicated the necessity to make the personal relationship — between patient and nurse — the focus of nursing.

In general it can be said that the dominant use in nursing, of the emerging knowledge and spreading interest in psychiatric and mental hygiene, was to enrich general nursing practice.[66] Bennett, in 1929, succinctly stated outcomes to both general nursing and public health nursing of the current emphasis; he also discussed the "general avoidance" by nurses of psychiatric hospitals as a work area and pointed out the "crying need" for adequate care.[67] Affiliations in psychiatric nursing were conceived,[68] and a three-month course for students from general hospitals was proposed and put into operation.[69] Although the care of the mentally ill was included, the dominant purpose of such basic education was explicitly stated as an orientation that would enrich general nursing.

In 1929, the "International Committee" recomended the inclusion of psychiatric-mental hygiene content in the training of Public Health Nurses.

Despite the interest in mental hygiene, and the emphasis on the use of the word and its meaning in nursing literature, the nurse does not seem to be included when the effects of the mental hygiene movement are considered. The 1930 edition of *Mental Hygiene* contains many articles in which this is true, including such journal articles as "Finding a Way in Mental Hygiene," "Changes in the Theory of Religion," "Changes in the Philosophy of Education," "Administration of Criminal Justice," "The Study of Personality," "Changes in the Philosophy of Social Work," "Achievements in Industrial Psychology," "Psychoanalysis and Psychiatry," and "Twenty Years of the National Committee for Mental Hygiene." Not one word about nursing! Farrar, in 1930, attempted to stimulate interest in the difference between general nursing and nursing in psychiatry.[70] He felt that there was a difference with regard to authority — the nurse in psychiatry must "control, guide, and restrain patients." He felt also that there was a difference in the treatment role of the nurse — that it was much larger than in general nursing. He said, "The doctor cannot give all the psychotherapeutics that is necessary. . .and unless the nurse has a good view, and certainly the same general view and the same general insight and discernment into the patient's mental activities as the doctor, such psychotherapeutic treatment as she may be expected to give cannot be given." Chadwick, seeing the problem from the standpoint of a nurse, stated that the nurse "is prescribed as a form of treatment" — her presence, personality, and attitude are suited to the need of the patient.

Experimentation in psychiatric nursing paralleled the dominant psychiatry of the times. Group nursing was tried, under the influence of Adolph Meyer, to offer patients more varied contacts with many nurses than was possible in contacts with a private nurse. Nurses spent one week with a group of patients and were then rotated to another group of patients. The patient's day was carefully planned to afford stimulation and relaxation,[71] and in some situations the entire day was planned and courses for nurses revolved around the actual care of a patient at a stated hour.[72] Occupational therapy,[73] bibliotherapy,[74] and the emphasis on cleanliness, proper elimination, adequate nourishment, and sufficient fluids, as well as the use of continuous baths, were indicated as part of the nurse's work in psychiatric facilities.[75] Symptoms were often viewed not as an expression of need but as serious traits, which "may make or wreck a person," and habit training was suggested to eliminate certain traits such as "stealing, cruelty, temper tantrums, sensitiveness, impertinence, and profanity."[76] Recreation was viewed as a part of nursing care.[77]

Application "to the whole nursing field, to public health nursing" and to making the nurse a better person[78] continued to be stated as the purpose of the experience despite serious unemployment among nurses in the early 30's. At one conference it represented "the matured conviction of the group of 50 or more nursing school directors and other leaders in the field of nursing," although one person "deplored the shortage. . .because of it, patients remain indefinitely" in psychiatric hospitals.[79] A serious oversupply of nurses was thought to exist and one study posed the problem that "nursing is growing far more rapidly than the general population."[80] Following in the footsteps of what had been done earlier in medicine, this study suggested that ". . .the problem would seem to be one not only of raising standards but of actually limiting the output (of graduate nurses) as well."[81] And at the same time, others within the nursing profession were suggesting that "tuberculosis and psychiatry were needing women of high type who can take the initiative in formulating and expanding nursing programs."[82] It was in this climate of unemployment, seeming oversupply, avoidance of work in psychiatry, that schools of nursing in mental hospitals received their greatest impetus; 67 schools of psychiatric nursing were accredited by the American Psychiatric Association in 1936. The aforementioned studymaker suggested, "If a school has opportunity to teach the nursing care of mental and nervous patients — really teach it so that its graduates can handle such cases skillfully and intelligently — it might admit as many students as its clinical materials warrant."[83] Moreover, post-graduate courses "in these nursing specialties where demands are still greater than the qualified supply" was suggested as "one way to deal with distribution in the face of unemployment."

Nurses everywhere in the country must have sensed a need for post-graduate training courses prior to 1929. There inevitably was some recognition that the brief, orienting exposure, while perhaps adequate for general and public health nursing in light of the extent of knowledge available at the time, was not adequate for the nurse workrole in psychiatric facilities. One leader stated in 1929 that "there have not yet been created the specialists in the various branches of nursing,"[84] and simultaneously a study of existing post-graduate courses revealed that there were 14 in psychiatric nursing in 13 different states, varying in length from two to six months.[85] It can only be speculated that the registered nurses who sought the additional training then offered in these courses were in firm agreement with Russell, who stated, "It is largely through the study of disease and its treatment that knowledge of its prevention has come."[86] Three years later (1931) there were still 14 post-graduate courses distributed over six states, indicating closure of some and opening of new ones in psychiatric hospitals.[87] It is to the graduates of these courses that doctors and hospitals turned for nurse practitioners, teachers, supervisors and administrators of nursing programs in psychiatric facilities. These courses served as an interim pattern for securing advanced training, and they persisted until in 1943 advanced programs began to be established in the various universities.

A concept that was soon to receive widespread acceptance was stated in 1932, namely, "All true post-graduate courses should be connected with and fully accredited and supported by a university."[88] Various categories of post-graduate courses, such as "supplementary," "reorientation or review," and "specialty or advanced courses," were soon differentiated.[89]

In 1933, Noyes, in a statement that is still pertinent, indicated emerging functions of the psychiatrically trained nurse.[90] He pointed out that the hospital was shifting from a custodial institution to an agency "for psychological study and treatment with specialized techniques." He urged that nursing education be geared toward preparing nurses to function as an "extension of the psychiatrists — a more participative associate of the psychiatrist in the care, guidance, and treatment of the mental patient." He viewed the nurse as "an active therapeutic agent" and as a psychiatric observer who would provide "descriptions (of what went on in hospital wards) rather than interpretations" which the physician could use. He suggested that the nurse had an important role in averting and mitigating trauma in ward situations. A paper delivered by a nurse, at the same meeting, suggested also that the nurse "must detect the meaning of the non-verbalized."[91]

Twenty years ago it was asserted again that psychiatric nursing "requires greater skill and more training than any other kind of nursing."[92] Through contact, management, and relationship with the patient the nurse was seen as "part of the treatment offered to the patient." The need for patience, understanding, and insight in relating to the "less tangible sick personality" (rather than a localized physical ailment) and the long-term nature of this relationship (there were no quick cures as in medical-surgical nursing) was recognized. The nature of the pathology, as partly a non-rational need of the patient to thwart the efforts of nurses and doctors — their efforts to foster improvements favorable for the patient — was also recognized. Indeed, Erickson remarked that "all good psychiatric nurses will make good general duty nurses but the reverse is not true." Stevenson,[93] too, was challenging the nursing profession, saying, "If the nursing profession desires to improve nursing standards and place general hospital graduates in mental hospitals, they must arrange such affiliations or post-graduate courses because without such additional training. . .the general hospital nurse is of less value in a mental hospital than the mental hospital graduate."

In 1933, a nurse recorded a shift — an enlargement — of the role of nurse.[94] Nind stated that the "early psychiatrist combined the role of physician and friend" as he moved leisurely from ward to ward, but that "social treatment" had, in the process of time, been shifted to other specialists delegated to carry out the ideals of the psychiatrist. She felt that the social treatment required more intelligent supervision on the wards by nurses. She suggested a "painstaking investigation to seek out the exact nature of nursing needs in state hospitals, qualitatively and quantitatively." Miss Nind concerned herself, in this paper, with the nature of needed education programs, the qualifications of mental hospitals having schools of nursing, and the need for improvement in the quality of the institution not only for nurses but for residents who received training as well.

Ten years earlier Wheeler pointed out that young women choose nurses' training in schools in mental hospitals in order to be financially independent of their families, inasmuch as a generous allowance is given.[95] She believed that there was ". . .a definite trend toward giving the student in the mental hospital some knowledge of psychiatric nursing; it is all too true that coincident with this awakening has come the entrance of the occupational therapist and a tendency in some hospitals to give her the scientific and interesting part of the work, while the student is left to do attendant's work or act as general custodian of the patient." Wheeler pointed out that "the recovery of patients who are mentally ill is always slow; this in itself is discouraging, and the nurse who is engaged in mental nursing is under much greater strain than the nurse who is taking care of patients suffering from physical conditions." She felt that nurses trained in these schools preferred general nursing because:

1. They would not amount to much if they remained in this field.
2. The public had a negative attitude toward mental hospitals.
3. There was no recognition of the importance of mental nursing.
4. Psychiatrists tended to see the nurse as an attendant.

The most serious reason was:

5. Nurses of mental patients failed to get recognition from their "professional sisters."

In 1933, Noyes, always a helpful and clarifying spokesman for the workrole of nurse in psychiatric facilities, made several statements useful to nurses.[96]

1. Progress in any movement concerned with human welfare may be measured by certain outstanding events in its development.
2. There should always be ways and means to make the nurse a more proficient co-worker —

that common objective of the supplementary professions of psychiatric nursing and psychiatric medicine.

3. The time of the pupil nurse should be largely devoted to receiving instructions and training rather than in rendering essential services.
4. The time has come when the psychiatric nurse may be a more apprehending and therefore, to some extent, a more participative associate of the psychiatrist in the care, guidance and treatment of the mental patient. The nursing education should be more carefully and thoughtfully planned so the nurse could become the continuation and adjunct of the psychiatrist on the ward, just as the social worker has become the extension of the psychiatrist in the community.
5. The nurse should have much knowledge of the psychological, social, and psychopathological factors that may operate to produce personality disorders.
6. The period of training of the psychiatric postgraduate school should not be for less than one year and should consist of carefully graded lectures, demonstrations, and practice.
7. One of the important forces in the evolution of the state hospital has been the fact that the art and spirit of nursing penetrated and pervaded it.

In this era the Grading Committee carried on its important work.

Burgess reported that psychiatrists were exceedingly "unhappy about the quality of nursing service their patients receive," in contrast to surgeons — who are more apt to be "happy." Comments on the psychiatric problem in this report are as follows:[97]

"The preparation of nurses bears a direct relation to the special interest of the hospital. In hospitals where most of the work is surgical — and there are apparently many such — it is natural for the graduates to be interested in surgical cases and to be better prepared to take care of them than to take care of cases of other types. Students who have had practically no undergraduate experience in psychiatric nursing are apt to share the popular fear of mental cases. The best bred and most intelligent girls in such hospitals are naturally attracted by the surgeons to the surgical cases and are not attracted to mental nursing because they know so little about it. The increased emphasis upon the importance and interest in psychiatric nursing, however, and the outstanding success of those high grade young women who have taken special training in this field would seem to offer sufficient evidence that the demand of psychiatrists for women as well prepared and of as high social and intellectual standards as those available in the best hospitals for surgical nursing is not an impracticable dream, but is one which could be met were proper courses in psychiatric nursing available."

The chief concern of the Grading Committee at the time was not primarily "How much (nursing care) do the people need?" but rather "How much can they be persuaded to buy?"[98] It is therefore not unusual that in answer to the question "Is there unemployment now?" the summary is concerned principally with the difficulties of registries in employing "specials" or private duty nurses and that nowhere in this work is the shortage of nurses in psychiatric facilities and the opportunities in this area considered.

The purpose of the Grading Committee, however, as stated in its final report was "the study of ways and means for insuring an ample supply of nursing service, of whatever type or quality is needed for adequate care of the patient at a price within his reach." Established principles which govern both nursing practice and education are summarized in the Appendix. Here it is stated that "The International Council of Nurses, The National League of Nursing Education, the Winslow-Goldmark Report, and the Report of the Canadian Survey" are in agreement on recommended clinical content — and "psychiatric and neurological" services are included in the stated content. Yet in a section entitled "Fields Open to Graduate Nurses" there is not a hint of the need for numbers of qualified nurses in psychiatric facilities.

This report states several conclusions on the functions of nurses. All professional nurses, irrespective of the special field in which they have elected to practice, should be able:

1. To give expert bedside care. They should also have such knowledge of the household arts as will enable them to deal effectively with the domestic emergencies arising out of illness.
2. To observe and to interpret the physical manifestations of the patient's condition and also the social and environmental factors which may hasten or delay his recovery.
3. All professional nurses should possess the special knowledge and skill which are required in dealing effectively with situations peculiar to certain common types of illness.

4. All professional nurses should be able to apply, in nursing situations, those principles of mental hygiene which make for a better understanding of the psychological factor in illness.

5. All professional nurses should be capable of taking part in the promotion of health and the prevention of disease.

6. All professional nurses should possess the essential knowledge and the ability to teach measures to conserve health and to restore health.

7. All professional nurses should be able to cooperate effectively with family, hospital personnel, and health and social agencies in the interest of patient and community.

8. Every nurse should be able, by means of the practice of her profession, to attain a measure of economic security and to provide for sickness and old age. It should be possible for her to conserve her physical resources, to seek mental stimulus by further study and experience, and to follow that way of life in which she finds those spiritual and cultural values which enrich and liberate human personality.[99]

In connection with conclusion number 4, it is noted briefly that "nurses have not as yet entered the field of institutional psychiatric nursing in any large numbers, though the potential demand for their services is admitted to be great," and that "the Committee on the Costs of Medical Care...has stated, in 1930, the combined bed capacity of the hospitals for mental and nervous diseases exceeded the total bed capacity of general hospitals."

At this time, the recommended NLNE standard was a two-month experience in psychiatric nursing services. The Grading Committee report notes that 88% of the students in schools of nursing received less experience than this, 5% received this amount, and 7% of the students received a longer experience. The second Grading study had reported that 73% of all students had not spent even one day in caring for a psychiatric patient. The report comments, "It is no wonder that physicians have difficulty in finding graduate nurses both competent and willing to undertake the nursing care of psychiatric patients." The report continues:

> "There is an enormous need for good nursing in mental hospitals; yet there are few adequate courses; and in spite of thousands of graduate nurses looking for work, there is still a serious shortage of graduate nurses prepared to take care of nervous and mental patients. Nursing schools are nearly (not quite) unanimous in neglecting to prepare their students for graduate service in this large and as yet practically unnursed field. All these basic needs for nursing training should be met by affiliation when the home hospital cannot meet them itself."

In summarizing the findings in answer to the question of "what most nursing schools are like," the report stated in part:

> "Although mental hygiene is coming to be considered desirable not only in care of psychiatric and neurological patients, but in care of all patients, most students receive little or no preparation in this field. Approximately half of all hospital patients in the United States are psychiatric, yet most of their nursing is being given by trained or untrained attendants, maids, orderlies, or fellow patients. There is an enormous need for trained nursing in mental hospitals."

The report continued: "Psychiatric hospitals should rarely attempt to give basic undergraduate training to student nurses; but wherever adequate theoretical instructions and proper teaching of nurses on the wards can be assured, psychiatric courses for graduate nurses should be encouraged." The Grading Committee, however, did not do more than specify types of post-graduate courses in clinical nursing, for the Education Committee of NLNE has been active since the mid-twenties in developing a plan along this line.

The proceedings of the Fortieth Annual Convention include a report of "The Committee on Nursing in Mental Hospitals."[100] It states that the Chairman and one other member of the Committee met with the Nursing Committee of the American Psychiatric Association in New York City on December 28, 1933. The meeting was held to discuss the development of nursing education in the mental hospital; no action was taken. Discussion revolved around such points as 1) survey of selected mental hospitals to determine which hospitals had potentialities of development of nursing education; 2) the suggestion that a nurse in each state department of welfare or mental hygiene become State Director of Nursing Education for mental hospitals; the need to select hospitals for schools and nursing and also hospitals suitable for affiliation programs. Questions raised included ones about 1) the calibre of graduate students; 2) criteria for selection of hospitals; 3) methods of supervising hospitals; 4) development of the male nurse; 5) the need to bring more nurses into mental hospitals.

Undergraduate education in psychiatric nursing education, as an aspect of basic professional education, had its roots strengthened and firmly planted in this era. It was not until the 1950's, however, that the preparation offered in the psychiatric experience was viewed as the preparation of nurses for the staff nurse in any nursing situation — including in psychiatric facilities. Instead, the purpose which generally dominated the thought of this era is stated succinctly by Thielbar in 1935.[101] She felt that the basic course in psychiatric nursing must contribute tools and develop understanding and tact; it must assist in the nurse's personal adjustment to her work. Moreover, it should be placed preferably in the second year so that "the student will have more opportunity to apply what she has learned to her general experience." Thielbar pointed out that the mental hygiene approach must be integrated into the whole course of general experience.

Phase IV

Initial Development of Graduate Education in Psychiatric Nursing 1936-1945

Interest in undergraduate psychiatric nursing education, and in supplementary post-graduate courses, paved the way for graduate education as it evolved in this era. Less than 50% of the schools of nursing offered undergraduate experience in psychiatric nursing, but in this era the trend continued as more and more schools thus strengthened the basic curriculum. More nurses expounded the purpose of such experience, each helping to clarify, refine, and expand what had been said before.

Willis suggested that the goal of "teaching psychiatric nursing" was "to force the student to see the patient as a person and to deal with him by developing herself."[102] She said, "We reach the patient through feelings. The course of conduct and the effects therefrom depend upon the nurse herself and her ability to handle well the situations that arise." These ideas were further developed by the author, who in 1947 published an important work that was to stimulate still further thought among nurses about the workrole in nursing situations in psychiatry.[103]

Myers felt that "the nurse, to be helpful in the care and treatment of mental patients, must have knowledge and understanding of the race, the functions of the mind in general, and of the mind of her patient; she must understand people in general, individuals in particular; she must be able to recognize and understand their deviations from normal."[104] Thus, a physician put before the nursing profession the proposition to which it had always subscribed, namely, that the broad general base of undergraduate education would, in the long run, best serve the needs of all patients through the practices of all nurses.

In 1937, NLNE issued the last of three "Curriculum Guides."[105] As can be expected, the objectives of the psychiatric nursing content in each reflected the prevailing views about people, the nurse workrole, explanatory concepts, and the like. In 1937, it is stated that "emphasis should be placed on interpretation of the behavior of patients and the underlying dynamics of behavior rather than on diagnosis. None of the behavior groupings is mutually exclusive; for example, an underactive patient may be anxious and apprehensive." The stated objectives of the course, which was to include 60 to 80 hours of instruction and 12 to 16 weeks of clinical experience, were:

1. To develop appreciation of the interdependence of physical, intellectual, and emotional factors characterizing an integrated personality.
2. To develop a basic understanding of the etiology, symptomatology, course, and treatment of the more common types of psychiatric disorders.
3. To acquire a basic understanding of the principles and methods employed in the psychiatric aspects of nursing.
4. To better appreciate social problems associated with mental illness and the community facilities for dealing with these problems.
5. To appreciate the nurse's responsibility in furthering a positive mental health program in the community.

In 1938, William Menninger expressed the opinion that "psychiatric knowledge seems even more important to the nurse than surgery or pediatrics or medicine, for the reason that it is fundamental to all of these."[106] He felt, too, that "it is desirable to explode the phrase 'mental nursing'...we do not speak of physical nursing and have no justification to speak of mental nursing. It is not synonymous with psychiatric nursing, which is a specialized branch of endeavor, just as is surgical or obstetrical or public health nursing." He pointed out the total nature of a person, the impossibility of divisions such as physical and mental. He stated:

> "Psychiatric experience teaches the nurse to take an objective rather than a subjective attitude towards mental symptoms, even psychotic behavior...by objective attitude is meant more than becoming accustomed to such behavior; the nurse learns to evaluate it, learns what it may mean for the patient and the doctor, and how she may most effectively help the patient to overcome it. Most of all she learns to accept it as an emotional response."

He believed that student nurses needed at least four months of actual contact and experience, and that this length of time was possibly too short.

A "Bibliography on Psychiatric Nursing and Allied Subjects" was prepared and made available by the National League in 1939. Watters suggested that "the nurse's contact with psychiatry should begin in her first year and continue throughout the time she is in training."[107]

From 1940 to 1943 a series of "Round Tables" was conducted at the NLNE conventions. These meetings provided an opportunity for the presentation of many viewpoints and for discussion from the floor, and they reflect the continuing concerns as well as individual practices which were described at the meetings.

Harvey asserted that "psychiatric nursing is an aspect of all nursing,"[108] but that this relation should be shown to the student; she described the New York Hospital program and the way in which psychiatric units in general hospitals could be used to provide the undergraduate experience for students. Edgar asserted that students should not be used for service.[109] She attributed the Allentown program to the influence of "having a very understanding nursing consultant in our State Department," Pennsylvania having been the only state to have such a person and position title before 1946. Edgar felt that the consultant assisted greatly in the interpretation of the educational aims of nursing. She believed that the time could be planned so that a student's experience on a service could be educative, and that students should not do more than supplement the work of graduate nurses.

Walsh, at Bellevue, had for years been trying out perhaps the most progressive methods in teaching students. At the 1940 Round Table she said:

> "Since but 1/15 of our nurses who receive education in psychiatric nursing at the Bellevue Psychiatric Hospital, select this field for graduate employment, it is evident that our teaching must be directed to the increasing understanding of human behavior which can be applied to all patients and personnel in any nursing situation."[110]

Walsh felt that all of the hospital resources should be used to meet student needs, and through them the patient's needs. She advocated that teachers "put the student in close contact with the patient, at the same time giving constant direction, explanation, assistance, and supervision." Describing her own program, she said: "We have no examinations. The final study of a patient and the last two weeks of service indicate the degree of understanding and nursing which the student has achieved."

In the 1941 Round Table, Stevenson advocated that every ward in a psychiatric institution be headed by a registered nurse. He spoke of the "unrecovered patients" and said, "We are entitled to this; they are our failures."[111]

At the 1942 Round Table, it was suggested that this was not the time to promote the psychiatric affiliation, to which May Kennedy, who presided at all four Round Tables, replied, "This is actually the time to promote affiliations because now we are going to see the psychiatric aspect of the person emphasized."[112] Mrs. Eugenie Spaulding informed the group present that federal aid could be obtained for post-graduate courses in psychiatric nursing but that there had been few requests for it.

By 1943, the participation in World War II commanded the attention of the nursing profession. Nevertheless, the last Round Table discussion took place on the topic, "Psychiatric Nursing in the Accelerated Program." The discussion covered four main points:

1. Psychiatric nursing should be included in nursing school programs as many of the men in the service would become mentally ill, and thus become wards of the government.
2. The acceleration in the student's course could be continued in the psychiatric clinical experience by:
    a. The elimination of repetitious material.
    b. Careful integration of class teaching with ward teaching and experience.
    c. Giving ward teaching the same careful consideration as planned classes.
3. "The State Hospitals must obtain good directors who can organize suitable courses in

psychiatric nursing for affiliating students."

4. Nurses with psychiatric training take better care of patients, gain in maturity and in understanding of people.[113]

In this period in the historical development of psychiatric nursing, there was a Committee on Mental Hygiene and Psychiatric Nursing appointed by NLNE. Reports of this committee appear in convention proceedings for the years 1940 to 1945. The name has been changed to Committee on Psychiatric Nursing for 1946-1947.

In 1940, the committee presented its first report to the convention.[114] It had sent out letters to State Committees suggesting that:

1. The states endeavor to establish a closer relationship between nursing organizations and the public welfare department of their respective states.
2. An effort should be made to extend the educational programs by planning:
   a. Single lectures for laity and nursing groups.
   b. A series of lectures for laity and nursing groups.
   c. Courses for graduate and undergraduate students.
3. Studies and surveys should be made of the following:
   a. Facilities available for study in the fields of psychiatric nursing and mental hygiene.
   b. Patient care in institutions, the number of hours of care per patient, and the number of graduates and attendants giving the care.
   c. General hospital courses giving courses in psychiatric nursing and mental hygiene.
   d. Number of nurses prepared to do psychiatric nursing.
   e. Number of nurses who have had courses in psychiatric nursing and mental hygiene as undergraduate students.

The committee expressed interest in "having a historical study of courses in psychiatric nursing and mental hygiene for undergraduate students" and suggested that the Board secure a person qualified and able to give full time to such a study.

The committee was unanimous in the opinion that "there should be a nurse in" the United States Public Health Service who could assist lay groups, nurses and organizations in promoting psychiatric nursing and mental hygiene.

The 1941 Report of the Committee shows discussion of the education of attendants.[115] Dr. Fitzpatrick reported that courses for attendants in the United States and Canada differ in length from 12 hours to six months, and for two institutions the course is three years in length. The Committee on Nursing, of The American Psychiatric Association, was reported as favoring extension of psychiatric nursing education for all student nurses and standardization of the curriculum for psychiatric attendants, and it endorsed cooperative studies with NLNE regarding the attendant curriculum. These steps were suggested as necessary before the A.P.A. would support legislation for state licensing of attendants. The Committee members agreed that the attendant was needed "but that great care must be taken that she does not in any instance take the place of the nurse."

In 1942, the committee reported that it had outlined "a course for attendants in mental hospitals,"[116] which was later approved by the Board of Directors. It subsequently was made available to state committees, as well as to directors of schools and nursing services in mental institutions seeking such guidance.

The committee felt that financial aid for the purpose of promoting psychiatric nursing was urgent; it sent a letter to Dr. Thomas Parran, USPHS, presenting such a request and asking how states could get such aid.

The committee took action with regard to the classification of nurses in New York State Mental Hospitals, by the Civil Service Commission, into the groups — professional (administrative and teaching) and sub-professional (head nurses and staff nurses). It recommended that the NLNE Board bring the matter before the Civil Service Committee of ANA. It deplored the classification as one that would "tend to under-rate the importance of the work of head nurses and staff nurses in state institutions," and that it would also influence interest in this field of nursing.

The Board of Directors of the League of January 25, 1942 voted "that guidance on a voluntary basis be given schools contemplating an affiliation in psychiatric nursing by having the Committee on Mental Hygiene and Psychiatric Nursing offer a consultation service through correspondence and visits, the institution making the request to assume the expense if a visit is necessary."

The committee urged league members to encourage nurse educators "to give more attention to psychiatric nursing," among other reasons, for this was the prediction that "this was a war of civilian population and a war of nerves. There is going to be a great strain on the mental health of people, and psychiatry will be needed more than ever as a part of the equipment of a nurse."

In 1943, the Committee reported as follows:

1. A program on psychiatric nursing was prepared to guide general hospital schools of nursing having affiliations with mental institutions. Stress was placed on the mental aspects of all illnesses.
2. Several recommendations were sent to the Board of Directors of NLNE:
   a. That the Board request that USPHS give consideration to the allocation of funds to schools of nursing and mental hospitals having an affiliation program.
   b. That the Board of NLNE authorize funds, from the budget of the Committee on Mental Hygiene and Psychiatric Nursing, to prepare a program which would be helpful in promoting psychiatric nursing in the various states and also to pay the expenses of someone to assist in the execution of such a program.
   c. That the President of the League urge hospital schools to add or to continue affiliations in psychiatric nursing.
3. The shortage of psychiatric nurses was discussed.[117]

In 1944, the report indicated that two meetings of the committee had taken place at the headquarters of NLNE; previously, members carried on their work largely by mail. On the request of the Committee on Education Problems in Wartime, a plan for a psychiatric experience for cadets was drawn up and presented. Even though service needs were stressed in the Cadet Corps, the committee emphasized that the educational needs should be stressed in the psychiatric experience. The committee had reviewed, condensed and revised "The Suggested Activities for State Chairman of Committee on Mental Hygiene and Psychiatric Nursing." The suggestions covered four categories:

1. establishing and maintaining relationships with that department of the state which is concerned with the care of psychiatric patients;
2. education of the public and nurses;
3. acting as an advisory committee;
4. obtaining information on psychiatric nursing on various aspects of psychiatric nursing in the state.[118]

In 1945, it was reported that commitiees were active in 14 states and Puerto Rico. A brief list of source materials on psychiatric nursing, which would be mimeographed for distribution, was planned.

Beginning in 1943, three university-sponsored courses in psychiatric nursing were started.[119] These programs received financial assistance from funds allocated under the Bolton Act. By 1945, these programs had graduated 126 students.

The continuing concern of the American Psychiatric Association for the nursing care of patients in psychiatric facilities, and a grant of funds from the Rockefeller Foundation led to a study which began in 1942 and was reported in 1944.[120] The objectives of this study were:

1. To evaluate the educational facilities for the preparation of nursing personnel with special emphasis on attendant and student nurse programs, including post-graduate groups.
2. To study adequacy of personnel as to quantity and quality.
3. To acquaint administrators and teachers working in the hospital field with what is being done in various mental institutions.
4. To give guidance in the development of programs for the education and preparation of nursing personnel in mental hospitals.
5. To formulate through the Psychiatric Nursing Committee of the American Psychiatric Association and the National League for Nursing Education standards for professional courses in psychiatric nursing.
6. To stimulate interest of the state and national nursing groups in psychiatric nursing.

This study led to recommendations for consideration of the A.P.A.:

1. Education of the public to the needs of mental patients so that funds will be available to raise the care of all mental patients to an acceptable level. This would be the means of promoting a standard of hours, wages, and living conditions for personnel comparable to those prevailing in the general hospital.
2. Establishment of relatively uniform training for attendants.
3. Strengthening of the basic schools of nursing in mental hospitals.
4. Increasing affiliations for student nurses.
5. Revival and establishment of post-graduate courses for nurses.

6. Provision for a uniform standard of care for all patients within a given mental hospital.
7. Recognition of the status of the registered nurse and the establishment of an administrative policy to use the services of nurses to the best advantage.
8. Centralization of all nursing personnel under competent nursing directors.

The report includes many findings, e.g., the ratio of personnel to patients varies from 1:3 to 1:2,864; in 1944 there were 32 schools of nursing in mental hospitals — 17 in New York State; there had been 41 in 1915 and 67 in 1936; "Psychiatric nursing is rarely required by law for nurse licensure; 13 states do not give a course of psychiatric nursing of any kind."

And the nursing profession was slowly making headway in realizing its goal of the preparation of all nurses for nursing in all types of facilities, including psychiatric ones. By 1939, 50% of all schools offered a basic experience — by 1944, 54%.[121] By 1955, nearly every school in the country offered undergraduate psychiatric nursing.

Through a grant from the American Journal of Nursing, a Committee of the League was appointed to "study. . .the basic principles necessary for the evaluation of advanced courses in clinical nursing."[122] This committee then worked out an "outline of an advanced course in psychiatric nursing." It is not clear from the references consulted but it seems that this committee continued for several years and may be the same one referred to in the following paragraphs.

By the end of this era, the climate of the nursing profession was more favorable for considering the pressing problems of psychiatric nursing in institutions and agencies of all kinds. "The Committee on Post-Graduate Clinical Nursing Courses" reported the expansion of its work over the previous years.[122] It stated these purposes:

1. To prepare a classification and description of types of clinical courses for graduate nurses;
2. To formulate guiding principles for the development of these courses and criteria for evaluation;
3. To construct outlines of advanced courses in various clinical areas in accordance with the principles;
4. To collaborate with the Committee on Measurement and Educational Guidance in the construction of achievement tests for advanced clinical courses.

In October, after two years of work, a "Special Committee on Post-graduate Clinical Nursing Courses" of NLNE issued Pamphlet No. 1 entitled "Courses in Clinical Nursing for Graduate Nurses: Basic Assumptions and Guiding Principles — Basic Courses — Advanced Courses."[123] A Sub-committee on Psychiatric Nursing, of this committee, issued simultaneously Pamphlet No. 2, "An Advanced Course in Psychiatric Nursing."[124] These materials provided guidelines for the rapidly developing advanced programs, which were to follow, as funds under the Mental Health Act were allocated to the various universities who applied for them.

Pamphlet No. 1 specified the urgency of the need for clinical preparation for public health nurses and for teachers and supervisors in such fields as psychiatry, tuberculosis, and orthopedics. It stated that these nurses "often found themselves in the difficult position of knowing something about how to teach without sufficient knowledge of what to teach." It expressed the need for nurses to become experts in bedside nursing — to stabilize nursing service programs and to assist in teaching the student nurses by demonstration. The purpose of this report, therefore, was to clarify the situation by "formulating certain guiding principles and setting up criteria related to them" and "to state these principles and criteria as briefly as possible."

The pamphlet defines basic and supplementary instruction, the purpose of both being to assist graduate nurses to fill gaps in the previous preparation or even to have a recent experience; neither is an advanced course. The general plan for such courses is drawn and includes requirements for admission, organization, duration, instruction and experience, clinical facilities, control and administration, finance, teaching personnel and equipment, and records.

The nature of advanced courses is also specified. Terms used in the report were defined as follows:

> "*Advanced course* in clinical nursing: The term refers to a broad and unified plan of instruction which has as its purpose the development of abilities essential for practice as a clinical nursing specialist. The course may be part of a program in advanced clinical nursing which includes, in addition to this specific clinical nursing course, various related courses which contribute to its content and enrich the background of the student.
>
> "*Clinical nursing specialist:* A clinical nursing specialist is a professional nurse who may be considered expert because she has attained broader knowledge, deeper insight and appreciation, and

greater skill in a given clinical area than can be acquired in the professional undergraduate course. She is therefore better able to analyze, explore, and cope with nursing situations in that area.

"*Nursing situation:* In a given clinical field a nursing situation exists whenever a patient requires nursing of any kind. Nursing includes all that can be done by the nurse to teach positive health, to prevent and to assist in curing disease, to relieve symptoms, to support the patient by physical and psychological means, and to help him to take as much responsibility as possible for his own welfare. Such nursing may be performed by the nurse either individually or in cooperation with the family and with community agencies. Every nursing situation involves the personality of the patient, his physical and mental condition, and the environmental factors which affect him."

Assumptions which are basic to the guiding principles stated in Pamphlet No. 1, were formulated as follows:

1. There exists in the field of clinical nursing a body of advanced knowledge, appreciation, and skill beyond that which can be attained during the professional undergraduate course.
2. This body of knowledge, appreciation, and skills can be acquired most effectively by means of an organized program of instruction and experience specially designed to develop the required abilities.
3. The fundamental purpose of the advanced course is the development of specialists in various fields of clinical nursing who will be capable of contributing to the continual improvement of nursing practice and nursing education.

The following principles were formulated and stated, and criteria — "statements concerning the conditions and practices which should characterize these courses" — are stated in relation to each principle, as follows:

I. "Advanced courses in clinical nursing should be either a part of a major program in nursing established in an accredited university or college or should be approved for credit by that university or college.

1. "The university or college in which the course is conducted is accredited by a regional educational accrediting body. The nursing division or department or school is approved or accredited by an appropriate professional accrediting or policy-making body.
2. "The organization and administration of the course is in accord with the general policies of the university or college, and contractual arrangements are made with hospitals and other cooperating agencies.
3. "The course is developed on a sound financial basis which assures stability, continuity, and satisfactory provision for education. Financial arrangements are made with cooperating agencies which enable them to offer an acceptable program of instruction and supervised experience.
4. "Eligibility for matriculation in the university or college and in its nursing department or school is a pre-requisite for admission to the course. The course is credited on the same general lines as other courses offered by the university or college.
5. "The administrative direction of the course is delegated to a nurse whose professional and educational qualifications meet the standards of the university or college as well as those of the cooperating agencies. Nurses who are members of the teaching and supervisory personnel have a schedule of hours comparable to that of the faculty of the college or university and in accord with the best present practice.

II. "An advanced course in clinical nursing should begin at a level of achievement equivalent to that attained upon the completion of a corresponding professional undergraduate course of approved standards. It should lead directly to the development of interests, abilities, and traits which are characteristic of a clinical nursing specialist.

"Evidence is available that candidates for the advanced course already have achieved that degree of competence which is expected upon the completion of the corresponding approved undergraduate course."

Pamphlet No. 2 specifies an advanced course in psychiatric nursing in accordance with the principles stated in Pamphlet No. 1.* The purpose of the advanced course is stated as the preparation of "the qualified graduate nurse to function as (1) a clinical nursing specialist in the care of psychiatric patients, (2) an exponent of the principles of mental hygiene, and (3) an agent to aid in community understanding of psychiatric disorders and their prevention." Five

*By 1947 there were pamphlets on pediatrics, tuberculosis, maternity and orthopedics.

c. Administration in a nursing service?

d. Consultation in a nursing service?

2. To what extent would preparation for teaching and supervision, administration, and "consultation" be dependent upon advanced study in a special field of (clinical) nursing service?

3. If preparation for teaching and supervision, administration, and consultation, through advanced study, presupposes a certain amount of "advanced" preparation in obstetric nursing, pediatric nursing, orthopedic nursing, psychiatric nursing, etc., to what extent, if any, should these two aspects of advanced study run parallel?

4. How should the nursing profession organize to promote most effectively the advanced education of nurses for special fields of nursing?

5. How should nurses in sections of the country (as, for example, states) and local communities organize to promote:

   a. Analysis of their needs for advanced preparation?

   b. Analysis of the facilities available for advanced preparation?

   c. Utilization of facilities available?

   d. Promotion of more adequate facilities?

6. To what extent should the "advanced" preparation of nurses who plan to function as "practitioners," teachers and supervisors, administrators, and "consultants" in hospitals and other community health agencies differ? Or, how much similarity and overlapping is there between the interest and needs of so-called "institutional" and so-called "public health" nurses?

7. To what extent is a group of common problems facing all clinical practitioners of nursing? To what extent is it possible for psychiatric nurses, surgical nurses, and pediatric nurses to study such problems in a "core course?"

8. To what extent is the professional accepting and acting on the recommendations of the Committee on Postgraduate Clinical Nursing Courses of the NLNE that such courses be on a collegiate level?

9. When advanced clinical courses are offered as part of a college program, can satisfying prerequisites be solved if colleges and universities must be depended upon to provide the immediate demand for large numbers of clinically expert nurses?

The conclusions of the round table discussion are of interest:

1. Preparation for specialized clinical practice has not been given proper emphasis, nor the need for it due recognition — that ultimately the teacher, the supervisor, and the consultant should be clinically expert practitioners in their chosen fields.

2. More effective organization on the national, state, and local levels is needed for the promotion of advanced nursing education, and for the development of standards in nursing specialization.

3. There is a great overlapping in the needs of so-called "institutional" and "public health" nurses in advanced nursing education, and an effort should be made to bring these two groups together in educational programs for graduate nurses. Some persons thought their interests and needs might be identical if their respective functions were broadly interpreted. Others thought that their programs of study should have some common and some special elements.

4. That a "core content" could be developed for all advanced clinical nursing courses was generally accepted.

5. Certain participants emphasized the importance of intensive study of advanced nursing education with relation to (1) effective overall planning, (2) development of vital functional courses, and (3) establishment of standards for clinical specialization as preparation for the practice of nursing, teaching, supervision, and "consultation."

In this same year, 1947, lists showing "clinical courses offered to graduate professional nurses" were prepared by NLNE and given wide distribution.

In the 1948 Proceedings, a "Symposium on Curriculum Concepts" is reported. Kalkman presented a paper entitled "Psychiatric Principles Applied to General Nursing Care." She reiterated the following: "the patient is a person," "the inseparability of mind and body," "certain kinds of behavior are symptoms," "the nurse is a therapeutic agent," and the need for "flexibility in adjusting oneself to recognize the needs of patients." Kalkman pointed out that there was no evidence in the literature of a serious attempt to reorient nursing practice, in the light of psychiatric principles. She suggested steps that might be taken in order to do this, as follows:

1. Affiliation with a program in a psychiatric hospital;
2. Integration of concepts in the curriculum prior to the affiliation;
3. Make psychiatric counseling available for students and as a consultative service to the school of nursing;
4. Education of the faculty of the school about psychiatric nursing;
5. Revision of the curriculum and integration of concepts of psychiatric nursing.

Kalkman pointed out that better prepared teachers of psychiatric nursing were needed as well as new teaching techniques and different attitudes, that psychiatric nursing was not exclusively factual information.

This was the era in which the G.I. Bill made it possible for World War II veterans to secure an education with government assistance. Many nurses who had served with the armed forces had become more aware of not only the need for nurses in psychiatric facilities but also the need for more knowledge. Many of these nurses went to the various universities seeking such preparation as would give them the desired "trained technique." Now there were students — students who were interested and could pay for their tuition. There were also Mental Health Act funds to support not only the training program — faculty salaries, travel, equipment, etc. — but also still other tuition money, in the form of stipends, was available. These factors and the initiative and curiosity of the students forced improvements in the university programs. Many of the program directors needed help, and needed most particularly to strengthen university programs through consultation with their colleagues and peers in psychiatric nursing. This urgent need was communicated to NLNE at the 1948 meeting to consider the Schmitt Criteria. Funds were then sought for the 1950 conference at Minnesota.

From April 3 to April 14, 1950 a "Conference on Advanced Psychiatric Nursing and Mental Hygiene Programs" was held by the National League for Nursing, in cooperation with the University of Minnesota, under a grant of funds from the Public Health Service.[132] This conference provided an opportunity for inter-program consultation, and for mutual discussion of needs and problems of nurse educators who were conducting some 22 programs in the universities represented. Areas of general agreement of the conference are reflected in reports of general sessions:

> "It was agreed that clinical specialization represents the base upon which special preparation for positions such as instructor, supervisor, etc., is built.
>
> "The goal toward which we are all working is that clinical specialization should be only on the master's level, and that the bachelor's degree should be a prerequisite for all advanced preparation."

In a discussion of "Shall We Prepare Nurses to do Psychotherapy" there was agreement among the participants that:

> "The nurse is a therapeutic force and her relationships have meaning in the treatment of patients.
>
> "The study of concepts of psychotherapy belong on an advanced level.
>
> "Nurses should move forward in the direction of being able to become participants in psychotherapeutic teams."

It was recommended that "a request be made to the National League of Nursing Education to form a Committee on Advanced Clinical Programs in order to review and revise the proposed guide for an Advanced Clinical Course in Psychiatric Nursing."

There was consensus of the following definition of psychiatric nursing:

> "Psychiatric nursing, as a branch of the art and science of nursing, is concerned with the total nursing care of the psychiatric patient through the development and guidance of interpersonal relationships, the creation of therapeutic situations and the application of other nursing skills used in psychiatric treatment, and with the prevention of mental illness and the promotion of mental health."

Three working definitions were accepted by the conference:

> "*Content* is all the experiences a student has in a designed program for which the university takes the major responsibility.
>
> "The experiences designed for the student include all the typical problems a psychiatric nurse faces - the ideas, principles, skills, and training experiences in relation to these problems.
>
> "Content for *basic and/or supplementary to basic*

programs includes what every general nursing practitioner needs to know about psychiatric problems in order to function in first level positions in any institution (as defined by institutional and/or standard setting bodies).

"Content for *advanced programs* in psychiatric nursing includes what selected nurses need to know in order to function in specialized positions in psychiatric nursing, to include clinical practice, teaching, supervision, administration, consultation, and research."

This conference was perhaps the most important of all of those held for nurses connected with graduate programs. It was an intensive 13-day conference, and those participants who were present, and are attending this 1956 conference, will attest that it was not only strenuous, interesting, and provocative, but also growth-provoking. It was not exactly a peaceful or formal type of conference.

One of the most important instruments which promoted change within the nursing profession was the Brown Report.[133] This report states unequivocally:

"We recommend that hospitals for the mentally ill still conducting schools of nursing consider means whereby they can relinquish their schools, and, as a substitute, make their clinical facilities more widely available for affiliating students. We recommend also that the nursing profession, both autonomously and in conjunction with the medical profession and the public at large, attempt to redress the imbalance resulting from long neglect of mental disease by assisting these and other similar hospitals to introduce substantial teaching programs for affiliation or internship, and to utilize in-service training for assistant personnel more extensively and effectively. We recommend particularly that ways be sought to stimulate interest among the health professions in wider practice in the field of psychiatry as contrasted with other diseases, and in wider research for its prevention and cure."

Also in 1948, a committee of twelve — of which only three were nurses (non-psychiatric) — provided another report.[134] This report states:

"Perhaps the greatest challenge to nursing still lies in the future. The increasing importance of psychiatry as a branch of medicine, and, even more important, the increasing recognition that emotional factors play in health and disease, presents a unique challenge and opportunity to the nurse. It is she more than any other member of the medical and health team who is in frequent and intimate contact with the patient. Hence she is particularly able to assess the subtle interplay of the psyche and soma. She not only becomes the eyes and ears of the doctor; she can also become an invaluable assistant in diagnosis and therapy."

The word "team" is defined as:

"...the systematic cooperation of a self-directing group of individuals in the performance of certain tasks, each of whom has a job to do and knows how to do it, whether independently or under supervision. The members of the team have a sense of responsibility to each other and toward the outcome of their efforts. Specifically, we refer to a number of associates, all subordinating personal prominence to the efficiency of the whole. The direction of the team comes from within, from its members."

The report also presents 45 findings and recommendations.

A third report on the nursing profession was made by Bridgman in 1953.[135] She states, "Among nurses giving psychiatric care, including those in a supervisory capacity, 24% have had no preparation in their basic program; 80% have had no education in psychiatric nursing beyond the basic course." The urgency of the need for a training program for attendants is also emphasized.

In 1950, the suggestion was made by Mary Schmitt that the plans of the structure of nursing organization, which were under study, be scrutinized as to the suitable place for psychiatric nursing. Accordingly, a group of nurses met informally for several sessions to appraise printed materials about the structure study, to confer with consultants from NLNE on this matter, and to determine a proposed course of psychiatric nursing to take in the organization. It was felt that opinions of nurses from other sectors of the nation should be secured. Consequently, a questionnaire was circulated asking nurses to indicate their opinions regarding various courses of action. These opinions were then tabulated and the findings prompted the nurse group to draft a petition for an Interdivisional Council on Psychiatric Nursing. Petitions other than this one also may have been sent to NLNE, as were letters disapproving the step recommended in the petition. Nevertheless, on June 21, 1952 the Board of NLN received and acted on the petition, and an Interdivisional Council on Psychiatric and Mental Health Nursing was formed. Early in 1956, there were 34 Councils in operation, as well as a newsletter, which is circulated by NLN.

The Newsletter followed an initial letter sent out by Ruth Sleeper, President, NLN under date of November 20, 1952. Miss Sleeper said, in part:

> "There has existed among nurses a prevailing tendency to think of basic education in psychiatric nursing as a means of enriching all nursing practice without due regard to its function in the preparation of nurses to give adequate care to the mentally ill. While this point of view predominates, nurses continue to graduate from our schools without ever having given real consideration to the possibility of choosing psychiatric nursing as a career."

It was also in 1952 that NLN initiated the "Integration Project" in collaboration with the New York Hospital-Cornell University School of Nursing; one phase of this project is related to psychiatric nursing. This proposal was blueprinted in 1951. In this same year, at the Council of State Leagues, the need for psychiatric nurses and other nurses to plan together was pointed out; Florence Wilson also suggested that NLN investigate what is being done in the field of prevention of mental illness.

In November 1950, Julia Miller was appointed as Executive Secretary of NLN, and her interest in the concerns of nurses in psychiatry proved to be not only genuine but timely, as events began to move more swiftly to coerce consideration of the many aspects of the complex psychiatric care problem by the League and the American Nurses Association.

Two "factual" studies made in 1950 were publicized in reports that were distributed widely. The Nowakowski study[136] was based upon a questionnaire submitted to 9,100 "professional registered nurses active in the field of psychiatric and mental hygiene nursing." These questionnaires represented 74% of the number originally submitted to 633 directors of nursing and returned by 600 directors of nursing in psychiatric institutions throughout the United States and its territories. The purposes of the study were as follows:

1. "To determine, insofar as might be possible, the present qualifications of psychiatric nurses in the United States and its territories.
2. "To determine the number and distribution of these nurses.
3. "To determine the types of positions of these nurses."

Because of the limitations of "time, personnel and finances available," it was necessary to delimit the study of "desirable qualifications for psychiatric nurses."

The second study, by Clark,[137] is a report based on 407 replies to a questionnaire submitted by psychiatric hospitals and facilities in the United States. The tables presented "facts and figures for 1950 concerning patient-personnel ratios, educational programs, responsibilities of nursing and attendants, and personnel policies as they pertain to psychiatric nursing personnel in mental hospitals of the United States."

These reports may be of help in determining whether there is a local, regional, or national shortage of nursing personnel in psychiatric facilities, and, where there is no shortage, to help locate areas where there may be problems more directly related to effective use of nursing personnel.

In 1951, two psychiatric nurses were appointed as members of the WHO Expert Advisory Panel on Nursing — Esther Garrison and Hildegard Peplau — for a five-year period. It was in this same year that the A.P.A. published its "Standard for Psychiatric Hospitals and Clinics."[138]

At the Minnesota conference, the recommendation was made that a similar conference be sponsored in the near future by NLNE. In 1951, the second conference was held at the University of Cincinnati, May 14 to 18.[139] The purpose of this conference was stated as to "...study and evaluate present practices with the view of improving psychiatric and mental health nursing education." The conference discussion focused around "six functional areas": the psychiatric nursing specialist, head nurse, instructor, supervisor, administrator of nursing service, and psychiatric nursing consultant. The functions and learning experiences stated are extensive and might well be reviewed for purpose of the 1956 conference. It was recommended that a similar conference be convened in the next year.

In 1952, the NLNE sponsored a conference at the University of Pennsylvania.[140] The following topics were considered: "The Basic Program in Psychiatric Nursing," "The Integration of Psychological Aspects of Nursing Care Through the Basic Program," and "The Psychiatric Aide and In-service Education." The conference recommended that NLNE seek funds to sponsor a conference of basic psychiatric nursing. It endorsed the recommendation made by the Advisory Committee on Psychiatric Nursing, to the Department of Services to School of Nursing, and to the Psychiatric Nursing Consultant of NLNE, "that the 12- to 16-week experience in psychiatry be continued as the recommended standard until evidence is obtained based upon research on (1) how and what to integrate and (2) the relationship between integration of psychiatric concepts and the purpose of the experience with psychiatric patients."

The "First Experimental Workshop on the Training of Attendants" was held in Peoria, Illinois, in 1951, under the joint sponsorship of the American Psychiatric Association and the National Association for Mental Health. This workshop was followed by a second similar one in Manteno, Illinois, January 11 to 13, 1952. These two conferences not only helped to spell out the felt difficulties of various personnel in psychiatric work with regard to nursing care, but they also provided opportunities for face-to-face relations and joint discussion of such problems by professional and non-professional workers in psychiatric services.

The outcomes of these conferences were reported to the Board of Directors of NLNE. The Board recommended "that a special committee be appointed to serve as an Advisory Committee to the Department of Services to School of Nursing and the Psychiatric Nursing Consultant, to explore further the questions raised in the report, including representation from the Joint Committee in Practical Nurse and Auxiliary Workers in Nursing Services." Headquarters staff also discussed steps that could be taken to implement positive action at an early date.

During 1952 the Advisory Committee met, as did others such as "Joint Committee on Practical Nurses and Auxiliary Workers in Nursing Service," "Sub-Committee to Study the Licensure of Non-professional Workers in Psychiatric Nursing of the A.N.A. Committee on Licensure," and so forth. A "Pre-Service Curriculum" for non-professional nursing personnel in psychiatric nursing services is in preparation.

In 1953, the Group for Advancement of Psychiatry appointed its first full-time nurse consultant to the Committee on Nursing, Mrs. Frances Lenehan. The GAP report on "Psychiatric Nursing," issued in 1952, had used nurse consultants on invitation rather than on a full-time working basis.

Within the overall National Institutes of Health, one of the seven institutes for specialized study is the "National Institute of Mental Health." These institutes opened in 1953. Mrs. Gwen Tudor Will was the nurse who initiated a design for the nursing program in the psychiatric portion of the Clinical Center in collaboration with the Chief Nurse.*

In 1953, NLN published a report of "A Study of Desirable Functions and Qualifications for Psychiatric Nurses" conducted by Claire Mintzer Fagin with the assistance of an Advisory Committee on the Psychiatric Nursing Project. The question, for which answers were sought in this study, was "What are the functions and qualifications of psychiatric nurses and what should they be?"

In Table I, this study suggests an "interrelationship among components of functions and qualifications" in the following manner:

*Mrs. Gwen Tudor Will's important contribution to clinical psychiatric nursing will appear in Mary Lohr's paper at the 1956 conference.

Table 1

FUNCTIONS	QUALIFICATIONS
Determinants	**Determinants**
Tasks	Personality
Duties	Experience
Problems of questions	Education
Patient's needs	Position demands
Hierarchy	Professional activities and attitudes
	Legal
	Physical characteristics
Operations	**Operations**
Roles assumed	Use of:
Activities carried out	Knowledge
	Abilities
	Interpersonal skills
	Technical skills
	Special skills

The studymaker made nine trips to eight census areas to confer with a total of 217 psychiatric nurses. These problems were specified in the individual and group conferences that were held:

- Lack of qualified personnel on all levels
- Lack of time
- Lack of teamwork, cooperation
- Lack of adequate facilities
- Lack of coordination between nursing service and nursing education
- Need for doing work not considered nursing or part of their particular job
- Difficulty in communicating with patients and personnel
- Inadequacy of basic preparation in psychiatric nursing
- Inadequacy of personnel policies, salaries, and atmosphere for attracting prepared people
- Lack of defined roles; misuse of professional nurse time
- Lack of dynamic in-service teaching programs

In the conclusions and recommendations of this report, the following functions were identified:

1. Establishing relationships with people, i.e., with patients, personnel, the public, members of the "team," etc.
2. Teaching, which involves helping others to become aware of ideas, techniques, and the like, through information and/or experiences.
3. Supervision, which involves participant observation, direction, counseling, and evaluation.
4. Administration, which involves management and coordination, liaison activities, and the like.
5. Consultation, which involves viewing overall problems and advising by suggesting new ways to view them and alternative means for solving them.
6. Research and participation in learning situations which involve investigating problems, learning new ideas and techniques, and the like.

In reviewing these six functions and the data collected in this project, the Advisory Committee interpreted the following four dynamic (operational) functions as desirable and properly within the province of psychiatric nurses.

1. Collecting significant data relating to identification of problems and steps toward their solution, e.g., observing behavior, recording observations.
2. Making inferences and/or judgments based on these data and leading to action, e.g., interpreting behavior of patients, seeking to understand the needs of patients, recognizing nurse roles in a situation.
3. Acting or intervening on the basis of inferences, e.g., clarifying with a patient the meaning of a procedure, discussing and acting to solve problems in a work situation.
4. Evaluating the entire process in terms of whether problems identified have been solved, e.g., evaluating experiences and learning with students.

Desirable qualifications are stated as follows:

"All psychiatric nurses should have:

1. "The intelligence, attitudes, and motivations required by work in a psychiatric facility, as determined by whatever established criteria are available;
2. "An attitude of inquiry into the thoughts, feelings, and actions of oneself and others;
3. "Trained capacity to make inferences and judgments in ways that are useful in the nursing role used in relations with patients;
4. "Ability to express warmth for people and appreciation of their difficulties;
5. "Ability to be imaginative and resourceful in limited situations;
6. "Good health and physical stamina commensurate to the job;
7. "Appreciations and understandings in the area of knowledge required for psychiatric nursing."

This report is a veritable compendium of information, in as much as pp. 44-100 itemize information and opinions about the various positions in psychiatric nursing, derived from the participants in the study, and the functions are classified in a variety of ways using the abstractions stated above.

In this era, there were many decisions which were made by the NLN Board of Directors and the ANA-NLN Coordinating Council which affect psychiatric nursing education and service.

January 20, 1953 — The basic professional program

should prepare nurses for beginning positions in the care of psychiatric patients, as it does in the case of medical-surgical, obstetric, and pediatric patients.

January 1953 — The statement was approved by NLN Board of Directors, submitted by NLN Interdivisional Committee on Practical Nursing and Auxiliary Nursing Services:

"It is the belief of the NLN that psychiatric aides are practitioners of nursing.

"We believe that there is a common core of principles basic to the practice of all nursing, whether that practice is performed by the professional nurse, the practical nurse, or the aide or attendant in special nursing fields. The professional nurse is prepared to perform all the functions of nursing. Other workers in nursing are prepared to perform parts of those functions with professional nurse supervision. Because there is a common core in nursing, the basic preparation of all nursing personnel should contain common elements. Implicit in the care of the special types of patients is the need for preparation in the specific clinical area.

"The nature of nursing is such that all who engage in the practice of nursing should be licensed under one law in each state.

"We believe that the scope and limits of the practice of the psychiatric aide in nursing should be defined as expeditiously as possible. When this is accomplished, legal regulations of the practice of this worker should be provided within nursing practice acts."

March 13, 1953 — ANA-NLN Coordinating Council (combined Boards of Directors):

To create a special committee to consider the means by which organized nursing can move in a concerted manner to meet the nursing needs of the mentally ill.

June 1953 — The ANA-NLN Coordinating Council accepted a recommendation of the Sub-Committee on Psychiatric Nursing to consider the means by which *organized nursing can move in a concerted manner to meet the nursing needs of the mentally ill.*

1. That nursing assume the leadership and responsibility for the training of all nursing personnel rendering care to psychiatric patients, and to look to the American Psychiatric Association and other professional, organized psychiatric groups for critical evaluation and psychiatric concepts that should be used in providing psychiatric nursing care and the training for that care.
2. That the whole problem of progression in nursing education be given continued study; not only of progression from practical nursing into professional nursing, but also from psychiatric aide training into professional nursing.
3. That the ANA and the NLN study the standards for psychiatric hospitals and clinics established by the American Psychiatric Association with a view to evaluating those standards which relate to nursing personnel.
4. That a report of this meeting and information regarding other activities of the national nursing organizations in the area of psychiatric nursing be transmitted to SNAs and SLNs.
5. That coordinating councils of state nurses associations and SLNs be encouraged to create committees similar to this committee in order that they may explore state and local problems in providing care for psychiatric patients and promote the coordination of programs in this area of common concern to both organizations.
6. That provision be made for the continuation of this committee, subject to annual review.

In June 1955, Esther Garrison, training specialist in psychiatric and mental health nursing, and Gwen Tudor Will, Chief, Psychiatric Nursing Service, Clinical Center, Bethesda, Maryland, attended the meeting of the WHO Expert Committee on Psychiatric Nursing in Geneva, Switzerland, August 29-September 3. Mrs. Will prepared for the meeting during the summer, visiting England, Scotland, Holland, Sweden, and Denmark.

The Expert Committee recommended:[141]

1. That national health administrations include, among their administrative officers, nurses with responsibility for the over-all planning of nursing service and nursing education, and that this planning include consideration of the nursing needs of mental hospitals and other mental-health programs;
2. That fellowships be provided for nurses to prepare them for advanced positions in psychiatric nursing;
3. That, on request, WHO make available consultant services in psychiatric nursing and research methods;

4. That an understanding of psychiatric nursing, mental health, and social and preventive aspects of nursing be extended nationally and inter-country;
5. That training programs for psychiatric nurses be developed to a professional standard as rapidly as practicable, following general educational principles such as the careful respect for the learning needs of the students in planning their course of study and clinical work, with nurses teaching the nursing aspects, and other modern educational practices;
6. That facilities be provided for psychiatric nursing students to be taught in their native tongue, and in any case, in a language that is well understood by them;
7. That programs of nursing education include the study of mental health and of social and preventive aspects of health, and that these subjects be integrated throughout the curriculum;
8. That in relation to further studies in psychiatric nursing:
   (a) administrative personnel in national and local positions encourage and facilitate studies on the subjects indicated in Section 4 of the report;
   (b) participation of nurses in research pertaining to psychiatric nursing, and inclusion of nursing with other disciplines in psychiatric research, be stimulated and encouraged;
   (c) advanced programs of study for psychiatric nursing include research methods;
   (d) WHO stimulate and co-ordinate studies in these fields.

In July 1955, Hildegard E. Peplau was appointed to the Council on Mental Health of the Southern Regional Education Board. An organizational meeting was held in Atlanta, Georgia July 11 and 12, at which time Marjorie Bartholf, Dean, School of Nursing, University of Texas, Galveston, was elected to the executive committee of the Council.

And in September 1955, Dorothy E. Gregg, coordinator of psychiatric nursing and mental hygiene at the University of Colorado, was appointed to the panel of consultants by the Western Interstate Mental Health Project.

In September 1955, Kathleen Black, Director, Mental Health and Psychiatric Nursing Advisory Service of the NLN, was appointed a member of the board of trustees of the Joint Commission on Mental Illness and Health, representing the NLN and ANA. The Commission includes representatives of more than 20 organizations interested in mental health. Its principal purpose is to survey all aspects of the problems of mental illness and mental health, and to formulate comprehensive plans and programs for improvement of diagnosis, treatment, care, and rehabilitation, and for the promotion of mental health.

In 1955, the American Psychiatric Association sponsored a conference on "Psychiatric Nursing Consultation" at Princeton.[142] The stated purpose of this institute was "To explore the present functions of psychiatric nursing consultant with a view to developing a more unified approach, and to clarify the purpose and direction of consultative work on problems related to the nursing care of the mentally ill." The institute provided an opportunity for 22 consultants and 10 faculty members to exchange ideas and to contribute toward clarifying the functions of psychiatric nurse consultant. The report points out that in 1955 there were 17 states having appointed consultants, with some emphasis in psychiatric nursing, including California, Illinois, Indiana, Maryland, Massachusetts, Michigan, Minnesota, New Jersey, New York, Ohio, Oklahoma, Pennsylvania, Texas, Virginia, and Wisconsin. Four states had the position established but unfilled — Kansas, Kentucky, South Carolina and Tennessee.

In this report Redmond defines the functions of the consultant in this way:

> "The consultant is generally regarded as a specialist who, by expert knowledge, skill, and wide experience, can help people discover and analyze problems, work out satisfactory solutions, and put those solutions into operation. . .she must be well informed in clinical psychiatric nursing, education, administration, and consultation."

This review of the historical development of psychiatric nursing can be brought to a close with a statement about the present conference, which was preceded by five regional conferences. The Newsletter describes this effort as follows:

> "Toward this goal, the Central Planning Committee of the NLN Psychiatric Nursing Conference Project will hold its first meeting September 29 and 30, 1955 in Washington, D.C.
>
> "Conference participants will represent many groups: directors of basic and graduate education in psychiatric nursing, deans of nursing schools,

directors of psychiatric aide training, supervisors and students in psychiatric nursing, psychiatrists, psychiatric social workers, social scientists, directors of public health nursing service, and administrators of psychiatric nursing service.

"The need for the conference is inherent in the nature of such typical problems as: the need for warmer and more supporting interpersonal relationships with patients and other psychiatric nursing personnel, the physical environment of large, highly populated, isolated mental hospitals, and the system of communications between nursing personnel and others.

"Those representing the various groups on the committee are: Luther B. Christman, South Dakota; Mrs. Lulu Wolf Hassenplug, California; Mrs. Ruth Perkins Kuehn, Pennsylvania; Pauline Lucas, Washington, D.C.; Marion E. Russell, Connecticut; Mrs. Mary Scott, Tennessee; Ruth Von Bergen, Minnesota; Richard York, Ph.D., Massachusetts; Ewald Busse, M.D., North Carolina."

Grant for Improving Psychiatric Nursing Care

A grant from the National Institute of Mental Health has made it possible for the NLN to sponsor a project to bring about improvement in psychiatric nursing education. The plan as outlined now includes a series of regional conferences which will precede a national conference on psychiatric nursing. The findings of these conferences will be published in a book to be widely distributed by the National League for Nursing.

Briefly, the objectives of the conference will be to define the nursing needs of the patients with mental and emotional illnesses and to determine and analyze the skills, attitudes, understandings, social situations and types of administrative organization of nurses and psychiatric aides with a view to developing certain qualities through education.

Many important events in psychiatric nursing which have aided its development and enlarged its significance in the whole of professional nursing education and service may have been omitted from this report. This is unavoidable when this paper is considered in the light of its title: A preliminary statement of some facts and trends.

References

1. Roberts, Mary M. *American Nursing: History and Interpretation,* N.Y., MacMillan, 1954.
2. *One Hundred Years of American Psychiatry,* Columbia University Press.
3. Deutsch, Albert. *The Mentally Ill in America,* N.Y., Columbia University Press, 1946.
4. See paper by Miss Brown, Massachusetts General, *Proceedings of the Fifth Annual Convention of the National League of Nursing Education,* 1889, p. 18.
5. *One Hundred Years of American Psychiatry,* p. 115.
6. Roberts, Mary, p. 5.
7. *One Hundred Years of American Psychiatry,* p. 203.
8. *Ibid,* p. 293.
9. Hunt, J. McV. *Personality and the Behavior Disorders,* Volume II, N.Y. Ronald Press, pp. 1119-1120 (Original work: Call, Annie Payson. *Power Through Repose,* Boston, Little, Brown, 1891, 1914.)
10. Jacobson, E. *You Must Relax,* N.Y., McGraw Hill, 1934; See also, *Progressive Relaxation,* Chicago, Univ. of Chicago Press, 1938, p. 134.
11. Rippon, T.S. and Fletcher, P. *Reassurance and Relaxation,* London, George Routledge, 1940.
12. *Proceedings of the Fifth Annual Convention of the National League of Nursing Education,* (see Maxwell) p. 21, 1899.
13. Snively, Mary Agnes (Canada) "A Uniform Curriculum for Training Schools," *Proceedings,* 1895, p. 24.
14. Drown, Miss. "A Consideration of Methods for the Protection of Training Schools for Nurses, from Applicants who have been discharged for cause from other schools," *Proceedings,* 1895, p. 49.
15. *Proceedings,* 1896, p. 17.
16. *Proceedings,* 1897, p. 59.
17. *Proceedings,* 1899, p. 8.
18. *Ibid,* pp. 15-21.
19. *Ibid,* p. 22.
20. McMillan, Helena M. "Affiliation of Training Schools," *Proceedings of the Twelfth Annual Convention of NLNE,* 1906, p. 144.
21. Paper by M.G. O'Brien, not given in convention proceedings, see: *Nurses Journal of the Pacific Coast.*
22. Lawler, Elise M. "Nursing of Nervous Diseases," *Proceedings of the Annual Convention of NLNE,* 1909, p. 43.
23. *Proceedings,* 1910.
24. *Ibid,* p. 104.
25. DeWitte, Katherine. "Specialties in Nursing,"*AJN,* Vol. 1, No. 1, 1900, p. 14.
26. Knight, Delia. "The Nurse and Psychic Factor,"*AJN,* Vol. 2, 1900, p. 111.
27. Gulick, Walter (MD). "Cathartics and Hypnosis" in *Treatment of Nervous and Mental Diseases,* Vol. 2, No. 1, 1902, p. 99.
28. Chapman, Mrs. "Asylum Nursing," *AJN,* Vol. 2, No. 3, Dec. 1901, p. 164.
29. Laird, S. Louise. "Nursing of the Insane,"*AJN,* Vol. 2, No. 3, 1901, p. 167.
30. *AJN,* 1900, p. 45.
31. Roberts, Mary, p. 264.
32. "Psychiatric Nursing Consultation," Report of the Institute of Nursing Consultants in Psychiatry, American Psychiatric Association, 1955, p. 39.
33. Taylor, Effie J. "Mental Hygiene,"*Proceedings,* 1914, pp. 187-190.
34. Tucker, Katherine. "Nursing Care of the Insane,"*AJN,* 1915, Vol. 16, p. 198.
35. *One Hundred Years of American Psychiatry,* p. 130.

36. Richards, Linda. *Reminiscences of America's First Trained Nurse,* Boston, Whitcomb and Barrows, 1915, pp. 108-110.

37. Parsons, Sara E. *Nursing Problems and Obligations,* Whitcomb and Barrows, 1916.

38. Bailey, Harriet. *Nursing Mental Diseases,* New York, MacMillan. First printing July 1920. See also Book Reviews in *AJN,* Vol. 20, Oct. 1919-Sept. 1920, p. 1007.

39. Roberts, Mary, p. 264.

40. *Standard Curriculum for Schools of Nursing,* National League for Nursing Education, 1917, p. 177.

41. *Ibid,* p. 111.

42. *One Hundred Years of American Psychiatry,* pp. 388, 403.

43. Sinclair, Helen. "What Constitutes a Course in Psychiatric Nursing," *Proceedings of the 29th Annual Convention of the National League of Nursing Education,* 1923, p. 203.

44. Williams, Helen C. "The Place of the Attendant in the Hospital for the Mentally Ill," *Proceedings of the 29th Annual Convention of the NLNE,* 1923, p. 214.

45. Taylor, Effie J., p. 216.

46. Roscoe, Maude H. "Should Every Nurse Have Psychiatric Training," *Proceedings of the 29th Annual Convention of the National League of Nursing Education,* 1923, p. 199.

47. Bowman, Carl (MD). "The Responsibility of the Psychiatrist in Interesting Nurses in Mental Nursing," *Proceedings,* 1922, p. 199.

48. A Curriculum for Schools of Nursing, Committee on Education, *NLNE,* 1927, pp. 17-46.

49. Holden, Alice (RN). "Advantages of Training in a Hospital for Nervous and Mental Diseases," *AJN,* 1924, Vol. 24, No. 10, pp. 809-810.

50. McLean (Steele), Katherine (RN). "Values of Psychiatric Training for Nurses," *AJN,* 1928,Vol. 28, No. 5, pp. 501-503.

51. Richards, Esther Loring (MD). "Mental Hygiene and the Student Nurse," *AJN,* 1928, Vol. 28, No. 2.

52. Whitney, Myra (RN). "The Value of a Brief Course in Psychiatric Nursing," *AJN,* 1928, Vol. 28, No. 5, pp. 503-505.

53. Faber, Marion J. "Mental and Physical Factors Essential for Good Nursing," *AJN,* 1929, Vol. 29, No. 2, pp. 206-212.

54. Taylor, Effie J. (RN). "Psychiatry and the Nurse," *AJN,* 1926, Vol. 26, No. 8, pp. 631-634.

55. "Revision of the Standard Curriculum" (two papers: "Psychology" and "Psychiatric Nursing"), *AJN,* Vol. 26, No. 2, pp. 140-146.

56. National League for Nursing Education, *Curriculum Guide,* 1927.

57. National League for Nursing Education, *Curriculum Guide,* 1937.

58. Neuman-Rahn, Karin (RN). "The International Committee on Mental Nursing and Hygiene," *AJN,* 1929, Vol. 29, No. 9.

59. McGibbon, Anna K. (RN). "Adaptation of the Standard Curriculum to Meet the Needs of a Mental Hospital," *NLNE Convention Proceedings,* 1926, p. 150.

60. Ruggles, Arthur H. "Psychiatry and the Nurse," *AJN,* 1926, Vol. 26, No. 5, pp. 357-361.

61. Pratt, George K. "Psychiatric Departments in General Hospitals," *AJN,* 1926, Vol. 26, No. 7, pp. 545-548.

62. Hubbard, L.D. (MD). "Nursing the Mental Patient," *AJN,* 1927, Vol. 27, No. 3, pp. 179-181.

63. Russell, William M. (MD). "The Place of the Nurse in Mental Hygiene," *AJN,* 1928, Vol. 28, No. 9, pp. 863-870.

64. Olsen, Marie (RN). "Mental Nursing, A Privilege," *AJN,* 1929, No. 9, pp. 1080-1084.

65. Richard, Esther Loring (MD). "Mental Hygiene Applied to Personal Relationships in the Field of Nursing Education," *NLNE Proceedings,* 1929, p. 173.

66. "In Louisville," *AJN,* 1928, Vol. 28, No. 7. A report of the Biennial convention indicates many papers on mental hygiene and the emphasis on getting training for understanding of the preventive aspects.

67. Bennett, A.E. (MD). "The value of psychiatric training," *AJN,* 1929, Vol. 29, No. 3, pp. 303-307.

68. Haydon, Edith M. (RN). "Teaching and Supervision of Mental Nursing," *AJN,* 1928, Vol. 28, No. 5, pp. 499-501.

69. How, Anne (RN). "Mental Hospital Affiliations for General Hospital Students," *AJN,* 1930, Vol. 30, No. 7.

70. Farrar, Clarence B. (MD) (Part 1) and Chadwick, Mary (RN) (Part 2). "Psychiatric Education," *AJN,* 1930, Vol. 30, No. 10, pp. 1260-1265.

71. Mullen, Bernadette (RN). "Group Nursing in Psychiatry," *AJN,* 1929, Vol. 29, No. 11, pp. 1287-1288.

72. McGibbon, Anna K. (RN). "Mental Hygiene and Psychiatric Nursing," *AJN,* 1932, Vol. 32, No. 3, p. 269.

73. Putnam, Mary L. (RN). "Occupational Therapy in Relation to the Pupil Nurse," *AJN,* 1920, No. 5, pp. 548-552.

74. Morrissey, Mary R. "The Library in a Mental Hospital," *AJN,* 1929, Vol. 29, No. 2, pp. 139-142.

75. "A Study in the Nursing Care Given to Mental Patients in the Cook County Hospital," *AJN,* 1929, No. 2, pp. 143-147.

76. Faber, Marion J. (RN). "The Value of Psychiatric Nursing as a Method of Teaching Mental Hygiene to Students," *AJN,* 1930, Vol. 30, No. 1, pp. 69-71.

77. Lewis, George M. (RN). "Schizophrenia," *AJN,* 1933, Vol. 33, No. 11.

78. Thielbar, Frances C. (RN). "Ward Teaching in a Mental Hospital," *AJN,* 1934.

79. Editorial "Conference on Nursing and Mental Hygiene," *AJN,* 1931, Vol. 31, No. 12, p. 1417.

80. Burgess, May Ayres. "Where Does Nursing Want to Go," *AJN,* 1928, Vol. 28, No. 5.

81. "Not our School," *AJN,* 1929, Vol. 29, No. 1, pp. 63-64.

82. Editorial *AJN,* 1929, Vol. 29, No. 1, p. 67.

83. Burgess, May Ayres. "The Distribution of Nursing Service," *AJN,* 1930, Vol. 30, No. 7, pp. 857-861.

84. Goodrich, Annie W. (RN). "The Responsibility of the Community for Nursing and Nursing Education," *AJN,* 1929, Vol. 29, No. 11, pp. 1349-1354.

85. Gray, Garoline E. (RN). "Post-Graduate Courses: A Study of Existing Post-Graduate Courses given in Hospitals and Exclusive of those in Universities," *AJN,* 1929, Vol. 29, No. 6, pp. 709-720.

86. Russell, William M. (MD). "The Place of the Nurse in Mental Hygiene," *AJN,* 1928, Vol. 28, No. 9, pp. 863-870.

87. "Courses Offered to Graduate Nurses," *AJN,* 1931, Vol. 31, No. 5, pp. 612-614.

88. Soule, Elizabeth (RN). "How Shall We Select and Prepare the Graduate Nurse," *AJN,* 1932, Vol. 32, No. 5, pp. 567-569.

89. Stewart, Isobel (RN). "Advanced Courses in Clinical Subjects," *AJN,* 1933, Vol. 33, No. 6, p. 583 (See also Vol.33, No. 4, p. 361).

90. Noyes, Arthur P. "What are the Nursing Needs in State Mental Hospitals from the Standpoint of Medical Superintendent," *AJN,* 1933, Vol. 33.

91. How, Anne (RN). "From the Standpoint of the Superintendent of Nurses," *AJN* (Greystone), 1933, Vol. 33, pp. 794-796.

92. Erickson, Isobel (RN). "The Psychiatric Nurse," *AJN,* 1935, Vol. 35, No. 4, p. 351.

93. Stevenson, George J. (MD). Statement at the American Psychiatric Association meeting and reprinted in *AJN,* 1935,

Vol.35, No. 1, p. 66.

94. Nind, Gretchen (RN). "What are the Nursing Needs in State Mental Hospitals from the Standpoint of the Superintendent of Nurses," *NLNE Proceedings*, 1933, p. 245.

95. Wheeler, Catherine. "The Reasons Why Nurses Specially Prepared in Psychiatric Nursing Choose General Nursing," *NLNE Proceedings*, 1923, p. 196.

96. Noyes, Arthur P. (MD). "What are the Nursing Needs in the State Mental Hospital from the Standpoint of the Medical Superintendent," *NLNE Proceedings*, 1933, p. 250.

97. Burgess, May Ayres. *Nurses, Patients and Pocketbooks*, A Study of the Economics of Nursing Conducted by the Committee on the Graduating of Nursing Schools, N.Y.C., 1928, pp. 451-452.

98. *Ibid*, p. 47.

99. Nursing Schools Today and Tomorrow: Final Report of the Committee on the Grading of Nursing Schools, N.Y.C., 1934, p. 16.

100. "Report of the Committee on Nursing in Mental Hospitals," *NLNE Proceedings*, 1934, p. 56.

101. *NLNE Proceedings*, 1935, p. 211.

102. Willis, Helena L. "Teaching Psychiatric Nursing," *NLNE Proceedings*, 1936, p. 260.

103. Render, Helena Willis. *Nurse-Patient Relationships in Psychiatry*, New York, McGraw Hill, 1947, p. 346.

104. Myers, Glen (MD). "Nursing the Psychiatric Patient," *NLNE Proceedings*, 1936, p. 261.

105. *Curriculum Guide*, 1937.

106. Menninger, William C. "Psychiatry in Nursing Education," *NLNE Proceedings*, 1938, p. 201.

107. Watters, Theodore A. "Psychiatry in Nursing Education," *NLNE Proceedings*, 1939, p. 191.

108. Harvey, Florence. "The Teaching of Psychiatric Nursing in the Psychiatric Unit of a General Hospital," *NLNE Proceedings*, 1940, p. 201.

109. Edgar, Helen. "The Teaching of Psychiatric Nursing in a State Hospital," *NLNE Proceedings*, 1940, pp. 205-211.

110. Walsh, Irene. "The Teaching of Psychiatric Nursing in a Psychiatric Department of a Municipal Hospital, *NLNE Proceedings*, 1940, pp. 211-213.

111. "Round Table on Psychiatric Nursing," *NLNE Proceedings*, 1941, pp. 179-188.

112. "Round Table on Psychiatric Nursing," *NLNE Proceedings*, 1942, p. 52.

113. "Round Table on Psychiatric Nursing," *NLNE Proceedings*, 1943, p. 273.

114. Report of the Committee on Mental Hygiene and Psychiatric Nursing, *NLNE Proceedings*, 1940, pp. 108-110.

115. Report of the Committee on Mental Hygiene and Psychiatric Nursing, *NLNE Proceedings*, 1941, pp. 71-73.

116. Report of the Committee on Mental Hygiene and Psychiatric Nursing, *NLNE Proceedings*, 1942, pp. 118-120.

117. Report of the Committee on Mental Hygiene and Psychiatric Nursing, *NLNE Proceedings*, 1943, pp. 67-69.

118. Report of the Committee on Mental Hygiene and Psychiatric Nursing, *NLNE Proceedings*, 1944.

119. Favreau, Claire H. "Existing Needs in Psychiatric Nursing, *AJN*, 1945, No. 9, p. 716.

120. Fitzsimmons, Laura W. "Facts and Trends in Psychiatric Nursing," *AJN*, 1944, Vol. 44, No. 8, Aug., p. 752.

121. "Nursing Specialties in the Curriculum," *AJN*, 1944, No. 7, pp. 680-683.

122. Goostray, Stella. "The Time is Now," *AJN*, 1944, No. 7, pp. 677-679. See also *NLNE Proceedings*, 1945, "Report of the Committee on Post-Graduate Clinical Nursing Courses," p. 89.

123. Courses in Clinical Nursing for Graduate Nurses, *NLNE*, 1945 (out of print). See *AJN*, June 1944, p. 579, Pamphlet No. 1.

124. Courses in Clinical Nursing for Graduate Nurses, *NLNE*, 1945, Pamphlet No. 2. See also *NLNE Proceedings*, 1946 and 1949.

125. *One Hundred Years of American Psychiatry*, p. 131.

126. "National Mental Health Act Passed," *AJN*, 1946, No. 9, p. 637.

127. Report of the Director of the NLNE-NOPHN Study of Advanced Psychiatric Nursing and Mental Hygiene, Programs of Study, 1949, *NLNE Proceedings*, p. 144.

128. *Manual of Accrediting Educational Programs in Nursing*, NLNE, 1949, "Additional Criteria for Evaluation of Advanced Programs of Study in Psychiatric Nursing and Mental Hygiene," pp. 67-84.

129. Report to the Advisory Council of the Committee on Psychiatric Nursing, *NLNE Proceedings*, 1946.

130. *NLNE Proceedings*, 1947.

131. *NLNE Proceedings*, pp. 325-327.

132. Mimeographed report of proceedings not available for distribution.

133. Brown, Esther Lucille. *Nursing for the Future*, N.Y. Russell Sage Foundation, 1948, pp. 136-137.

134. Committee on the Function of Nursing, *A Program for the Nursing Profession*, N.Y., MacMillan, 1948, pp. 42-43.

135. Bridgman, Margaret. *Collegiate Education for Nursing*, N.Y., Russell Sage Foundation, 1953, p. 25.

136. Inventory and Qualifications of Psychiatric Nurses, Aurelie J. Nowakowski, National League of Nursing, 1950.

137. Clark, Dorothy (RN). Psychiatric Nursing Personnel, American Psychiatric Association, 1950.

138. "Standards for Psychiatric Hospitals and Clinics," American Psychiatric Association, Washington, D.C.

139. Report of the Conference on Advanced Programs in Psychiatric and Mental Health Nursing, *NLNE*, 1951.

140. "Report of Conference for Directors of Advanced Programs in Psychiatric Nursing," 1952, University of Pennsylvania, Mimeographed.

141. "Expert Committee on Psychiatric Nursing," World Health Organization, 1956, (Columbia University Press, International Documents Service, New York City).

142. *Psychiatric Nursing Consultation, Report of the Institute for Nursing Consultants in Psychiatry*, American Psychiatric Association, 1955.

Additional References

Phase I: 1773 — 1881

No additional references.

Phase II: 1882 — 1914

McMillan, Helena M. "Affiliation of Training Schools." *Proceedings of the Twelfth Annual Convention of the National League of Nursing Education*, 1906, pp. 144.

Hall, Manuel J. "Manual Work as a Remedy." *Proceedings of the Sixteenth Annual Convention of the National League of Nursing Education*, 1910, pp. 196.

Neff, M.L. "Successes and Failures in the Employment of Occupation for the Treatment of the Insane." *Proceedings of the Sixteenth Annual Convention of the National League of Nursing Education*, 1910, pp. 183.

Dow, Arthur Wesley. "How Art May Aid in this Field." *Proceedings of the Sixteenth Annual Convention of the*

National League of Nursing Education, 1910, pp. 204.

Noyes, Clara D. "Some Problems Arising in Affiliations between Nursing Schools." *Proceedings of the Seventeenth Annual Convention of the National League of Nursing Education*, 1911, pp. 82.

Arnold, Sarah Louise. "Cooperation of Educational Institutions with Training Schools for Nurses." *Proceedings of the Seventeenth Annual Convention of the National League of Nursing Education*, 1911, pp. 173.

Phase III: 1915 — 1935

Ansted, Ida J. "Problems and Possibilities in State Hospital Training Schools." *Proceedings of the Twenty-Second Annual Convention of the National League of Nursing Education*, 1916, pp. 208.

Taylor, Effie J. "Why Does the Nurse in the General Hospital Need Training for Mental Work?" *Proceedings of the Twenty-Second Annual Convention of the National League of Nursing Education*, 1916, pp. 195.

Thomson, Elnora. "Mental Hygiene Movement and Preventive Measures." *Proceedings of the Twenty-Second Annual Convention of the National League of Nursing Education*, 1916, pp. 215.

Walsh, Adelaide Mary. "Laws Pertaining to the Care and Commitment of the Mentally Ill." *Proceedings of the Twenty-Second Annual Convention of the National League of Nursing Education*, 1916, pp. 221.

Ambrose, Edith M. "Where and How Should Attendants be Trained." *Convention of the National League of Nursing Education*, 1917, pp. 171.

Taft, Jessie. "Demands Which Mental Hygiene Makes Upon the Graduate Nurse." *Proceedings of the Twenty-Third Annual Convention of the National League of Nursing Education*, 1917, pp. 69.

O'Brien, M. Grace. "Training, Licensure and Supervision of Attendants." *Proceedings of the Twenty-Fourth Annual Convention of the National League of Nursing Education*, 1918, pp. 217.

Strong, Anne Harvey. "The Attendant." *Proceedings of the Twenty-Fourth Annual Convention of the National League of Nursing Education*, 1918, pp. 158.

Swainhardt, Blanche. 'Supervised Attendant Service." *Proceedings of the Twenty-Fourth Annual Convention of the National League of Nursing Education*, 1918, pp. 193.

Barnsby, Marietta D. "School for Attendants, Hospital Affiliations." *Proceedings of the Twenty-Seventh Annual Convention of the National League of Nursing Education*, 1921, pp. 234.

Shepard, Katherine. "School for Attendants, Organized Independently." *Proceedings of the Twenty-Seventh Annual Convention of the National League of Nursing Education*, 1921, pp. 227.

Bryan, Edith S. "How Can the Education of the Nurse be Directed Toward Preventive Work and Health Promotion." *Proceedings of the Twenty-Eighth Annual Convention of the National League of Nursing Education*, 1922, pp. 210.

McKibben, William. "White Cross Campaign Against Narcotics." *Proceedings of the Twenty-Eighth Annual Convention of the National League of Nursing Education*, 1922, pp. 199.

Earl, Mary Goodyear. "Mental Testing." *Proceedings of the Twenty-Ninth Annual Convention of the National League of Nursing Education*, 1923, pp. 220.

Williams, Helen C. "The Place of the Attendant in the Hospital for the Mentally Ill." *Proceedings of the Twenty-Ninth Annual Convention of the National League of Nursing Education*, 1923, pp. 214.

Stearns, Warren. "Community Need for Nurses with Psychiatric Training." *Proceedings of the Twenty-Ninth Annual Convention of the National League of Nursing Education*, 1923, pp. 189.

McGibbon, Anna K. "Adaptation of Standard Curriculum to Meet the Needs of a Mental Hospital." *Proceedings of the Thirty-Second Annual Convention of the National League of Nursing Education*, 1926, pp. 150.

Faber, Marion. "Present Use and Future Possibilities of Mental Tests in Schools of Nursing." *Proceedings of the Thirty-Fourth Annual Convention of the National League of Nursing Education*, 1928, pp. 157

Densford, Katherine J. "An 'In Service' Program of Staff Education." *Proceedings of the Thirty-Fifth Annual Convention of the National League of Nursing Education*, 1929, pp. 115.

Richards, Esther Loring. "Mental Hygiene Applied to Personal Relationships in the Field of Nursing Education." *Proceedings of the Thirty-Fifth Annual Convention of the National League of Nursing Education*, 1929, pp. 173.

Eldredge, Adda. "Responsibilities of State Boards of Nurse Examiners in Requiring Affiliations." *Proceedings of the Thirty-Sixth Annual Convention of the National League of Nursing Education*, 1930, pp. 163.

Hall, Carrie M. "Responsibilities and Problems of a School Sending Affiliating Students." *Proceedings of the Thirty-Sixth Annual Convention of the National League of Nursing Education*, 1930, pp. 158.

Muse, Maude B. "Problem of Selecting Applicants for Schools of Nursing." *Proceedings of the Thirty-Sixth Annual Convention of the National League of Nursing Education*, 1930, pp. 206.

Muse, Maude B. "The Importance of Psychology in Schools of Nursing." *Proceedings of the Thirty-Sixth Annual Convention of the National League of Nursing Education*, 1930, pp. 206.

Burton, William H. "Principles of Administrative Organization." *Proceedings of the Thirty-Seventh Annual Convention of the National League of Nursing Education*, 1931, pp. 186.

Bigler, Rose. "Educational Resources of the State Mental Hospitals." *Proceedings of the Thirty-Ninth Annual Convention of the National League of Nursing Education*, 1933, pp. 259.

How, Anne. "What are the Nursing Needs in State Mental Hospitals from the Standpoint of the Superintendent of Nurses?" *Proceedings of the Thirty-Ninth Annual Convention of the National League of Nursing Education*, 1933, pp. 240.

Nind, Gretchen E. "What are the Nursing Needs in State Mental Hospitals From the Standpoint of the Superintendent of Nurses?" *Proceedings of the Thirty-Ninth Annual Convention of the National League of Nursing Education*, 1933, pp. 245.

Noyes, Arthur P. "What are the Nursing Needs of the State Mental Hospitals from the Standpoint of Medical Superintendent?" *Proceedings of the Thirty-Ninth Annual Convention of the National League of Nursing Education*, 1933, pp. 250.

Potts, Edith Margaret. "The Use of Psychological Tests in the Selection of Students." *Proceedings of the Thirty-Ninth Annual Convention of the National League of Nursing Education*, 1933, pp. 174.

Thielbar, Frances C. "Clinical Experience of Psychiatric Nursing." *Proceedings of the Forty-First Annual Convention of the National League of Nursing Education,* 1935, pp. 211.

Phase IV: 1936 — 1945

Peterson, Edna E. "Another Cooperative Program for Revising the Nursing School Curriculum." *Proceedings of the Forty-Fourth Annual Convention of the National League of Nursing Education,* 1938, pp. 195.

Faber, Marion. "Facilities for Preparation of Nurses in Psychiatry." *Proceedings of the Forty-Fourth Annual Convention of the National League of Nursing Education,* 1938, pp. 209.

Draper, Warren F. "The National Health Program and the Nurse." *Proceedings of the Forty-Fifth Annual Convention of the National League of Nursing Education,* 1939, pp. 242.

The Work of Clinical Specialists in Psychiatric Nursing

Hildegard E. Peplau, R.N., Ed.D.

Dr. Peplau is Chairman, Department of Psychiatric Nursing, College of Nursing, Rutgers - The State University of New Jersey, 18 James Street, Newark 2, New Jersey.

This paper was presented May 1, 1959.

More rapid improvement of direct nursing care of the mentally ill may depend in large part upon the development of "clinical specialists in psychiatric nursing" — a new trend in the nursing profession.* Such expert practitioners would work directly with patients. These "clinical specialists" would try out, demonstrate, and in other ways indicate the form and substance of new patterns of nursing care. The expert practitioner, therefore, would be the growing edge of clinical practice in nursing. The current need is great for nurses who can grasp and apply the rapidly enlarging body of new knowledge being developed by the various basic sciences. Equally great is the need for deriving additional knowledge from empirical observations in nursing practice. In order to meet these two needs — in ways that favor the recovery of patients and that help to speed up improvements in the practices of all generalized practitioners of nursing — a new position and job title, with new functions, is being considered.

In 1955 a master's level program in advanced psychiatric nursing was initiated at Rutgers.** This program prepares "clinical specialists" *only* and serves also as a basis for a study of the functions, content, and process of training — which will be reported in 1961.*** While at the outset the faculty had a conception of functions, and of placement of the "clinical specialist" in the current ladder-type hierarchical progression of the established positions, (from attendant, practical nurse, staff nurse, head nurse, supervisor, director of nursing), this new position was then non-existent. A need was apparent for knowing the opinions of others on this provocative subject. Consequently, the opinions of twenty-three nurses and fifteen doctors were sought with regard to a first draft description of "nurse specialist (in psychiatric nursing)." These opinions were analyzed and a second draft job description will be prepared from them. A questionnaire based upon this second draft description will be sent out to a larger, representative sample in order to secure a wider view of professional opinion.

The job description was intended as a statement of the clinical functions which the clinical specialist would carry out in giving direct care to psychiatric patients, as seen by the faculty.**** The respondents were asked to give their opinions on "the completeness and usefulness of the stated functions;" the feasibility of including such a position as a budget item and personnel category; the salary that should be offered for this position; and the problems foreseen as connected with the position as described.

With regard to the "completeness and usefulness of the stated functions," 10 respondents endorsed the statement; 18 cited omissions; 4 stated criticisms; and 8 (2 included in endorsement above) offered restatements. The omissions suggested were largely restatements of the given content of the job description; the criticisms included statements that the functions were "generalities" or overlapped with the work of the supervisor. In addition, an "overall impression" of the idea of preparing clinical specialists was clearly indicated in many of the covering letters. While no such impression was indicated by 8 nurses and 3 doctors, 15 nurses and 8 doctors definitely approved of the idea; 2 doctors indicated ambivalence and 2 doctors disapproved the idea as

*While this is a new trend, the actions of the House of Delegates of the American Nursing Association, June 1958, in adopting the report of its Committee on Current and Long-term Goals, indicates widespread interest in this trend represented in the following two goals that were adopted: "*Goal One:* Stimulate efforts by nurses and other specialists to identify and enlarge the scientific principles upon which nursing rests, and to encourage research by them in the application of these principles to nursing practice. *Goal Two:* Establish ways within the ANA to provide formal recognition of personal achievement and superior performance in nursing."

**The College of Nursing received a training grant from NIMH under the Mental Health Act which supports this program. The College of Nursing submitted its application for a grant in December 1954. It is of interest, from the standpoint of timeliness of the idea, that the Regional and Williamsburg Conferences of NLN in 1956 focussed upon this subject. See: "The Education of the Clinical Specialist in Psychiatric Nursing," National League of Nursing, 10 Columbus Circle, New York City, 1958.

***There are twenty-six master's and doctoral level programs in various colleges and universities, several of which have been in existence since 1947. While these programs all include some clinical training, their focus in 1955 was upon preparing teachers, supervisors, administrators, consultants and/or researchers. The master's programs tend to be 10-12 months in length.

****For a more complete discussion, see League Exchange Pamphlet No. 26, "Aspects of Psychiatric Nursing," Sections A: Concepts of Nursing Care, B: Therapeutic Concepts, C: Administration, and D: Education, National League for Nursing, 10 Columbus Circle, New York City.

"unrealistic" and "difficult to conceptualize in a state hospital."

The question of the feasibility of including a "clinical specialist" title as a budget item and personnel category was not clearly answered by the respondents. Only 8 of the 38 respondents replied directly and of these, the stated difficulty in finding financial support was outstanding. Five respondents stated that "clinical specialists" could be employed on an experimental basis as a pilot project; 7 felt that it can and should be done; 3 stated that the "clinical specialist" was a non-feasible luxury; 1 stated that it could not be done in a state hospital; 1 stated that it could not be done in a teaching hospital; 3 respondents believed administrative understanding and acceptance must first be gained.

No clearcut suggestion as to salary that might be commanded by the "clinical specialist" emerged. Half the respondents suggested salary levels comparable to or above such established positions as clinical instructor, supervisor or director; 9 specified a salary range of $4500-5500; 4 indicated $5500-7200 as the range.

Many problems were stated by the respondents as those foreseen if "clinical specialists" are employed in existing psychiatric facilities. Some of these were reactions against the idea or the functions stated in the job description. *The work of the clinical specialist* as seen by the faculty at the College of Nursing, Rutgers includes direct work with individual patients and with groups within the ward setting, including interviewing (nursing therapy) patients, preparing some patients for long-term medical psychotherapy, serving as a resource person to ward personnel, making sociological studies of a ward, and reporting findings at staff meetings. The job description also stated that the nurse would keep confidential records of data secured in her work. The job description *did not* state that the clinical specialist would administer a ward, do formal teaching of any kind, or supervise the work of others — *all functions were stated in the form of giving or demonstrating direct care to patients.* (There have been so very many complaints that nurses do not want to give direct care, or that they must and do move upward in the nursing service hierarchy in order to earn more money that it was anticipated that this lateral promotion and "return to the bedside" would be quickly seen and appreciated.)

The problem of who should state the functions of clinical specialist — a local agency, a university faculty, ANA, a specialty board, or regional groups — was raised.

The problem of whether nurses and the nursing profession should decide upon the need for "clinical specialists" *or* whether other disciplines should be the major determining factor was raised.

The problems suggested by the respondents clearly indicated that the differences between a clinician and a teacher were not seen. The need for teachers who "know their stuff" clinically is so great that 7 respondents gave lengthy statements on the need to make the "clinical specialist" a teacher of other nursing personnel. This can be interpreted as unwitting negation of the idea of "clinical specialists"!

Moreover, the difference between a clinical practitioner and a supervisor was also not seen. This is not to say that a supervisor — in the foreseeable future — ought not have advanced clinical training also. But the respondents more often than not suggested taking the specialist away from direct care and giving her, instead, the functions of supervisor.

A more basic problem, relevant to the direct care given by a clinical specialist, is whether she would be a qualified psychotherapist or merely use a therapeutic approach in her clinical work. One respondent argued that the length and quality of training would determine resolution of this problem.

The job description stated that data secured by the nurse would be treated as confidential, i.e., revealed to others only with the permission and knowledge of the patient. Some respondents read into this statement a lack of sharing of data by the clinical specialist; some questioned while others argued strongly that the nurse should have the right to treat patient data as confidential.

The outstanding problem was in relation to the placement of these clinicians within the administrative structure. Only 1 of the 38 respondents would have the "clinical specialist" administratively responsible to the director of nurses; others place her under the physician, nursing education department, nursing supervisor, or head nurse. The adverse effect of placement upon salary of the specialist was suggested.

The need for acceptance of the skilled practitioner — who is a "rare bird" — was suggested as essential. That doctors, psychologists, and social workers might take exception to the nurse as therapist, functioning as described, was pointed out. Many of the respondents wrote long letters on the kind of "spade work" that would be needed to permit such a nurse to do the work for which she was prepared. The concerns revolved around threats to other disciplines, rivalries among other nurse personnel, institutional resistance, restriction and sabotage of her work based upon maintenance of the current stereotyped conception of nursing in psychiatric facilities, and the like. Many respondents pointed out that "clinical specialists" would have to interpret, "sell," and survive the onslaught of misunderstanding of their work. Needless to say, the coercions of nurse shortages were mentioned as equally great forces which would mitigate against the specialist working as a clinician for very long.

If the work of expert clinicians in psychiatric nursing is seen as a promising development that will speed up improvements in nursing care, then surely the nursing profession is upon the horns of a dilemma. There is the task of demonstrating the need and proving the worth of the clinicians while this pioneer effort is barely beginning. The idea is an answer to the general criticism that nurses want to and do leave the direct care function to less well prepared, non-professional nursing personnel. The idea involves a lateral rather than upward movement as the nurse becomes more educated. But, the idea is also a threat — the clinician would be a model who could demonstrate what can be done, but this very demonstration may be an unwelcome reminder to current nursing staff that their efforts are not equally useful. Several respondents believed that reduction of the workload of current staff, better in-service education, or the use of existing position titles such as head nurse would be less upsetting to everyone concerned.

I would suggest that perhaps ten years of experience in training and in placement of such "clinical specialists" will give a wider view of the possibility of bringing to fruition this development.

Facilitating Student Learning Through the Teacher's Use of Self

Catherine M. Norris

Miss Norris is Assistant Professor of Psychiatric Nursing, University of Colorado School of Nursing.

This paper was presented at the 1957 Curriculum Conference, National League for Nursing, 2 Park Avenue, New York 16, New York

We have all heard teachers say, "I give my students a thorough grounding in physiology," or "I don't have enough time to give my students all the theory they need in obstetrics." The concept of give in this context says that the teacher "gives" knowledge. This concept does not have meaning or validity to me because I cannot spell out the teaching process involved in helping students grow and develop through the teacher's self-involvement or giving of self in participation with students. I would like to share some of the results of my struggle with you this afternoon with the understanding that this is only a beginning, and that other educators have contributed considerably to my interest and study in this area.

A student's learning about herself and her capacities takes place within her relationships with people. As teachers we have a responsibility to function in ways that help the student grow and develop.

The content of any subject or the content of many books will not provide the answers to the questions who am I, what can I do, and where do I want to go. It is not a matter of learning a set of principles and applying them in one's life experiences, including clinical nursing experience.

One of the greatest contributions a teacher can make in her work with a student is to help the student find out who she is, what she can do, and where she wants to go. This might be considered the mental health aspect of any teaching job. Mental hygiene in nursing is not a list of principles to be learned and applied in clinical situations. The theory of content of mental hygiene or psychiatry is voluminous and is increasing at a rapid rate. In other words, a thorough knowledge of content or facts may have little relation to one's ability to be imaginative and creative in nursing. We have all been aware of this at one time or another when we have said about someone, "She certainly knows her theory but she can't apply it." We have also been aware that some nurses who have little knowledge of theory are quite skillful in handling their own problems constructively and are creative in relationships with patients. This kind of intuitive functioning is exciting to observe. The only problem with it is that any performance carried out at the level of intuition cannot be taught to anyone else since the process involved in the helping role is not spelled out or identified. It might be said that the nurse who functions intuitively has had certain life experiences that have helped her become understanding, insightful, perceptive, respectful, and useful in relationships.

Our job in nursing is to identify these experiences that promote development of this kind of person and then, as teachers, to spell out our role within the realm of all of teaching to provide these experiences for students. In my experiences as a teacher, I have come to some general conclusions about what kinds of experiences students need. (1) Students need experiences with teachers who use authority rationally; (2) they need experiences in which they are respected and accepted; (3) they need experiences in which they know the limits and can learn to set limits for themselves; (4) they need someone to listen to them; (5) they need someone to be concerned about how they feel; (6) they need someone who can help them examine their participation with patients and others, and they need someone to support them to try out nursing care plans; (7) they need someone to support them when they fail, and someone to help them get satisfaction out of their experiences in nursing; and (8) they need experiences in which they can visualize their own potential.

Students need help in finding out who they are. This involves assisting the student in studying many questions about herself such as: Why did I choose nursing as a career? Why did I choose to deal with people who are helpless and in bed rather than choosing a career in which I deal face to face with people? Why did I choose a career that always involves helping others? Do I need to be needed? Do I need to have others dependent on me? Do I need to feel powerful in relation to others? Why didn't I choose a field in which I would have to compete more? Why did I choose a career that involves watching people suffer? Do I enjoy seeing others suffer? Was I really just curious about life and morbidity? What satisfactions do I expect to get out of nursing? Is it possible to get these satisfactions in nursing? What are the rational or real satisfactions in nursing? They will need assistance also in answering such questions as: What kinds of situations with patients or others make me tense, angry, embarrassed, afraid or helpless? How much tension can I tolerate in a situation? What values do I have that prevent me from understanding and being helpful to others? What do I respect in myself? What do I respect in others? How do I communicate respect? How do I communicate disrespect? What kinds of skills do I need to develop? How can I use the teacher to develop these skills?

These questions cover a broad area and could be very threatening to students if asked in the form that I have given them to you. I would expect the teacher to raise the questions that I have been raising within the context of daily nursing problems which the teacher and student examine together. In this way, the student deals with only a small part of the big question at a time. To cite an example:

A student told the teacher that a patient complained that the nurses on the ward didn't like him. The student told the patient that the nurses liked him, that they were just busy. The student went on to say that she had really not known what to say and felt quite uncomfortable. The teacher at this point has the data that the student interpreted what the patient said as a complaint; that the student defended the nurses, that she denied the possibility of the patient's observations being valid, and that she prevented him from exploring the problem further. The teacher will want to help the student recognize why she doesn't know what to say, why she interpreted the patient's remark as a complaint. The teacher speculates with the student about the student's identification with nursing getting in the way of her being able to recognize how the patient feels in a situation in which he feels disliked. The teacher will want to help the student look at whether she felt the patient was blaming her by implication. The teacher and student will want to get clear on what really threatened the student. Then the teacher will want to help the student identify how the patient was feeling and what his problem was. She might do this by asking the student about how the patient must have felt being on a ward where he felt disliked or rejected. The teacher will also want to help the student identify what the nurse's role in helping might be like. Would it have been useful if the nurse could have been concerned about how it would feel to be the patient, and would it have been useful if the nurse had been able to express some concern that he feels as he does? The teacher will want to help the student identify what kinds of data she and the patient need to get the real problem identified. The student might have explored with the patient the events that led up to the conclusion he came to. The student might have helped the patient get clear on whether the conclusion he came to was a valid one, and how to deal with it if it is correct. These are not the only possibilities here, but what I am describing here is a day by day kind of work with students that, day by day, over the course of a school program, get the big questions which I raised earlier answered.

Because we are all teachers, I would like at this point to spend the remainder of my time discussing the roles of teachers in which teachers use themselves to promote the goal of personal development of students. These roles describe the teaching process, and I stress this not to the exclusion of content, but I am aware that the content in any specific area is more readily available to you in literature than is a description of the teaching process.

The first teacher role that I would like to describe is that of the *authority role*. I think that sometimes in nursing we have been in conflict about this role. In our efforts to be a good authority figure and to use our authority rationally in our efforts to be permissive, we have become laissez-faire. In our efforts to be fair, and for fear of traumatizing the student, we deny our authoritarian responsibilities. Others of us, in our insecurity about teaching or insecurity about our job situations, demand perfection of the students. Others of us tell our students that we are democratic or permissive and then become dogmatic and manipulative in our relationships with students.

First, as teachers we need to accept the fact that, in relation to the student, we are authority figures and are viewed by students as such, along with all the distortions that they may have about people in authority. We also need to accept the fact that the moment the young student dons a uniform and enters a clinical situation, she is an authority figure in relation to the patient. The student as an authority will participate with the patient in terms of the way she has experienced authority in the past. If the student's experience with the teacher is that the teacher decides what is useful and non-useful, and if the student must accept the teacher's methods and values, then the student in her relationship with the patient will decide what is good for him and will expect him to accept her values.

What are the bases for rational authority? It is not the inspiration of awe in the student. It is not motivation of students in terms of the vested interests of authority. It is not deciding what is right and wrong for students. It is not the denial of potentiality of students and it is not praising and blaming in which the student learns only how to stay safe. It is not getting one's own personal needs met through the manipulation of students. This may seem like strong language to some of you, but each one of us could cite many examples from our own experience and observation that would illustrate the irrational use of authority. I would like to cite two examples of problems in the use of the authority role.

A student, in checking a post-operative plastic surgery patient, found the patient, who was coming out of anesthesia, gasping and cyanotic. The student, deciding that the patient must have a mucous obstruction, called another student who helped her get the foot of the bed up on a straight chair she had pulled from the side of the bed. She instructed the other student to get help and then ran for the suction machine. After suctioning the patient for a few minutes the patient's color became more pink and she began to breathe normally. The student's tension lessened and she began to feel good about herself and the way she had handled the emergency. At this point the instructor appeared at the bedside and saw the expensive new chair, just purchased for the unit, holding a heavy bed on its padded seat. She spoke sharply to the student and repeated the proper procedure for elevating the foot of the bed. The student, who was unsure about herself in the role of nurse, felt that she should have been more adequate in the situation. She also felt resentful that she had had no opportunity to tell the instructor about what had happened. The possible learnings for this student have been that "no matter how helpful one seems to be, one could have done it better," that "others evaluate your performance without adequate exploration of the problem," and that "teachers blame you instead of trying to help you." How was authority used irrationally? The teacher's values about the new chair may have gotten in the way. The student's performance as a reflection of the teacher's teaching may have gotten in the way. At any rate, something prevented the teacher from respecting the student enough to consider that there might be a reason for what she saw as she walked in. Something got in the way of the teacher helping the student get satisfaction out of the experience, helping the student recognize her potential for handling emergency situations, and helping the student examine her performance to see whether there were alternate choices in the situation.

The second example I would like to relate to you concerns a teacher who communicated to her students that the class would be conducted in terms of the expressed needs of the students. During the first class period the teacher gave the students a course outline, an assignment sheet, a bibliography, and the objectives of the course in order to save time in getting down to the work of the course. During the course the teacher helped the students at any point where it seemed that they might make an error or might not remember what to do. If patients became upset emotionally, the teacher, if she were present, always protected the student at the time and would deal with it herself. If students were late in getting their work done, either in the clinical area or for class, the teacher held conferences with them to urge them to work harder. The teacher was very interested in the students' getting a wide variety of experience, and if an interesting patient came into the clinical center on a day when the students did not have class, the teacher would call the students and ask them if they would like to get the useful experience. If the students didn't want to take advantage of this experience, the teacher would explain to the students that it was only for their own learning that she had called and weren't they interested in getting all the experience they could. If the students had made other plans, she reminded them that education should take precedence over other activities.

In this situation we see a teacher who states that she would like to function democratically. She may even feel that she does. However, we can observe that she is unable to respect the potential of the students to say what they need and to get down to work immediately. We can observe that the teacher cannot permit students the freedom to struggle with nursing problems. For some reason she must protect the student from getting into a problem and from dealing with it if it occurs. She cannot leave the students free to take the responsibility for meeting the course requirements or let them fail if they cannot assume responsibility for their own functioning, and she cannot help them look at why they cannot assume responsibility for their work. She cannot leave the students free to decide what is useful and important to them in their leisure time. Her values about education get in the way of her identifying other activities which have significance in the life of the student. She doesn't help the student examine the meaning of her experience with either the patient or the teacher, but intervenes in such a way that the student can only imitate or make decisions that keep her safe in her relationship with the teacher.

Rational authority is based on knowledge and ability in an area. It is based on understanding, including the understanding of one's self. It is based on respect for others and the ability to grow. It is based on the respect that others can think through and deal with problems that are presented to them. It is based on give and take in which the participation of both the authority or teacher and the student can be examined. Rational authority says that you do not need to do what I do or believe what I believe, but you need to know why you do what you do and believe what you believe. In teaching, rational authority is represented not in the student becoming a reflection of the teacher, but in the student becoming a person in her own right with the ability to think for herself, to become creative in her own ways and to further her own growth. The student who is dependent on the value system of an authority will search in vain all her life for a perfect authority in order to become a more perfect reflection.

The second teaching role that I would like to outline is that of *acceptance*.

The premise underlying the role of being accepting is that present performance is accepted or tolerated or respected and represents the best the individual can do at any given moment. The performance is accepted, however, not unconditionally but with the expectation that there will be change. Much of the functioning in this role is communicated nonverbally through tone of voice and posture. Communication of the role is also done by the way one listens to the person and the problem. Verbally the role is carried out by the non-blaming response to the student who is experiencing the problem. This means that one is not feeling like blaming and one is not thinking in blaming terms. It also means that the teacher has to be pretty clear about herself and what kinds of things or situations she can tolerate without blaming. If the teacher, in this role, feels blame, she will communicate it in some way and cut the student off from exploration of the problem. The student gears her behavior to staying safe in a situation where there is blame. This role also involves waiting for change in the other person. This wait may be in terms of minutes, days, months, or years. This may be the most difficult aspect of the role because it seems sometimes as if the change will never come, or it is difficult to tolerate the other's behavior as it repeats itself over and over, or because one might begin to wonder about one's effectiveness as a teacher.

I would like to cite an example from the experience of a teacher of medical-surgical nursing: A senior student who was married, had a husband in the army, and was four months pregnant, made three errors in medication over a two-week period. The student was asked to see the instructor and came to the conference angry and somewhat belligerent. She stated that she had never made an error before and that these were not serious errors, that she was aware of why she had made the errors, that is, what steps in the procedure she had not followed, and that she did not see why everyone was getting excited. The teacher explained that she was not excited but was concerned because these errors represented a real change in the student's functioning as a nurse. The student remained defensive about her errors, stating that anyone can make an error. The teacher recognized that this was true and that she wasn't as concerned about the errors, as such, but concerned about their meaning in the student's functioning as a nurse. For 45 minutes the student defended her errors, attacked the head nurse and staff nurses, and repeated that she knew how she had violated the principles of administration of drugs. The teacher focussed on helping the student examine other factors that might have accounted for the change in the student's performance. Finally, the student said, "It *isn't* like me to make so many errors and it isn't like me to be so argumentative. I think I have been tense and worried since I heard that my husband is going to have to go overseas before the baby comes." The teacher asked when she had found this out and the student replied, "About three weeks ago." Two days later the student came in and stated that she had decided to leave the school a month earlier than she anticipated in order to be with her husband. She decided that she would function more effectively now that she knew she could join her husband. She stated that she needed his support during her pregnancy and this need interfered with her putting her heart into her student role in the school.

The third role that I would like to comment on is that of *limit setting*. The premise underlying this role is that problems can be worked through most usefully or effectively within certain kinds of relationships. Stating expectations is one way of developing structure within a relationship. Further limitations may be set in terms of what kinds of needs or what kinds of problems can be dealt with in the relationship. An example of this might be that the teacher will deal only with problems that the student has that prevent her from functioning as a nurse, and cannot deal with problems that are strictly personal in nature. If limits are not adhered to, they can be restated. If a student, over a period of time, used the time with the teacher to socialize or joke, limits would need to be set in terms of the use of conference time. If students try to get the teacher to handle a problem with another student, the teacher can redefine her role as that of helping the student to work with the problem herself. Broken appointments and frequent unplanned conferences sometimes have to be dealt with in terms of the student's avoidance or overdependence. The amount of attacking or hostility in the relationship may need some limitation. The teacher who respects herself does not permit the student to act out her hostility in ways that are destructive in the relationship. Within this role the teacher can communicate, "I respect myself and set limits with you in terms of this respect. You can learn to set limits and make demands on others in keeping with developing respect for yourself." Another communication might be that "I will not be manipulated by avoidance behavior or deal with problems that are not related to my role with you." If you need to avoid or manipulate, our task is to find out what it means. Limit setting is not punishment or discipline. Irritation or anger involved in the limit setting requires the teacher to examine whether the limit was set because of her own needs or because it promoted a better working structure. If anger is involved, the student learns that people retaliate when she makes demands or tries to get her needs met.

It may sound to you as if the roles of limit setting and accepting are in conflict with each other. One of the problems of teachers is to clarify what they can accept as individuals and as teachers. Beyond this, they set limits. If one really doesn't know how the limit contributes to the improvement of the student-teacher relationship, or if one only rationalizes to explain the limit that the student has with the patient, a colleague, or the teacher, it is accepted. How she dealt with the problems is accepted. However, if the student continually avoids examining her participation in the problem situations, or if she avoids the teacher, has temper tantrums, or cries every time she is asked to examine a problem, limits are set in terms of the overall goals of teaching. If the student tries to get her personal problems solved with the teacher, this is another area where limits may be set in terms of the purposes of the educational program. Some limits are set in terms of limits of the school policies and some in terms of the clinical situation. The use of the authority role influences this role also. Teachers who need to feel powerful or important go to extremes in limit setting without examining the rationale of the limit. From time to time all limits need to be examined in terms of whether the limit prevents creativity in planning nursing care or prevents the personal growth of students and teachers. Some examples of unsound limit setting were those that had to do with standing, door holding, hair off collar, lipstick, and finger nail polish.

The fourth role that I would like to discuss is that of *support*. The premise underlying the supporting role is that each individual has worth and potential which can be developed. This development can be facilitated by experiences with a helping person who is interested, concerned and understanding. In this role the teacher is involved in finding meanings and in trying to understand the performance of the student. Even if the meanings cannot be understood, the feelings of the student in the situation can be appraised. The teacher uses herself in that she is concerned that the student is anxious, feeling helpless, or in conflict. She uses herself in that she can communicate that she is concerned that the student is anxious. Another facet of the role is to recognize when a student is too anxious to deal with a problem. The teacher supports her by deciding on a course of action that will lessen the student's anxiety to the point where the problem can be dealt with. Still another facet of the role is that of respecting student decisions and plans and encouraging the student to try out new plans or ideas that the student may have. This encouragement and respect is usually not in terms of "I think this is good," which only tells us about the teacher's values, but is rather in the tenor of "Would you like to try it?" or "Have you thought of trying that out?" If the student fails, the teacher helps her look at the failure in terms of what it means to have taken the risk in the first place, and helps her look at the failure not only in terms of why it happened but also in terms of what can be learned from it and how little creativity there would be if no one ever tried anything new. The teacher supports the student to try again.

Sometimes support means helping a student look at herself a little differently. If a student who does well constantly denigrates herself as a nurse, the teacher might say "What gets in the way of your being able to see your real worth as a nurse?" or in a different situation she might say "I wonder if you are looking at your real worth as a nurse?" or in a different situation she might say, "Now that you have looked at all the negative aspects of your performance, can you look at some of your useful functions?" I don't think that quotes are very helpful because all people would function somewhat differently in the role in any specific situation. A good deal of judgment based on the data of the problem situation is necessary in order to determine what would be most useful and what is most needed at this moment by the person seeking the help. For example, the communication "What gets in the way of your seeing your worth as a nurse" could be very threatening to one person in a situation and very supporting to another person in a similar situation. Sometimes just helping a student explore a problem can be very supportive if she is having a difficult time talking about something. Listening can be very supportive since attentiveness might communicate "You are worth listening to." Availability of the teacher can also be supportive.

The last role that I would like to describe is that of *participation or intervention.* It includes two activities. It is based on the promise that students, who have an opportunity to examine with a teacher their participation with others, become more aware of how they function and how they need to function in order to participate usefully in nursing situations. It is also a promise that students can translate the experience they have with teachers into experience which they, as students, can provide for patients.

The first activity that I would like to describe is that of listening. Listening is not a passive activity but, as I use it here, involves great activity. Listening involves being alert to the ideas expressed in the verbal productions of others. It involves being alert to the words selected by others to express these ideas. It involves speculating on the reasons for the student's choice of words to express the ideas. It may involve identifying the literal meaning of figurative expressions and the figurative meaning of literal expressions. Listening means being alert to the feelings expressed in the words, in the tone of voice, hesitations, slips of the tongue, eye movements, and other gestures that have communication value. Listening involves sorting and grouping what is heard and what is seen. It may involve resorting and regrouping as more is seen and heard about a problem. Listening involves interpretation of what is heard and seen. Listening goes further than interpreting what was meant and felt. It means that the interpretations are arranged in such a way that some kind of a formulation can be made about the interpersonal dynamics of the problem. It may mean that several formulations are made as possibilities when the problem cannot be clearly seen. Listening involves identifying what else the teacher and student need to know in order to define the problem. Listening means making judgments about whether to ask for more data, and if so, when and how to ask for it. The listener makes judgments about when to interrupt, when to limit digression, when the student needs support to go on, when to raise questions, when to express concern, and how to express it usefully.

Listening skill is related to what is heard and this is a problem for all of us. We all hear things that we want to hear and all interpret what we hear in terms of our previous experience. As teachers, we are aware of this when we get written work from students. Sometimes it is almost unbelievable how what we said was heard. It takes literally years of practice to develop skills in observation and perception and to develop the necessary intellectual skills, and years of experience in living to appreciate or understand the feelings of others. Except for the rare individual, it requires the help of a skillful teacher. The task is never complete, but with effort the rewards of becoming increasingly useful to students in their development are great. The second activity under the teaching role that I have called participation is that of helping. Not that all the activities that I have been describing aren't helpful — they are — but this is the role where action is directed toward doing something about the problem.

In the listening role I have described the problem solving process up to the point where a problem is identified, clarified, and stated. The role of the teacher at this point is to help the student identify the possible courses of action that would bring about a possible solution. Some of these courses of action the student will identify and some may be identified by the teacher. The next phase is one in which the teacher and student examine the limitations, risks, and the possible outcomes of the courses of action. They may also need to examine them in terms of what would be most reasonable and useful. At this point the student may choose a course of action, or she may decide to think further about it, or she may even bring additional data to bear on the problem that will involve restating it. The student may need support in carrying out the course of action she has chosen. This does not mean that the teacher agrees with the action or that she thinks it is right. It means that the student has the right to make her own choices within the limits of the structure. It means also that the teacher recognizes that the student is different in intellect, skills, values and goals, and as such will make choices that are different than the teacher's. If the student fails, the teacher helps the student get clear on the reasons and the meaning of the failure to the student. There are satisfactions to be gotten from failure. It may be necessary to go through the whole problem solving process again. It may involve helping the student change her goals or accept only a part of what she wants to accomplish. It involves, and this I think is important, helping the student get satisfaction out of her experience for herself. It also involves making judgments about whether to let the student struggle with a problem, or to help her, or to take over in a situation.

Time doesn't permit me to give an example of this complex process, although I recognize that it might be helpful to you.

I have tried to briefly outline five teaching roles in which the teacher uses herself as a person to promote the growth and development of students. I believe that if nursing is to be a profession in which every nurse-patient relationship is creative, it will be because of teachers who can use themselves in these ways.

A Definition of the Hallucinatory Process: A Review of the Literature and Clinical Investigation

Cynthia A. Rector

This is a summary of a thesis by Cynthia A. Rector based on a report developed by the Committee on Psychiatric Nursing of the Group for the Advancement of Psychiatry with the collaboration of Mrs. Gwen Will, RN (representing The American Nurses Assocation), Miss Kathleen Black, RN (representing the National League for Nursing), Mrs. Frances Thompson Lenehan, RN, and Mr. Gordon Sawatsky, a psychiatric aide. We gratefully acknowledge their help. This report was prepared under the chairmanship of Elvin V. Semrad, M.D. It was presented at Rutgers — The State University in 1964.

Introduction

Hallucinations have puzzled mankind for many centuries. The experiences of those who perceived things which others did not notice have often mystified and terrified their fellows. The origin of these perceptions has been the object of a great deal of speculation and study.

Recently there has been increasing investigation of hallucinations in terms of a possible organic cause or precipitating factor. Nevertheless, the hallucinations of the schizophrenic patient are still unexplained, and one promising avenue of exploration seems to be in the area of interpersonal relations.

The problem of the patient who hallucinates is a very real one for the nurse planning care. Because hallucinations tend to create awe or fear in others, this patient may receive no help, and perhaps harm, from those who should offer encouragement and definite assistance in dealing with the problem. The objective of this research study was to formulate, through an investigation of the literature and clinical data, a definition of the process of hallucinations to be used as a beginning base in designing testable nursing practices for intervention into the pathological process of hallucinations.

Editor's Note: This paper is an exception to the stipulation that only materials written prior to 1963 be included in this book. The reasons for this exception are 1) the ideas for the research project upon which this summary is based predated the project itself by more than a year, 2) the clinical significance of the topic warrants inclusion in the book, and 3) the substance of the study has never been published.

The Problem

What were the phases and steps in the hallucinatory process as demonstrated through investigation of the literature and of clinical data from schizophrenic patients?

The Sub-Problems

1. What stressful events in the patient's life had preceded the development of the hallucinations?
2. What was the patient's method of choice in dealing with the stressful events which preceded the hallucinations?
3. In what way were the interpersonal relationships of the patient changed and/or disrupted prior to the development of the hallucinations?
4. What was the patient's reaction to the hallucinations?
5. What were the types of hallucinations and what was the content of the hallucinations experienced by the patient?

Review of the Nursing Literature

A review of the nursing literature revealed a general lack of information on the subject of hallucinations. In the *American Journal of Nursing* since 1940, one article has appeared on the subject of hallucinations.[1] In *Nursing Outlook* and *Nursing Research* there were no articles on this subject. There was a descriptive study of the hallucinations of one patient by Isani,[2] and the book, *The Nurse and the Mental Patient,* had a chapter which offered some constructive pointers for supportive care of the hallucinating patient.[3] Three nursing textbooks were reviewed,[4,5,6] and while each discussed the occurrence of hallucinations, nursing intervention was not formulated.

The most helpful formulations about hallucinations in the nursing literature were by Gravenkemper, Clack, and Peplau. Each of these formulations aided in the development of the definition of the hallucinatory process presented and tested in this research project. Gravenkemper explored the development of hallucinations as a product of the self-system and interpersonal relationships of the person.[7] Clack presented a theoretical formulation of the basis for hallucinations by examining the development of the self-system and by looking at the phases in the hallucinatory experience as it develops, and she used clinical data to illustrate the steps in intervention.[8] Peplau described the hallucinations of the schizophrenic patient as "an adaptive response to new conditions in the individual's psychosocial field."[9] The suggested phases and steps in the hallucinatory process are outlined in this article.

Review of the Medical Literature

Medical literature contained many references to hallucinations. In 1932 Mourgue[10] reviewed more than one thousand publications, and since then much interest in hallucinatory phenomena has been aroused by the studies of the hallucinogenic drugs[11,12] and of sensory deprivation.[13,14] The literature pertaining to neurophysiology[15,16] and the theories of the self-system[17] or ego[18] pertaining to the development of hallucinations were reviewed. Much of the literature was descriptive or dealt with only one dimension of the phenomenon, and therapeutic intervention was not specifically formulated.

Process Definition of Hallucinations Occurring in Schizophrenia

Following the literature review, the proposed process was formulated as follows:

Phase I: An Adaptation to Stress Occurs

Steps:

1. The individual experiences a situation of great stress (disruption of interpersonal relationship).
2. Anxiety increases.
3. The individual thinks of a person who might be helpful in this situation.
4. The individual thinks about the way in which the recalled person would help.
5. Anxiety decreases.

Phase II: Stress Continues and Adaptive Behavior Recurs

Steps:

6. The individual continues to experience a situation of stress.
7. Anxiety increases.
8. Steps 3 and 4 of Phase I are repeated.
9. Relief is felt and anxiety decreases.
10. In order to increase the periods of relief from the stress condition, the individual begins to set up situations to provide more opportunity for reveries about the helpful person.
11. The individual begins to be anxious about whether the reveries of the helpful person can be recalled at will.
12. The individual does not wish the reverie process to be interrupted by real persons and activities, so they are avoided.

Phase III: Withdrawal from People and Difficulty with Control of Focal Awareness Occurs

Steps:

13. As the individual spends more time in autistic reverie, there is a beginning loss of control over focal awareness.
14. Because of the loss of control over focal awareness, the individual behaves in an inappropriate manner (i.e., talks to self or voices) in the presence of other persons.
15. The inappropriate behavior results in shame and embarrassment.
16. Anxiety increases.
17. The individual returns to Step 10 of Phase II, and anxiety decreases for the moment.
18. As more time is spent in reverie, the individual begins to be aware of the loss of ability to choose the contents of awareness, and anxiety increases.
19. To avoid further shame and embarrassment, the individual begins to actively reduce contacts with real people to a bare minimum.

Phase IV: Loss of Ability to Control Focal Awareness and Inappropriate Behavior Occurs

Steps:

20. Someone (e.g., family member or person at work) tries to intervene in the individual's isolation.
21. Anxiety increases because of the threat of further shame and embarrassment.

22. The individual tries to repeat the pattern of Step 10, Phase II, but fails because of the loss of control of the content of awareness.
23. Inappropriate behavior occurs and there is more shame and embarrassment.
24. Anxiety increases further — to the point of panic or terror.
25. Usually hospitalization occurs at this point, and the individual is further cut off from familiar situations and persons.

Phase V: Hallucinations Become Vivid and Must be Dealt With

Steps:

26. The loss of control of awareness increases and the anxiety level remains high (terror or panic).
27. The individual's thoughts are no longer controlled by the self.
28. The hallucinatory phenomena are regarded as "real;" external perceptions and real persons are avoided.
29. The individual makes promises to the hallucinatory voices and/or figures and reaches some "compromise" about living with them.
30. Anxiety decreases.
31. The individual attempts to identify and explain, by some means, the hallucinatory phenomena.
32. The individual accepts his hallucinations as a part of his life and becomes involved with them.

Collection of Clinical Data

A combination of the focused interview and clinical interview as defined by Selltiz[19] was used to obtain clinical data in an attempt to validate the hallucinatory process. Five patients were selected for inclusion in the study on the basis of the following criteria: they were diagnosed as schizophrenic by the medical staff of Hospital X; they had no known organic pathology of the central nervous system; they had received no electroconvulsive therapy within six months preceding the study; and they had had and/or were having hallucinations which they were willing to discuss with the researcher.

The data were collected in four interviews of one hour each in a two-week period of time. During the interviews, notes were taken verbatim, or a tape recorder was used. In the initial interview with the patient, the researcher asked for names of two persons who might be contacted for information about the patient's illness. The researcher specified that the name of "the person who was closest to you" and the name of "the person who understood you best" were desired. The persons so named by the patient were contacted for interviews of one hour each. *All patients,* without exception, indicated that no one really understood them, but then gave a name of someone they thought was satisfactory. There was a total of ten significant others named by the patients; however, only eight were interviewed, as two could not be contacted in the month allowed for this purpose.

Analysis of Clinical Data

A jury of two clinical specialists in psychiatric nursing was used to test the reliability of the selection of data to substantiate the hallucinatory process. In addition, the descriptive analysis of each set of data was submitted to a clinical specialist in psychiatric nursing for correction and validation of the researcher's description of the findings.

Each verbatim interview was typed in triplicate, names were deleted, a code letter was assigned to each patient, and each interview with the patient and significant other was numbered. Each set of interviews consisted of four interviews with the patient and two interviews with the significant others named by the patient. A form containing the steps in the hallucinatory process with space left for filling in the data was used. The data from each set of interviews which applied to the steps in the process were inserted in the appropriate space. The data taken from the interview to substantiate the steps in the process were marked and numbered so that they could be easily identified. Each set of data was used to fill in one form containing the hallucinatory process. Discrepancies in the data from the patient and significant others were noted. The forms of the hallucinatory process containing the clinical data were compared to see if the process was substantiated, if the steps were in proper sequence, or if steps were missing.

Clinical Findings

The clinical data substantiated the majority of the

steps in the hallucinatory process. The steps in the process not substantiated are those dealing with the reverie process the individual goes through as hallucinations develop.

In Phase I: An Adaptation to Stress Occurs, the clinical findings support Steps 1 and 2, but they do not support Steps 3, 4, and 5. Each of the patients experienced disruptions in interpersonal relationships, but none of them indicated that reverie about helpful persons was used to cope with the stress situations.

For Phase II: Stress Continues and Adaptive Behavior Recurs, Steps 6, 7, 10, and 12 are verified, but Steps 8, 9, and 11 are not verified by data. Each patient indicated a number of stresses which he had experienced, but as in Phase I, the data do not support use of a reverie process to deal with the stress. However, each patient or the significant others stated that the patient spent increasing amounts of time alone as the illness progressed, and what went on during the withdrawal, which provided opportunity for reveries, was not obtained.

In Phase III: Withdrawal from People and Difficulty with Control of Focal Awareness Occurs, there are clinical data to support Steps 13, 14, 15, 16, 18, and 19. Step 17, which deals with the reverie process, is again the unsupported aspect of the process. Each patient indicated that he experienced some loss of control of his thought processes and that inappropriate behavior resulted.

Steps 20, 24, and 25 of Phase IV: Loss of Ability to Control Focal Awareness and Inappropriate Behavior Occurs, are substantiated by the clinical data. Steps 21 and 23 are each supported by two patients, and Step 22 lacks support. Each patient indicated that his anxiety reached the point of panic or terror and then hospitalization occurred. Four patients noted that someone tried to intervene when their isolation became noticeable. Again, the reverie process, Step 22, lacks confirmation.

In Phase V: Hallucinations Become Vivid and Must be Dealt With, there are data to corroborate all the steps, but the data to corroborate Step 30 are given by only two patients. The findings from clinical data in this phase of the process are consistent with the types of description of hallucinations found in the literature review.

Conclusions

This exploratory study answered some important questions and raised many more. The following statements represent trends suggested by the findings in the review of the literature and the clinical investigation:

1. Disruption of a significant interpersonal relationship, as defined by the patient, precedes the hallucinations by not more than two years. The patients experienced other disruptions before and after the named significant relationship was disrupted. No specificity of stress situations to the development of hallucinations (vs. schizophrenia) was established.
2. The disruptions in relationships result in an increase of the patient's anxiety.
3. Hallucinating patients utilize methods of dealing with stress which do not involve relationships with other, "real" people.
4. There was no support in the clinical data for the role of reverie as defined in the proposed hallucinatory process, but there were data which suggested that reverie might occur.
5. All data about the withdrawal of patients from contacts with others came from significant others rather than from the patients. This suggests that the patient is unaware of the withdrawal which he unwittingly used to protect himself.
6. The data are highly suggestive of the loss of control of the thought process resulting in inappropriate behavior. After the inappropriate behavior occurs there is an increase of anxiety, and shame and embarrassment occur. Because the patient is unable to control his thought processes and hence his behavior, more shame and embarrassment occur with a corresponding increase of anxiety to the point of terror or panic. Hospitalization usually occurs at this point.
7. All patients in this study attempted to explain their hallucinations in some manner, unscientific and inaccurate though it may be.
8. There were insufficient data to revise the phases and steps in the proposed definition of the process of hallucinations at this time. The proposed definition may be used as a tool for further study of the hallucinatory process.

References

1. Field, William E., Jr., "When a Patient Hallucinates," *American Journal of Nursing*, 63:80-82, February, 1963.

2. Isani, Rebecca S., "The 'Veil' Phenomenon in an Hallucina-

ting Schizophrenic," in *Some Clinical Approaches to Psychiatric Nursing*, edited by Shirley F. Burd and Margaret A. Marshall, The Macmillan Company, New York, 1963, pp. 189-196.

3. Schwartz, Morris S. and Shockley, Emmy L., *The Nurse and the Mental Patient*, Russell Sage Foundation, New York, 1955, pp. 113-138.

4. Hofling, Charles K. and Leininger, Madeleine M., *Basic Psychiatric Concepts in Nursing*, J. B. Lippincott Company, Philadelphia, 1960, pp. 154-155, 301, 304, 306, 317.

5. Kalkman, Marion E., *Introduction to Psychiatric Nursing*, Second Edition, McGraw-Hill Company, Inc., New York, 1958, pp. 136-137, 283.

6. Noyes, Arthur P., Haydon, Edith M., and van Sickel, Mildred, *The Textbook of Psychiatric Nursing*, Fifth Edition, The Macmillan Company, New York, 1957, pp. 63- 65.

7. Gravenkemper, Katherine H., "Hallucinations," in *Some Clinical Approaches to Psychiatric Nursing*, edited by Shirley F. Burd and Margaret A. Marshall, The Macmillan Company, New York, 1963, pp. 184-188.

8. Clack, Janice, "An Interpersonal Technique for Handling Hallucinations," in *Nursing Care of the Disoriented Patient*, American Nurses' Association Monograph Series, No. 13, 1962, pp. 16-26.

9. Peplau, Hildegard E., "Interpersonal Relations and the Process of Adaptation," *Nursing Science* 1:272-279, October-November, 1963.

10. West, Louis J., *Hallucinations*, Grune and Stratton, New York, 1962, pp. 74, 275-292.

11. Malitz, Sidney, Wilkers, Bernard, and Esecover, Harold, "A Comparison of Drug-Induced Hallucinations with Those Seen in Spontaneously Occurring Psychoses," in *Hallucinations*, edited by Louis J. West, Grune and Stratton, New York, 1962, pp. 50-63.

12. Feinberg, Irwin, "A Comparison of the Visual Hallucinations in Schizophrenia with Those Induced by Mescaline and LSD-25," in *Hallucinations*, edited by Louis J. West, Grune and Stratton, New York, 1962, pp. 64-76.

13. Solomon, Philip, *et al.*, "Sensory Deprivation: A Review," *American Journal of Psychiatry* 114:357-363, October, 1957.

14. Kubzansky, Philip E. and Leiderman, P. Herbert, "Sensory Deprivation: An Overview," in *Sensory Deprivation*, edited by Philip Solomon *et al.*, Harvard University Press, Cambridge, 1961, pp. 221-238.

15. Scheibel, Madge E. and Scheibel, Arnold B., "Hallucinations and the Brain Stem Reticular Core," in *Hallucinations*, edited by Louis J. West, Grune and Stratton, New York, 1962, pp. 15-35.

16. Marrazzi, Amedeo S., "The Action of Psychotogens and a Neurophysiological Theory of Hallucinations," *American Journal of Psychiatry* 116:911-914, April, 1960.

17. Sullivan, Harry S., *The Interpersonal Theory of Psychiatry*, W. W. Norton and Co., Inc., New York, 1953, pp. 161-163, 349, 379.

18. Rapaport, David, "The Theory of Ego Autonomy: A Generalization," Bulletin of the Menninger Clinic 22:13-35, January, 1958.

19. Selltiz, Claire, *et al.*, *Research Methods in Social Relations*, Revised Edition, Holt, Rinehart and Winston, New York, 1962, pp. 263-268.

National Mental Health Training Program in Nursing

Esther A. Garrison

Ms. Garrison is Chief, Nursing Section, Training and Manpower Resources Branch, National Institute of Mental Health, Bethesda, Maryland

This paper is based on material presented at a workshop for Registered Nurses from mental institutions in the Southern Region, the National Institute of Mental Health training program in psychiatric-mental health nursing at the University of Maryland, August 1964.

Historical Background

The Training Program of the National Manpower Resources Branch was established under authority contained in the National Mental Health Act passed by Congress in 1946. This legislation authorized expenditure of Federal funds for research, training, and community services in the mental health field. A major objective of the training program was to alleviate the acute shortage of *qualified* persons in the mental health field, and grants were authorized to universities and other training centers for the purpose of increasing the number of qualified personnel (specialists) in this field for clinical and community services, teaching, research, and administration. In addition, efforts were to be made to increase content from psychiatry and the social and behavioral sciences in basic curricula of medical schools, graduate programs in schools of public health, and in basic collegiate education in nursing.

Training objectives, in accordance with the purposes of the Act, were established at the outset, and it was recommended by the National Advisory Mental Health Council that *high priority* be given to the improvement of *quality* of training in the generally recognized core mental health disciplines of psychiatry, clinical psychology, psychiatric social work, and psychiatric nursing. Funds would be used as authorized in the legislation to establish, expand, and improve training programs in the mental health field. Funds would also be used to provide stipends for trainees.

In the beginning, training efforts concentrated on the training of clinical specialists. The program has broadened over the years to include training of specialists and research personnel in the core disciplines, research personnel in the social and biological sciences related to mental health, career teachers, and special training in such areas as juvenile delinquency, mental retardation, geriatrics, and alcoholism. There are other areas of support for which there is insufficient time for discussion.

I should like to point out, however, that the basic purpose and philosophy of the program have not changed since its inception — namely, to increase through quality training the number of mental health workers to improve the mental health of the people of the nation. High standards of education are not only expected but required in the approval of training institutions (training centers) for grant awards. Funds are approved for *full training* of health workers — the professionals — and for less than full training in mental health in such fields as general education, law, and religion. Training grants are awarded as recommended by the National Advisory Mental Health Council.

The Program in Nursing

In 1947 (fiscal year 1948), nine universities received grants to develop, improve, and expand programs in psychiatric nursing for graduate nurses. At the time, funds were approved for graduate training only. Since nursing had no clinical programs of study, and only a few nurses were prepared to study at the graduate level, an exception was made which permitted the support of "advanced" training in psychiatric nursing at the baccalaureate level.

In 1947, about 5,000 registered nurses were known to be in psychiatric nursing teaching and service positions (for patient care) in mental hospitals, about 500 of whom were assumed to have had some preparation beyond that obtained in a preservice diploma program in nursing. As you can see, by today's standards their preparation for work with psychiatric patients was minimal. It was clear that nursing must begin by preparing, as best it could, first-level practitioners and teachers in programs leading to the bachelor's degree.

A total of nine universities was awarded grants in fiscal year 1948 to develop clinical nursing programs in this specialty. During this period, four of the nine participating schools admitted students to undergraduate "advanced" and graduate programs, the latter providing more advanced clinical training and some preparation in teaching, supervision, or administration. None of these programs — graduate or undergraduate — was advanced as measured by

Editor's Note: Although material in this paper was presented in 1964, the history of federal support for programs in psychiatric nursing began in 1946. This paper, although "post-1963," reviews that support and is therefore included because of its significance.

current educational standards. Nor would more than one or two meet present criteria (1946) for national accreditation. Nonetheless, they provided the base for subsequent program development.

As proportionately larger sums of money for training became available and funds allocated to nursing increased — from approximately a quarter of a million dollars in 1947 to roughly 7.3 million dollars in 1964 — educational programs in nursing increased in number and kinds of training. Two broad areas of grant support are provided in nursing at the present time. The first of these provides grants to schools of nursing to support graduate education preparation for expert clinical practice teaching, administration, research and consultation in a variety of settings and mental health services. The second provides support to undergraduate collegiate schools of nursing. The primary purpose of this aspect of the program is to equip nurses with the knowledge and skill to deal with the emotional aspects of health and illness, and to increase the potential pool of nurses interested in graduate preparation in psychiatric nursing.

Programs of Support: Graduate Education

Masters Education

Currently there are roughly 40 graduate programs leading to a master's degree in *adult* or *general psychiatric nursing* and *nursing in child psychiatry* offered in universities throughout the country. Programs in general/adult psychiatric nursing vary in length from one year to two academic years and a summer term in length. While emphasis and program content vary in these training centers, all include sound preparation for expert clinical nursing practice. Some programs, as indicated above, continue to include course content in functional areas such as teaching, supervision, and administration. Nearly all include research courses appropriate to this level of study. In addition, training for community mental health is rapidly being incorporated into both graduate and undergraduate collegiate nursing curriculums.

The programs in nursing in child psychiatry differ considerably. All require a minimum of one year for completion. Some, as is the practice in the training of child psychiatrists, require completion of a graduate program in adult or general psychiatric nursing for admission to this specialized area of study; others require no advanced preparation in psychiatric-mental health nursing for admission. The latter group, while focusing on the child, also includes study and work with adults. A third curriculum pattern combines nursing of psychiatric and emotionally disturbed children and public health nursing. Students were first admitted to this program in the fall of 1963. In addition to the areas of study noted above, support is available to the psychiatric nurse who wishes training in a school of public health and to the public health nurse who wishes mental health training in a school of nursing or a school of public health.

Doctoral Education

Students wishing to pursue doctoral education in this clinical specialty or in a behavioral science related to mental health are eligible for support under this program. The intent of this program is to prepare psychiatric-mental health nurses for leadership positions in nursing, more specifically for teaching, research, and consultation. More than fifty psychiatric nurses are currently enrolled in doctoral programs in nursing or a behavioral science related to mental health including anthropology, sociology, psychology, and growth and development.

Post-Doctoral Education

The senior stipend is a special category of training and is intended to meet the special training needs of professionals. These stipends are intended for *specialists* in the mental health disciplines and for individuals from other fields who seek training in a mental health discipline in preparation for work in this field. Senior stipend awards are intended for study at the postdoctoral level. Senior psychiatric nursing educators have been awarded senior stipends for postdoctoral research training.

Trainee stipends, plus tuition and registration and laboratory fees, are available to nurses for study in these graduate programs. Annual stipend rates are as follows:

Year of Graduate Training	Level	Annual Rate
1	3	$2400
2	4	3000
3	4	3000
4	5	3600
5*	5	3600

*Available to students studying for the doctor's degree in a basic science related to mental health.

Programs of Support: Undergraduate Education

Grants are made to collegiate schools of nursing to *expand and improve* the teaching of psychiatric and mental health content from the behavioral sciences in the undergraduate curriculum. The *purpose* of this program as noted above is to better prepare all nurses completing the basic collegiate program or a general nursing program leading to the baccalaureate degree to deal with the emotional aspects of health and illness, and to increase the potential pool of nurses interested in graduate training in psychiatric-mental health nursing. This program of support was initiated in 1955 when two very small grants were made to the University of Colorado and Yale University Schools of Nursing to explore and develop undergraduate content and teaching methods. One hundred nineteen schools are currently participating in this program. A recent review of this program revealed a remarkable change in content and teaching methodology and marked improvement in the ability of students and graduates of these programs to deal with the preventive treatment and rehabilitative aspects of patient care.

Trainee stipends of $1800, plus tuition and fees, per year are available to basic undergraduate and graduate nursing students interested in a career in the field of mental health to complete the final two years of prebaccalaureate study. To be eligible for these trainee stipends, candidates must have an above-average academic record and potential for admission to graduate study and an aptitude for psychiatric-mental health nursing, and must plan to enroll in a graduate program upon completion of the baccalaureate program. Two hundred thirty-five undergraduate stipends were awarded in 84 nationally accredited schools this year (for the year July 1, 1964 to June 30, 1965). The selection of students for these stipends is a function of the college or university.

Special Programs of Support

Career Teacher

Career teacher grants are intended to encourage students with exceptional ability and potentiality to choose careers in teaching and provide support for them during the training period. A substantial number of trainees in nursing choose teaching of psychiatric- mental health nursing as a career. The career teacher program offers an *additional opportunity* for *highly selected candidates* preparing for teaching and educational leadership to study and work in a university under the careful supervision and guidance of master teachers in psychiatric nursing education. These programs are especially designed by the training centers to meet the individual candidate's training objectives and needs. A maximum of two years of support, adjusted to the beginning teacher salary in the university, may be provided for the student. Between six and nine or ten nurses are selected each year from a number of candidates applying for these stipends.

Pilot and Special Projects

Pilot Project grants are made in the psychiatric mental health disciplines and in the mental health-related behavioral sciences to eligible training centers. The purposes of these grants are:

1. To stimulate the development of new and experimental methods of teaching in the field of mental health;
2. To support projects to evaluate teaching and training methods in the mental health disciplines;
3. To support training programs in special areas where there is great need;
4. To develop training programs for persons whose roles or functions may be related to mental health; and
5. To develop training programs for new types of mental health personnel.

Pilot Projects in nursing encompass intensive training programs of varying types and extent; the greatest emphasis perhaps has been on the identification of psychiatric-mental health content for incorporation in the undergraduate curriculum and the development of appropriate instructional methodology. Other projects of considerable note are in the areas of mental retardation, community mental health, social psychiatry, and short-term, time-limited, special training programs such as the workshop in which you are currently enrolled.

Short-term programs may be supported if the basic requirements of a pilot project are met. Evaluation is one such requirement, and the plan must provide for collection of the necessary data for determining the real value or effectiveness of the endeavor. The basic rationale for support of short-term training, whether in a university or in a service-based hospital or agency, is to improve and upgrade clinical nursing care of patients.

These programs may be offered during summer months or at other periods, depending upon the availability of faculty time, clinical training facilities and other essential educational resources. Such endeavor is often directly related to the regular training activities of the school's psychiatric nursing faculty and graduate students. In some universities, extension divisions are charged with full responsibility for the development and administration of educational programs which do not fall within established program offerings leading to the degree. In addition to the programs sponsored by universities, a few service-based programs are approved for support. These, too, are time limited, also required to meet the rather rigorous criteria of sound training to qualify for support.

Special projects grant awards are made to support such mental health activities as conferences, institutes, workshops, demonstrations, and surveys. An occasional short-term training project qualifies for support under this grant mechanism.

Concluding Remarks

The National Institute of Mental Health training program is broad indeed. Its accomplishments and implications for the future are many. Support under this program has led to remarkable progress in nursing. And while the number of nurses seeking advanced preparation continues to be considerably less than in the other core disciplines, there is evidence of increasing interest in this clinical field.

Of considerable importance is support for in-service and continuing education for nurses employed in various psychiatric and mental health settings. The need for "refresher courses" to keep abreast with new knowledge and practice, and for short-term intensive training to upgrade and improve patient care, cannot be overemphasized. This aspect of the program is one of the many training program developments of special interest to the National Institute of Mental Health staff and its advisory committees and council.

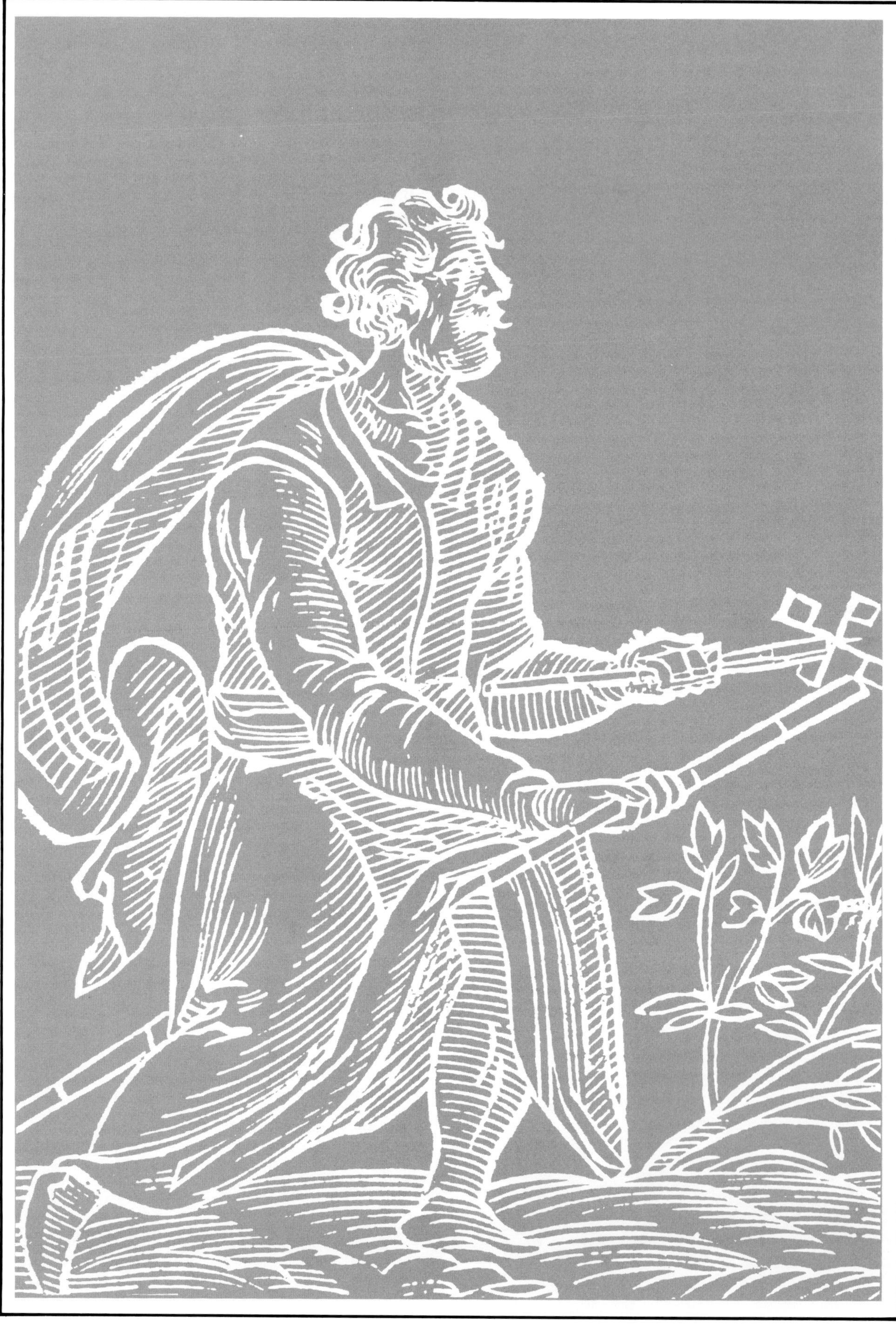

Selected Publications Significantly Contributing to the Field but Not Readily Available, or Not Widely Disseminated, When Originally Published

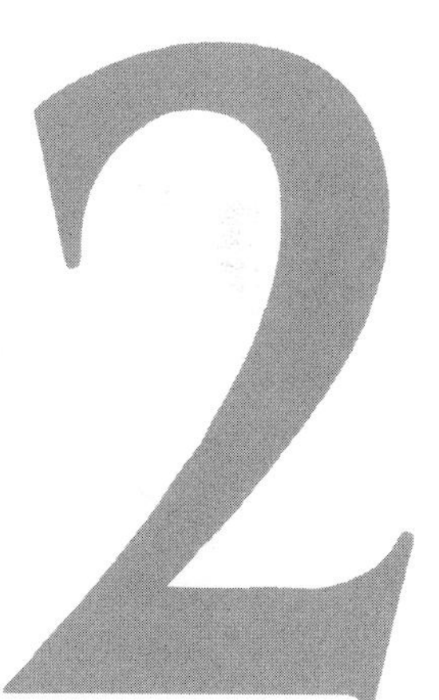

Introduction

The papers in this section provide an opportunity for today's psychiatric nurse to observe the hopeful tone of psychiatric nursing's direction in the 1950s. The Mental Health Act of 1946 had long been passed; graduate programs in psychiatric nursing were being initiated. When *Action for Mental Health* appeared in 1960, advising full development of all psychiatric manpower, psychiatric nursing had already been on the move in the areas of program, intellectual, and clinical development. The papers reproduced here testify to the seriousness with which the leaders of the day approached their task. The task was to treat patients; to do so meant to educate psychiatric nurses with substantive content developed and presented in the best possible ways, and to make the treatment process understandable and available.

Therapeutic Use of the Self: A Concept for Teaching Patient Care

Committee on Psychiatric Nursing of the Group for Advancement of Psychiatry

This report was developed by the Committee on Psychiatric Nursing of the Group for the Advancement of Psychiatry with the collaboration of Mrs. Gwen Will, R.N. (representing The American Nurses Association), Miss Kathleen Black, R.N. (representing the National League for Nursing), Mrs. Frances Thompson Lenehan, R.N., and Mr. Gordon Sawatsky, a psychiatric aide.

This is a reprint of Report No. 33 of the Committee on Psychiatric Nursing of the Group for Advancement of Psychiatry, June 1955.

Contents

I. Introduction

An understanding of the behavior of the mentally ill patient, and an appropriate response to it by nursing personnel (a) is necessary for the therapeutic effectiveness in the day by day care of the patient.

This communication deals primarily with psychiatrically oriented concepts which will assist in the better interpretation of the patient's manifest behavior. As a consequence we should have better recognition of the patient's emotional needs, awareness and use by nursing personnel of supporting and corrective responses to his emotional needs, appreciation of some aspects of interaction between patient and nurse, and its meaning and application in the therapeutic effort.

We wish to discuss these concepts as current working formulations and to offer a dynamic orientation for persons, by whatever title designated, who participate in the daily 24-hour care of the mentally sick.

We hope that these concepts will be transmitted into daily action and thus help the leader, supervisor, teacher, or administrator to make his job assignments and conferences and classes more purposeful, so that personnel may become more aware of the patient's needs, and therefore more successful in treating him. In particular, we direct this communication to those concerned with instruction of psychiatric aides, professional nurses, orderlies, practical nurses, attendants, psychiatric technicians, and others who perform similar duties.

A hierarchy of personal relationships exists in every mental hospital, private or public, large or small, well-staffed or not. It is not our task, and it would be presumptuous, to prescribe for each institution how the director and the directed, teacher and student, supervisor and supervisee, nurse and patient should put these concepts into operation. We prefer to call attention to this ubiquitous and complex problem, and offer some suggestions toward assessing it. We hope thus to define the meaning of personal relationships and of the forces involved. These relationships are sensed by all. Too often they are left anxiously unscrutinized or are defensively assigned to "roles" that nurses "should" assume.

The earlier survey (b) of training programs for psychiatric nursing personnel suggested only limited awareness of the problem of nurse-patient relationships. We do not believe that this indicates an absence of concern regarding this complex problem but rather that it indicates a lack of clarity about conceptual goals, an imperfect focus on which area of patient behavior to scrutinize, an inadequate comprehension of emotional processes, and an incomplete understanding of the anxiety-provoking nature of the behavior of the mentally ill.

A patient enters a psychiatric hospital because he has experienced difficulties in living in the outside world. Whatever the nature and expression of these difficulties, they invariably include a breakdown in relationships with other people. The hospital must serve as a smaller, limited world wherein new experiences in living, and new personal relationships, produce minimal anxiety and maximal support. Thus, the patient gradually may be helped to feel that living with others is less threatening and a

(a) The term nursing personnel or nurse will be used throughout the text to include all persons, by whatever title, who are involved in the 24-hour care of the mentally sick patient.

(b) G.A.P. Report No. 22, "The Psychiatric Nurse in the Mental Hospital."

less forbidding experience.

We assume that the behavior of the patient has meaning; that his behavior affects the behavior of those who care for him; and that the behavior of those who care for him affects the patient.

The patient's hospitalization should enable him to learn to live more effectively with other people. Every mental illness includes the problem of the patient's particular way of relating himself to others and participating with others in activities. When a patient enters a mental hospital he has already established patterns of behavior intended to facilitate his withdrawal from anxiety-provoking relationships. Withdrawal may be variously expressed. In the attempt to cope with his anxiety, the patient chooses that form of expression which, in his past experience, has been most effective in maintaining distance from others for his subjective comfort.

In the hospital, new personal relationships must gratify the patient's needs, facilitate his communication with others, and enhance his social participation. It follows that the nursing personnel, which has the longest and most intimate contact with the patient, is deeply involved in these processes. Every contact with the patient, whether in the performance of "official nursing care" or in a less directed capacity, involves patient-nurse relationships. The relationship can be therapeutic or harmful. If these relationships remain essentially therapeutic, the patient-nurse relationship can become an integral part of the patient's whole therapeutic regimen. It is important for nursing personnel to understand and to be aware of the feelings, thoughts, and actions of the patients. They should have a similar understanding of their own thoughts and actions in any situation. Such awareness is acquired gradually and depends upon collaboration with the psychiatrist, conferences with supervisors and co-workers, and repeated experiences with patients.

II. General Comments

To extend the common awareness of anxiety, and of reactions and defenses to anxiety, we should like to elaborate, first on the theme of *regression* with symptoms of *dependence* which is part of every illness, mental and physical. Next, we wish to re-examine the *changes in object-relationship* that invariably ensue when chronic and intense dependency are expressed.

To illustrate these two main inter-dependent dynamic concepts of every mental illness we have chosen to discuss the following dysfunctions: 1)Disturbance of Productive Activity; 2) Inability to Control Basic Impulses; 3) Changed Moral Standards and Conventional Attitudes; 4) Diminished Integrative Capacities; and 5) Disturbances of the Function of Reality-testing.

These phenomena are readily available for continued observation in daily behavior. They are manifestations about which society has ideas of "normality," concepts of good and bad, and of morality and immorality. They deal with problems whose mastery is the concern of patient as well as nurse.

This report will not allude to structure, etiology, and genesis of the basic conflicts. The understanding and resolution of these conflicts in the patient are essentially the task of the psychiatrist. This demands orientation and techniques which are not available to the nurse. Although nursing personnel and psychiatrist may well have different goals and techniques, it cannot be sufficiently emphasized that whoever works with the mentally ill must face and react constructively to the phenomena of regression and altered, decreased capacity for object relations.

The recognition of these processes and the understanding of their dynamic significance can become the common denominator of all the different "therapies" to which the patient is invariably and unavoidably exposed. The understanding of these concepts should offer a basis for communication among the various participants in patient care. It is only through such communication in the hierarchy of personnel that consistency and direction can be brought to the total therapeutic regimen. The understanding of these concepts should further facilitate the definition of different roles for personnel, and of the various levels and areas wherein each person can make his contribution toward a plan of treatment.

III. Specific Considerations

1. Regression with Symptoms of Dependence. Regression is a return to earlier (childhood) methods of solving personal conflicts. It occurs when physical or emotional stress is too severe to be integrated in the usual (adult) manner. Each individual, in his ordinary relationships with people, at one time or another finds the need to return to earlier modes of behavior. For instance, sleep is the universal form of regression following the tiring activities of the day. Often, under the influence of group situations, an individual may allow himself activities which are regressive in nature; for example, the mischievous, childlike behavior frequently observed as part of activity at a class reunion of old alumni, or at a business convention.

To understand the process of pathological regression, it is necessary first to understand the effects of progression, as manifested in the growth toward maturity in the formative years. The infant is endowed with capacities, instincts, and drives that propel it steadily toward growth, development, and maturity — physical and emotional. The normal development of this process can be envisioned as a complex progression. Various stages of development are clearly recognizable in the maturation of the organism.

However, at any time during the course of that maturation, the individual may find himself faced with insurmountable conflicts. To cope with the anxiety produced by these conflicts, and despite his propensity for growth, the individual may be forced to return to an earlier level of development in which he felt more protected, and therefore safe. This return to earlier modes of behavior is the characteristic of regression.

The regression will take on the features of the developmental stage to which the individual returns. The more profound the regression, the more childish and infantile will be the behavior of the patient. The depth to which he regresses will depend on a number of variables such as the intensity, duration, and severity of the conflict which he has had to face in the present situation; the nature of the conflicts which he has faced during his maturation process; and the similarity between the conflicts experienced by him as an adult and those conflicts experienced by him as a growing child. Following are examples of the operation of each of these variables:

a. The soldier in combat, overwhelmed by fear, fatigue, hunger and low morale, may regress to very primitive modes of behavior. These may be characterized by inattention to basic physical needs. He may lie mute and disinterested in his surroundings.

b. An individual in childhood had had repeated demands for performance, which have been a source of intense, chronic anxiety. He enters into a relatively benign work situation. Intellectually he has the capacity to perform this job successfully. Because of his chronic anxiety and his fear of failure, he constantly seeks reassurance from his employer. At home he demands special attention and sleeps a great deal.

c. A child may have felt unloved and deprived of essential emotional relationships. As a man he may react to a minor loss of love, such as a girl friend's refusal of a date, by behavior including temper tantrums, crying or petulance.

When regressive behavior appears, the individual, though an adult, will seem more childish in his behavior. His usual mature ways of handling problems will be changed. Instead, he will come to depend increasingly on others. He will become indecisive. He will expect more care and attention both physically and emotionally. He will refuse responsibility, or when he attempts to deal with problems he will do so in an inadequate and childlike manner. Following are two examples of such behavior:

a. The patient hospitalized for a minor surgical procedure has an uneventful post-operative course. However, on the day he is able to be ambulatory, he says he cannot get up, and rejects the nurses' attempts to help him. During the next several days, he repeatedly rings his bell and refuses to help himself in any way. It is important to understand this behavior (regression) as a response to the patient's anxiety. If this situation is to be handled in a therapeutic way, the nurse should avoid labeling him as uncooperative and demanding.

b. On the ward one observes a carelessly dressed, unshaven patient. He never washes, shaves, or changes his clothing unless the nurse reminds him to do so and assists him. He seems unable to make the most minor decisions for himself. He repeatedly asks the nurse for favors. Yet before his illness this patient was a fastidious, self-sufficient business executive.

The degree of regression with resultant dependence may vary from the simple increase of demands for physical care in a person with an organic illness, to that of a completely dependent individual who no longer assumes responsibility for the most basic functions of the organism, such as eating or control of bowel and bladder function. Thus, his dependence is an attempt to cope with the threats from the physical and emotional environment (defense).

Thus far we have discussed regression and resulting dependence as if they occurred in pure form. However, as in any disease, the organism attempts in some way to overcome or deny the occurrence of the process. As a result other responses are set in motion. These are in the form of mechanisms that attempt to hide from others and from himself the severity and type of disturbance taking place in the personality. We may have, then, the type of reaction in which the individual simply seeks oblivion from the presence of the process. This is an example of simple *Denial*. On the other hand, the person may go one step further than simple Denial and impute the dependence to someone else. This is *Projection*. Or, again, he may attempt to cope with the conflict by using actions and expressions that are contradictory and thus ineffective in solving the problem. This is an example of *Reaction Formation*. In some instances, the organism is able to function fairly well by becoming aggressive in helping others or in caring for others as he would like to be cared for. In this way he may overcome somewhat successfully the anxiety provoking process. This is an example of *Overcompensation*.

It is useful for nurses to understand the patient's need which is expressed by the defense and that against which he defends. It is important to point out here that attitudes, reactions, and roles cannot always be prescribed for the patient's needs as they are understood in the framework of his whole personality. It is frequently necessary to respect and support the defense and to make it operable as such. At other times, it is more helpful to support that which is defended against, than to implement the mechanism used by the patient. The following are examples:

a. A group of patients is going out for a scheduled activity. At the last minute Mrs. Smith, a new patient, complains she has cold feet, feels cold all over, and returns to her bed. The nurse, though aware that this is a defense against the patient's anxiety, responds directly to this expression by covering the patient, getting a hot water bottle and staying with her. In this instance, the defense is respected and supported.

b. At a later time in Mrs. Smith's hospitalization, it may be more therapeutic to anticipate anxiety-provoking situations and to give support and help in these, thereby decreasing the necessity for Mrs. Smith to develop the previously mentioned type of defense. In other words, the nurse may discuss the activity with Mrs. Smith and help her to identify her feelings and fears about them.

In addition to the decision to support the defense, or that which is defended against (never a complete either-or proposition) an estimation of the degree of support and timing of support is necessary. Furthermore, there must be a readiness to modify degree and timing of support. We may categorize these concepts as follows:

A patient with a mild degree of dependence may require support of his dependence until he is able to accept more responsibility.

A patient with a moderately severe problem of dependence may need gratification of the dependence by the nurse. At the same time, other members of the team may help the patient toward insight that would enable him to assume more responsibility.

A patient with severe problems of dependence may require the nurse's tolerance of complete regression. The nurse must offer kind, understanding support and love over a long period of time before the patient can accept some responsibility.

The most common nursing problems demand insight and therapy to some degree, but deal chiefly with supportive attitudes and activities.

Nurses not infrequently display overindulgence, rejection, or punitive control of the patient. With awareness, however, the nurse can be sympathetic, supporting, accepting, permissive and firm in her guidance of the patient.

It is quite obvious that the nurse by herself cannot make the decision for the most effective plan of treatment. Communication through conferences and discussions should formulate the general therapeutic attempt. Further supervision should be available to help each nurse to assess her part in the accepted therapeutic effort.

The patient may withdraw from participation in living by regression and symptoms of dependence. This prevents his having many experiences that would contribute to strengthening relationships with people. For example, the patient may refuse to eat by himself, bathe and dress, and may become completely dependent on nursing staff for physical survival. The nurse may easily assume the role of a person on whom the patient is dependent. The patient may come to feel comfortable when fed, bathed, and dressed. The nurse needs to understand why this kind of participation is a comfortable one for the patient, and also must be aware of her own feelings about having someone dependent upon her. Otherwise, the nurse may be uncomfortable about giving the sort of care which may be helpful to the patient at this point in his illness. This involves some understanding of the patient's past experiences which have necessitated his dependence, and also some understanding of the nurse's feelings about dependence.

A serious problem may arise when the nurse actually receives a great deal of satisfaction from working in a situation in which the patient is dependent on her. In such instances, the behavior of both may become fixed at this point, the nurse actually fostering continued dependent behavior on the part of the patient. Such fixation on dependence is contrary to goals in nursing. When present many cues are missed that might lead to experiences that would lead away from dependent or regressed behavior. The patient may reach for the spoon to feed himself, but this cue is not observed or used. The necessity to maintain the patient's dependence reflects, then, the nurse's need for satisfaction and security, and discourages the patient's first timid attempt away from dependence.

2. *Areas of Dysfunction.* The following five sections illustrate various mechanisms involved in personality change. These sections focus on essential areas of dysfunction of the personality that are associated with the ever-present regression and dependence and concomitant disturbed relationship to other persons.

a. Disturbance of Productive Activity. Every mature individual has at his disposal sufficient amounts of energy in his usual daily activity. The energy is used for physical activities which include his work and recreation. Additional amounts of energy are drawn upon in the solution of the emotional or intellectual problems which arise as part of the daily routine. The individual can also draw upon reservoirs of energy if emergency situations arise. In the integrated individual there is, then, an availability of energy to be used in productivity.

The growing and adult individual constantly exchanges energy with his environment. In infancy there are great demands for energy made on the environment, since the organism must use energy for growth. As growth progresses and becomes slower, there is increasingly more energy available for the use of the individual in productive activities. In the adult there is enough available energy so that some can be transmitted to others in the form of physical, emotional, or intellectual support. Energy is also available for productive and creative activity. Finally, energy will be used in procreation and in the rearing of children.

Wherever conflicts are met in life-situations, a certain amount of energy is used in an attempt to solve the problems inherent in the conflicts. This energy must be drawn from that which normally would be used for productive activity. A patient who is in constant conflict uses large amounts of energy in attempting to solve his problems. It follows, then, that there will be very little, if any, energy available for productive activity.

As a result, the patient may display a general decrease of activity, both physical and mental. He may, in extreme situations, appear stuporous, and therefore, unable to use any energy in productive activity related to his environment. The regressed schizophrenic is using much energy attempting to solve problems in an unrealistic (autistic) manner. In the less severe stages, we may see a patient who to some degree can participate in ward activities, but who soon tires and must be excused. This is quite apparent in the depressed patient who spends much time in self-contemplation, and in whom expenditure of effort is followed by almost complete exhaustion. Again, a patient may be using large amounts of energy in what seems to be productive activity, but on closer examination it becomes apparent that this is being used to deny the presence of internal conflicts. This activity is only a facade which is easily discernible. This type is most commonly seen in the manic patient who is overactive in an attempt to deny an underlying depression. His overt behavior shows that he is expending great amounts of energy, but examination of his productivity indicates that a host of projects is started enthusiastically but the work does not go beyond that stage.

The problems posed for the nurse who is in relationship with these patients are ones which center on the expenditure of energy. The recognition that the patient is using energy in attempts to solve internal conflicts will direct the nurse to keep the patient's activities within the limitations of his available energy. She will then be able to accept the patient's fatigue as real and not react to what is an apparent but not actual laziness. On the other hand, these patients tend to demand a great deal of energy from the nurse. This becomes a source of irritation and resentment if the nurse allows herself to go beyond her available energy.

b. Inability to Control Basic Impulses. Before considering this aspect, there must be some understanding about what the basic impulses are, how they function, and how they are normally controlled.

At the time of birth the child's energy is released by a constant discharge of varied and random impulses. This can be seen in the apparently purposeless movements of the muscles of the body. Any minor frustration is reacted to with massive impulsive responses; the crying of the baby involves his entire musculature. Again, when the bowels are filled, the baby responds immediately by evacuation. Hunger is responded to with desire for immediate gratification associated with a crescendo of crying.

In the process of growing from a baby to an adult, the individual learns different patterns for controlling his basic impulses through the relationships with his parents and other people. To gain love and approval he learns to postpone immediate gratification of such impulses as eating, evacuation of bowels and bladder. He learns that responses to minor frustrations by violent temper outbursts bring loss of love and approval, and therefore, he institutes controls. Later, when the sexual impulse becomes more manifest, the child shows early lack of control, just as with other impulses, but gradually and for the same reasons, he learns to control these impulses. By these experiences he learns to delay gratifications in accordance with the wishes of people with whom he lives and in keeping with the demands of society.

When a patient comes to a mental hospital, because of the regression inherent in his illness, we see the re-emergence of these basic impulses with the learned patterns of control removed in varying degrees. The patient immediately responds to his impulses. If he is hungry, he demands food, and if he is frustrated, he may respond with violent temper tantrums. He may no longer be able to control his bladder and bowels. He may void, soil, and smear on the ward, when and where the impulse emerges. In the sexual sphere the same response is apparent. The patient attempts to obtain immediate gratification.

The patient may respond to this loss of control by attempting to set up a variety of defenses. One example is seen in the patient who, constantly faced with sexual impulses which he cannot control, finds a solution by saying that those around him are making sexual approaches to him, or that voices tell him to masturbate (projection).

Another more direct solution for the patient is to participate on the ward in such a manner that he forces the nursing staff to place controls on him. For example, he may constantly tear off his clothing, and as a result of his nudity gets himself confined to his room. He may become so combative during his rages that those in the situation must use physical control of his behavior. His lack of bladder and bowel control may lead to his being dealt with as one would deal with the young child during toilet training. The patient thereby gets the nurse to help him control his impulses.

Another method of handling this problem can be observed when the patient deals with these impulses by incessant and vigorous denial. By this emphasis on the denial, he actually is giving the clue to his concern about his impulses.

When through illness there is a loosening of the inhibitions, and an inability to control the basic impulses as described above, the patient naturally experiences certain emotional disturbances. The whole process impairs the individual's confidence in himself and his security. We see here the emergence of anxiety. The very anxious patient often has a fear of some impending disaster such as death or loss of control. He usually hides these extreme fears, but gives clues to them in his actions. He may attach anxiety to things or situations that, in the immediate surroundings, can justify such emotion. The demand for frequent contact with the doctor or nurse may amount to the same thing. Anxiety arising from fear of loss of control may lead to a frenzied, or even panic state.

The threat of loss of control of basic impulses, especially those that might call for aggressive action toward others, may lead to anger. Anger, also, may come as a result of disappointment in the self. It is often closely related to, or intertwined with, anxiety because the patient fears his aggressiveness. Hostility is readily recognized when it is directed toward others, but not infrequently, in a more disguised manner, it may be directed inwardly, and the patient may show his feelings by denying virtues to and by criticizing the loved one, or by condemnation of himself as an unworthy individual.

Depression may be foremost as a reaction to the inability to control impulses, but usually it is coexistent with anxiety and hostility; sometimes it is less manifest. Occasionally the depression is so profound that all other emotions are blanketed or "snowed under." More often, anxiety and hostility will break through and show themselves in agitation and rebellion against those near the patient, against rules, regulations and reason.

This type of dysfunction may present a difficult nursing problem. The patient's own discomfort about this behavior and the anxiety about it may incite many negative responses. The patient may refuse to dress in what is considered appropriate clothing. She may allow her blouse to fall in such a way as to expose her breasts, or she may wear a skirt in such a way as to exhibit her genitals. In addition, she may act toward the nurse in a very seductive manner, or may withdraw to a corner of the ward and indulge in open masturbation. Such behavior on the part of the patient may make relationships very difficult with others on the ward. Even though it may be looked upon as the patient's attempt to gain some love and attention from others, nurses may experience great difficulty in maintaining any sort of relationship with the patient as this behavior is not acceptable to them. Here the understanding and awareness of their feelings toward their own basic impulses is significant. When nurses are able to discuss freely how they feel about this sort of behavior, rather than merely to focus on the "right and wrong" aspects of the behavior (people should not masturbate, people should wear clothing, etc.), they are much better able to handle the problem. Their anxiety and discomfort in such a situation does much to sustain this behavior in the patient. When expressed fairly openly, their discomfort decreases, and the patient may be helped to handle his problem in a more useful and mature way.

c. Changed Moral Attitudes and Changed Conventional Attitudes. In our culture, one way of securing approval and love is by being good. Patients often find such a pattern of behavior in their relationships with others successful when nothing else seems effective. However, the price of this is high. Self-expression, creativity and growth of the individual suffer. The person who pays this price often comes to harbor intense resentment against those who respond to his conventional "good" patterns. He may rebel against convention itself. Direct expression of resentment is not possible for this person as it may bring disapproval and loss of love. These resentments and fears find expression in behavior which deviates markedly from what is usually considered "proper" or acceptable in domestic or social situations. It is behavior that is usually expressed at the expense of some other person, has a retaliative quality, and very often is an implicit bid by the patient for punishment.

Respect for moral standards and conventional attitudes expresses itself in conformity. Social conformity is the result of a compromise between a person's need for affection and an inherent urge for independence. The need for parental affection is the young child's most fundamental incentive toward domestication and social conformity. In later childhood, incentive to social conformity comes from the desire for the respect of one's fellows. Opposing this need for the parent's affection is a strong human desire for independence and a resentment of control. This struggle ordinarily reaches its peak in adolescence. A conflict occurs when there is inadequate affectionate response from the loved ones, parents or others. Anxiety and insecurity which are part of this conflict may lead to attention-gaining behavior. This behavior defies the moral standards and conventional attitudes of the loved ones. Society commonly calls this bid for attention "misbehavior." Attention-getting tendencies are common means of fulfilling a common childhood need, yet evoke punishment and threats. These, in turn, lead to resentment. A conflict ensues, namely, resentment versus a desire for affection.

Some handle the conflict (resentment versus desire for affection) by an attitude of filial devotion (maintaining the moral standards and conventional attitudes of the parents) which, in turn, assures affection and security. Such a happy solution may not always be present. There are often periods of open resentment and a flouting of conventional and moral standards. The same series of events may result when a conflict is set up by frustrations of the natural propensities of a child.

Symptoms reflecting changes in moral standards and conventional attitudes deal essentially with the mechanisms of distortion and denial. These are generally ineffective defenses that try to reduce dissatisfactions experienced in being inadequate, and resentments associated with feelings of lack of affection. The distortion may vary in degree, harbor elements of "make-believe," and in their severest form, may appear as symptoms of delusions and hallucinations. The resentments translate themselves into a "don't mind," "don't care" attitude which then gives permission to ignore or defy standards and conventions. These mechanisms expressed in asocial, amoral, anticonventional behavior becomes a difficult problem to the patient, as his already handicapped ability to relate effectively with others will now be additionally threatened by disapproval, contempt, or open retaliation on the part of other patients and nurses. The nurse, however, has the opportunity to assess his behavior for what it implies, and can avoid adding fuel to fire.

Such conflict and anxiety is often demonstrated on the hospital ward by a change in the patient's moral standards and conventional attitudes; for example, a complete disregard of conventions, or rebelling against them. The patient may refuse to conform to any routine or control. He may be insulting, disrespectful of others, distort the truth, become boastful and tell long tales. This disregard of conventions and acting out behavior are often focused on the nurses, as they may assume the familiar roles of the patient's past, which seemed to the patient so unloving and ungiving except in response to "good" conventional behavior. Now all the resentment and anxiety are directed toward those caring for him.

In the setting of symptoms of outspoken resentment, acted-out resentment, distortion or denial, the patient usually finds himself in a recurrent state of helplessness. In spite of feeling helpless, the patient is compelled to use the very same or similar defenses which in the first place made him feel inadequate and ineffective. He may be chagrined or embarrassed about it and strives to minimize his helplessness by brazenly flaunting appeals made to him for moral and conventional conformity. He may welcome the invalid state with varying degrees of regression, such as not minding, denying, avoiding issues involving moral standards and conventional attitudes in order to achieve what is more important, namely, self-consolation. This invalid role may be very difficult for some patients to accept. In others an aptitude for invalidism is great and is the nurse's main problem. In these the tendency to welcome invalidism represents only the need to escape from a temporary but unusually harrowing set of anxieties. In either case, it is useful for her to evaluate the patient's sense of responsiblity and his capacity to tolerate it, as well as his capacity to tolerate anxiety. Here, again, is the need to understand the psychological and physiological functions of anxiety and various human reactions to it.

There are clinical syndromes in which the etiological factors are impersonal (e.g. organic brain disease). It is clear that some organic dementias may be more determined by brain disease, but nevertheless the problems of care entail the same considerations and implications as found in regressed patients.

The recognition that the symptoms of changed moral standards and changed conventional attitudes are (reaction to a need) namely, a need for human affection, can serve as an incentive to make bodily and social control worthwhile. The patient in his development has already experienced interference with carrying out skillful functions. In the past, such failure caused great resentment against the interferers (parental figures) who also were the persons upon whom the patient was dependent. It is the person upon whom he now is dependent who is involved in the struggle and becomes the object of revenge. It is from this person that the patient seeks punishment for flaunting the rules of the game.

The problem of the nurse's feeling which arises as a reaction to the patient's feelings (countertransference) can very seriously impede the patient's care. For example, he may become so uncomfortable that he may withdraw from the patient by involving himself busily in administrative or housekeeping tasks. On the other hand, this sort of acting-out by the patient may call forth punitive behavior on the part of the nurse. Overt forms of counter-aggression may be acted out by putting patients unnecessarily into packs, or confining them to isolation. Somewhat more subtle forms of aggression are conveyed through disapproving gestures, facial expressions, and the spoken word. All of this may tend to perpetuate the patient's pattern of acting-out against conventional attitudes and the usual moral standards.

It is important to help nurses develop

awareness and understanding that they may be unwittingly aiding the patient to break all the rules. This understanding will be greatly facilitated by group experience wherein the nurse has an opportunity to compare her own experience with that of others and thus become aware of the deviants in her feeling toward conventions. She may thus learn what resentments he harbors and what the rewards of "being a good child" are.

d. Diminished Integrative Capacity. Every person has some ability to act in life with a sense of control within himself. This sense of control arises from the maintenance of a harmonious equilibrium between the basic impulses and controlling forces. The process involved in this effort toward harmony we shall call integration. Some of the primitive forces within the individual are of a vehement and ruthless nature. They seek gratification in a selfish manner. If the forces were left unleashed, the person would tend toward disintegration. Such threats imposed upon others would arouse retaliation.

These forces are restrained early in a person's life. Prohibitions and limitations, primarily through parental attitudes, impinge upon the wishes for primitive gratification. It is the struggle between the inner desires and the prohibitions (other person, or later, self-imposed) that is sensed as conflict. Integration deals with the factors that implement mastery of the ensuing tensions.

The development of mastery begins in early life. It demands a gradual and appropriate weaning from the early feeling of power (omnipotence). This feeling of power is gradually relinquished under the supporting experience of obtaining satisfaction, of being loved and approved. Guidance that sets up pertinent limitations is essential. This helps the child to survive the ensuing struggle-for-power period of the first years of life. Gradually, a feeling of personal self-strength (ego-strength) is developed. This is implemented as the child is helped to delay immediate gratification in favor of long-term pleasurable experiences; to learn to make decisions; to accept disappointment and frustration; to tolerate varying degrees of anxiety; to engage in reevaluation of standards arbitrarily imposed upon him; and to refine reality-testing. Furthermore, reactions and defenses are developed to serve as buffers and to reduce the tensions if a more complete mastery is not immediately possible.

The development of ego-strength brings with it an ability on the part of the individual to meet stresses and strains in such a way that they are integrated (incorporated) into the fabric of his personality. However, integration is never complete, nor is it ever static.

In the course of life experiences, the individual may meet situations sufficiently traumatic to tax his capacity for re-establishing the harmonious balance. This occurs either because of the intensity, or of the duration of the stresses. Repeated experiences of trial and error, of satisfaction and disappointment, leave traces or residues of old conflicts. New situations that cannot be mastered may thereby recall feelings of anxiety attached to these residues. The new situations reinstate the earlier conflict. This will be apparent in a decreased ability to relate to others.

The individual whose capacity for integration is currently intact, can meet the ordinary stresses of the day to day experience without undue anxiety or loss of equilibrium. A friend's sarcastic or angry remark, for instance, will be resented briefly, but before long will be recognized as a sign of irritability or of momentary jealousy, and will be replied to either in kind or with friendly tolerance, and soon will be forgotten.

Often a patient who is ill is not able to integrate experiences or feelings which occur in accordance with learned patterns of behavior. He will participate on the ward in a less adequately integrated manner. For example, he may come to feel confused, doubtful, hesitant and afraid, and may be unable to resolve these feelings. These unintegrated feelings are often transferred to members of the nursing personnel with whom he associates in his daily living. These transferred feelings and behavior toward the staff may effectively create fear, doubt, hesitation, and hostility in return. This reciprocal response makes the nurse uncomfortable and anxious with the patient. In extreme situations, the nurse may withdraw from the patient, or almost completely isolate him.

The understanding of the nurse's feelings about problems of impaired integration needs to be explored and clarified. Nursing skills are often enhanced by participation in patient-oriented conferences and informal discussions.

e. Disturbance of the Function of Reality Testing. One of the most important examples of personality dysfunction is the impairment of reality-testing. In the child there is little ability to recognize what sensations originate from within. He is unable to recognize the boundaries of his own body. The environment is conceived of as continuous with himself. As the child grows, he learns to delineate himself from his environment. As a result, he is able to recognize what sensations are coming from within himself and what sensations are coming from without.

We may recognize varying degrees of impairment. These may include the complete breakdown of a psychosis in which impaired reality testing may be expressed by the patient's conviction that he is influenced by magic or electrical forces, or psychoneurotic disorders in which the patient may deny that physical complaints can be caused by emotional problems. He may be unable to rid his mind of disturbing fears or obsessive thoughts. The presumably normal person under stress may misinterpret other people's attitudes and intentions.

This impairment of reality-testing may be maintained by the use of a variety of defenses. The use of these prevents the patient from seeing things and people as they really are. His feelings do not correspond with the external reality. These defenses may include *denial,* when the patient maintains that a dead person is not dead; or *distortion* of reality, when the patient regards friendly persons as hostile; or *evasion,* when the patient seems quite unaware of a disturbing reality. This impairment of reality-testing follows the inability of a person to tolerate, without serious loss of self-esteem, a reality which is threatening or unsatisfying.

Mentally ill patients often experience difficulties in recognizing the origins of sensations as a result of the inevitable regression accompanying their illness. The patient may, as a result, appear unable to care for himself, while another patient may be unrealistically confident that he needs no help. Still another may create in fantasy a situation which does not exist, as in delusions and hallucinations.

The effort of the patient to create his own world, frequently without consideration of his family and community, provokes hostile, anxious retaliation from family and community, which may lead to his being forcibly removed from the community and placed in a mental hospital.

It is useful that the hospital provide a more tolerant, protective environment, compared with the disturbing, anxiety-provoking situations from which the patient came. It is to a large extent the nurse's attitude which provides a "world reality in miniature" that the patient can accept without anxiety. To be more specific, when a patient is extremely uncomfortable or anxious in his relationships with people around him, he may see or perceive ward situations and people on the ward quite differently from what they are in reality. This type of protective or defensive reaction on the part of the patient serves to create a safe distance between him and people around him, and thus decreases his discomfort and anxiety. At the same time, this distance or temporary loss of relationship leads to a peculiar effort to have some relationship with the people about him. For example, if the patient can distort the ward situation to the point that he believes all people to be against him, and can hear them talking about him, he may then become involved listening to these people, protecting himself against them, and thus withdraw to a marked degree from contact with people in his daily living on the ward.

The nurses, who are in reality the "people around him," may become uncomfortable through repeated expressions on the part of the patient regarding nurses' plans to do away with him. They may be so disturbed by their own discomfort that they may stay farther and farther away, and thus reinforce the patient's anxiety. Such a situation makes it difficult to focus on the real problem of how to provide experiences in which the patient does not feel so uncomfortable, and through which reality can, little by little, come within range for him.

3. *Decreased Capacity for Mature Object Rela-*

tionships. Some form of emotional interchange with others is characteristic of people. This interchange, which is not exclusively verbal, depends also on gestures, facial expressions, tears, laughter and more subtle physical signs such as turgor of skin, tone of voice, brightness of eyes, blushing, sweating and posture. These compositely reflect the individual's emotions. Feelings of anxiety, fear, anger, contentment, gaiety, calmness, puzzlement, to name only a few, can be discerned. The recognition of some of these emotions is easy; others take more sensitivity to grasp. It is of utmost importance to those working with the emotionally disturbed to learn to recognize unusual, peculiar, conflicting, often ineffective, seemingly purposeless ways of expression.

Emotional interchange between people is motivated by a need to express oneself, to reduce inner tensions, and to obtain a response from the other person. This response is important, since it leads either to gratification or frustration. When an anticipated gratifying response does not occur, the relatively healthy person can decide whether he has not made himself understood, or whether the other person could not respond appropriately. After making such an evaluation, he may try a different approach. The results of trial and error gradually develop the ability to grasp relatively accurately the effect of one's own emotions on others.

The process is complicated as conscious and rational feelings occur simultaneously with unconscious irrational feelings and expressions of these feelings.

It becomes clear that this complex interplay between individuals requires personal integration, and leans heavily on intact ability for reality-testing. It demands control of basic impulses. Evaluation of moral standards and conventional attitudes of the given cultural and social milieu are reflected in this process.

The essentially "normal" development of the capacity for emotional interchanges with other people is a complex, uneven, hazardous progression. This progression can be assigned arbitrarily to three periods in the individual's development.

First comes the early, completely dependent (biological and emotional) infant period when the necessity to receive appropriate recognition and gratification of needs is very high. The means of denoting satisfaction or countering frustrations are diffuse and undifferentiated.

Later, a semi-cooperative period evolves in which receiving gratification, guidance, tolerance, and support are essential. The response in this period can be expressed as active aggression, attack, nonconformity, refusal, withdrawal, or opposition. Satisfaction can be registered in words, compliance in behavior, outbursts of loving affection, and a host of other ways. This is a period of tentativeness wherein the strength of needs can quickly dispel the cooperative participating efforts.

A still later period eventuates in which the individual gradually embarks on a more reciprocal emotional level. Perceptions and feeling-into (empathy) the needs and feelings of others modify to some extent the demands made on others. Anticipations and expectations become more accurate. The subtle balance of obtaining gratification and of satisfactorily giving becomes refined. This period deals repetitiously in testing out the internal and external appropriateness of expression of feelings and the response obtained. The relatively objective assessment of this interplay is an expression of maturity. At best, there is unevenness, success and failure, for every person. To the most mature come experiences of stress and anxiety, both from within and without. The way equilibrium can be sought and obtained, the time in which this can be accomplished, and the maintenance of relative intactness of the person while he meets these stresses denote the state of mental health.

Certain life stresses can impair the individual's capacity to relate with other people. Such experiences include severe organic changes resulting from toxic or mutilating agents; severe and continued deprivations such as starvation, exposure to extreme temperatures; disorganization of familiar personal relationships because of death or separation; unconscious revival of unmastered inner conflicts, such as feelings of guilt about unrecognized destructive wishes, or anxiety over unconscious temptations of a sexual nature. Every illness, physical or emotional, decreases the individual's capacity for mature (object) relationships. The sick person makes bids for relationships with others, but his approaches may be clumsy, bizarre and inappropriate.

A patient's conflicts may be such that he no longer can repress thoughts of attacking or killing another person. In coping with the resulting anxiety, he may ascribe these feelings to another person and accuse the other person of his own wishes (projection). Irrational as this is, anxiety is thereby partially reduced and a relationship with another person is attempted. The response of the nurse to this behavior is of utmost importance. If the nurse responds with hostility or withdrawal, she may reinforce the behavior. If the nurse, however, can understand this behavior as a defense, achieve clarity about her (the nurse's) own feelings toward aggressive feelings and actions, the first step has been taken toward helping the patient to become less anxious and to facilitate a change in his behavior.

A retarded and withdrawn patient may give the impression that he is unaware of his surroundings, and does not care to relate to others. Such an assumption is erroneous. His extreme passivity is a form of human contact at the level on which he can participate in relationships at this time in his life. Passive participation on the part of the nurse is the first step in breaking the wall of non-communication. Nurses may be hampered by their feelings that one has to be actively doing something in order to help a patient. Sitting with the patient, saying nothing, may be the only sort of relationship in which the patient can be comfortable at this time.

A patient who has regressed to very infantile levels may use his need to be fed, or to be cleansed after soiling as a bid for help, for physical closeness to another, for love and affection, for encouragement. He may desire such responses to offset deep feelings of inadequacy, fear of loss of control of his emotions, possibly feelings of shame and humiliation. He is frightened and wants reassurance that he will not be abandoned. If, in addition to meeting these expressed needs in an understanding manner, the nurse through repeated experiences with the patient becomes alert to cues that indicate his readiness for a more mature relationship, the patient's anxiety may be greatly diminished. The sick person's emotional reactions give evidence that the "healthy" part of himself is trying to relate to others. Repeated failures may overwhelm the threatened person so that he will reach a "point of no return."

The nurse may tend to treat the patient as essentially a rational person. In common social intercourse, attack can be averted or met with attack, argument with argument. Withdrawal, annoyance, unresponsiveness may well be met with indifference or counter-withdrawal. The essentially healthy person soon will erect defenses that will bring a tolerable equilibrium to the tense situation. Anxieties, fears, hostile or erotic feelings can be managed in appropriate time.

When the nurse comes into contact with human behavior that is unfamiliar to her, she is tempted to take the expressions literally, using familiar values. The sick person's attempt to relate to the nurse may arouse anxiety, hostility, fear or contempt. These emotions then demand defensive attitudes and actions on the part of the nurse. The nurse who becomes overwhelmed by the patient's primitive and crude expressions may be unable to hide her feelings and may retaliate physically. In other instances, she may become oversolicitous. The patient's sexual behavior may become provocative and arouse in the nurse responses similar in kind and intensity. The nurse may become terrified as she becomes aware that she, too, may harbor feelings and impulses not dissimilar to those of the patient.

Conflicts, once well buried, may be revived under the impact of dealing with psychotic patients. The more the nurse defends herself against anxiety aroused by these conflicts, the less chance she has of helping the patient, and the less chance she has of using the relationship effectively. She may abandon the patient by overemphasizing her so-called administrative responsibilities. She may become overly interested in impersonal treatments, as diets and laxatives, or in time-consuming linen counts. She may argue with the physicians that the patient should have shock therapy and maintain that the physicians do not know what they are doing. She may become angry when the patient does not show his appreciation by getting well quickly. She may prevent the patient's discussing what is important to him. The nurse may act passively through failure to carry out working arrangements for the patient. She may not insist on regular schedules or may fail to remind patients of appointments. By such methods the nurse diminishes the likelihood that a therapeutic relationship can be developed with the patient.

Cogently directed patient-nurse relationships are therapeutically effective. The nurse's awareness of the patient's needs, and the nurse's increased conviction of her own adequacy in meeting these needs, will be reflected in her relationships with patients. Excellent opportunities for the development of these relationships are offered by necessary nursing care. The nurse can become aware of the meaning and significance of her very presence in relationship to the patient. The nurse will become increasingly able to carry the responsibility of being the person who conveys strengthening, supporting attitudes to the patient.

IV. Conclusion

We recognize that there is no easy answer to the problem involved in the selection and adequate training of specific individuals to provide the relationships needed by emotionally ill patients. Ideally, the curriculum should offer planned, supervised clinical experience which makes it possible for the nurse to increase her understanding of patients.

The instructor of nursing personnel has, in her relationship with her students, a royal opportunity to help students in their relationships with patients. The instructor, too, has to evaluate her own use of defenses against anxiety. One of the most common defenses observed is the zeal with which the various "ologies" are taught. Knowledge and memory are emphasized. Nursing routines are laboriously checked. Close relationships, living relationships are avoided.

We probably can teach didactically very little of value to the nurse in terms of dealing with patients. We can, however, provide situations in which she herself can learn with a minimum of anxiety. The nurse may gradually reach a high point of tolerance of anxiety because of her own self-knowledge. With experience she may learn not only to appreciate the dilemmas of her patients but also to help them through their disparate efforts to cope with them.

Selected Reading

1. Astryke, M., Women Aides to Care for Male Psychiatric Patients, Am. J. Nursing, 52:966, 1952.

2. Baer, W.H., The Training of Psychiatric Students, Am. J. Psychiatry, 109:291-295, 1952.

3. Barrabee, P., A Study of a Mental Hospital: The Effect of Its Social Structure on Its Function, unpublished Ph.D. dissertation, Dept. Social Relations, Harvard University, 1951.

4. Behymer, Alice F., Interaction Patterns and Attitudes of Affiliate Students in a Psychiatric Hospital, Nursing Outlook, 1:No. 4, 205-207, April, 1953.

5. Bennett, A.E. and Engle, B., Psychiatric Nursing and Occupational Therapy, Chapter 35, Progress in Neurology & Psychiatry, Vol. VIII, 1953.

6. Bettelheim, B. and Sylvester E., Therapeutic Influence of the Group on the Individual, Amer. J. Orthopsychiatry (1947), 17:684-692.

7. Bettelheim, B., On Institutional Group Therapy, Bull. of American Psychoanalytic Association, Vol. 6, No. 2, May, 1950.

8. Black, K., Appraising the Psychiatric Patient's Nursing Needs, Am. J. Nursing, 52:718-721, 1952.

9. Blasko, J., Problems in Training Today's Psychiatric Aide, Ment. Hospitals, 3:9, 1952.

10. Boston Psychopathic Handbook - Group Project, Jan.-March, 1952.

11. Boyd, R.W., Baker, T. and Greenblatt, M., Ward Social Behavior: An Analysis of Patient Interaction at Highest and Lowest Extremes, Nursing Research, Vol. III, No. 2, 77-80, Oct. 1954.

12. Brown, E.L., Nursing for the Future, New York, Russell Sage Foundation, 1948.

13. Bullard, D.M., Problems of Clinical Administration, Bull. Menninger Clinic, 16:193-201, 1952.

14. Caudill, W., Redlich, F.C., Gilmore, H.R. and Brody, E.P., Social Structure and Interaction Processes on Psychiatric Ward, Am. J. Orthopsychiatry, 22:314-334, 1952.

15. Caudill, W. and Stainbrook, E., Some Covert Effects of Communication Difficulties in a Psychiatric Hospital, Psychiatry, Vol. 17, No. 1, Feb. 1954.

16. Cook, L.C., Cunningham, E., and Maclay, W.S., Geriatric Problems in Mental Hospitals, Lancet, 1:377-382, 1952.

17. Deming, D., Careers for Nurses, New York, McGraw-Hill, 1952.

18. Department of Medicine and Surgery Information Bulletin, Oct. Administration, Feb. 1950, I.B. 10/5/18.

19. Devereaux, G., The Social Structure of the Hospital as a Factor in Total Therapy, Amer. J. Orthopsychiatry (1949) 19:492-500.

20. Dumack, H., Rooming-In Pediatrics, Am. J. Nursing, 52:47, 1952.

21. Frank, J.D., Corrective Emotional Experiences in Group Therapy, Am. J. Psychiatry, Vol. 108, No. 2, 126-131, Aug. 1951.

22. GAP Report No. 22, The Psychiatric Nurse in the Mental Hospital, Group for the Advancement of Psychiatry, 3617 W. Sixth Ave., Topeka, Kansas, May, 1952.

23. Gentry, M.E. and Swanson, F.L., Psychological Approach to Weight Control, Am. J. Nursing, 52:849-850, 1952.

24. Gilmore, Helen, The Psychiatrist's Part in Nursing Education Programs, Nursing Outlook, Vol. 1, April, 1953.

25. Ginsburg, Eli, A Program for the Nursing Profession, Macmillan, 1949. (New York)

26. Goldberg, N. and Hyde, R.W., Role-Playing in Psychiatric Training, J. of Social Psychology, 1954, 39, 63-75.

27. Gregg, D.E., Anxiety — A Factor in Nursing Care, Am J. Nursing, 52:1363-1365, 1952.

28. Hall, B.H., A Colleague Looks at Psychiatric Nursing, Nursing Outlook, Vol. 2, Feb. 1954.

29. Hall, Bernard H. et al., Psychiatric Aide Education, New York, Grune & Stratton, 1952.

30. Handbook on the Structure of Organized Nursing, Committee on the Structure of National Nursing Organizations, 1949.

31. Heidgerken, L., The Nursing Student Evaluates Her Teachers, Philadelphia, Lippincott, 1952.

32. Henry, J., quoted in Reference 15 as a personal communication.

33. Huntting, I., Semrad, E.V., More Specific Prescribing of Occupational Therapy, Am. J. Occ. Therapy, Vol VI, No. 6, Nov.-Dec. 1952.

34. Hyde, R.W., Factors in Group Motivation in a Mental Hospital, J. Nerv. & Ment. Dis. Vol. 117, No. 3, March, 1953.

35. Hyde, R.W., Greenblatt, M. and Boyd, R., Authority in Attendant-Patient Relationships, accepted for publication by J. of Nerv. & Ment. Dis., Vol. 117, No. 2, p. 166, Feb. 1953.

36. Hyde, R.W., Kandler, H.M., Altruism in Psychiatric Nursing, Chap. 25 of book "Forms and Techniques of Altruistic and Spiritual Growth." A symposium edited by Pitrim A. Sorokin, Beacon Press, Boston, 1954, pp. 387-399.

36a. Hyde, R.W., "Experiencing the Patient's Day," published by J.P. Putnam & Sons.

37. Hyde, R.W., Research in Occupational Therapy, Bull. of Mass. Assoc. for Occ. Therapy, Vol. 24, No. 1, April, 1950.

38. Hyde, R.W., Scott, B., The Occupational Therapy Research Laboratory, Occupational Therapy and Rehabilitation, 30:3, June, 1951.

39. Ingram, M.E., Principles of Psychiatric Nursing, Philadelphia, Saunders, 1949.

40. Jones, M., The Therapeutic Community, New York, Basic Books, 1953.

41. Kaldeck, R., Group Psychotherapy by Nurses and Attendants, Diseases of Nervous System, Vol. XII, No. 5, 138-142, May, 1951.

42. Kalkman, Marion E., Introduction to Psychiatric Nursing,

McGraw-Hill, 1950.

43. Kalkman, M.E., What the Psychiatric Nurse Should Be Educated to Do, Psychiat. Quarterly Supp. 26:93-102, 1952.

44. Kandler, H., Behymer, A.F., Kegeles, S.S. and Boyd, R.W., A Study of Nurse-Patient Interaction in a Mental Hospital, Am. J. Nursing, 52:1100-1103, 1952.

45. Kandler, H.M. and Hyde, R.W., Changes in Empathy in Student Nurses During the Psychiatric Affiliation, Nursing Research, Vol. 2, No. 1, pp. 33-36, June, 1953.

46. Kandler, H.M., Studying a Problem in Psychiatric Nursing, Am. J. Nursing, Vol. 51, Feb. 1951.

47. Kline, Nathan S., Characteristics and Screening of Unsatisfactory Psychiatric Attendants and Attendant Applicants, Am. J. Psychiatry, 106:573-586, Feb. 1950.

48. League Letter, N.L.N. Educ. No. 34, 1952.

49. Lenehan, F.T., In-Service Education Programs in State Psychiatric Hospitals, Nursing World, June, 1953, Vol. No. 27.

50. Lenehan, F.T., How One State Improves Psychiatric Nursing Care. Personal Copy.

51. Lentz, E., "Morale in a Hospital Business Office," Human Organization (1950) 9:17-21.

52. Lolli, G., Treatment of Alcohol Addiction, Quart. J. Stud. on Alcohol, 13:461-471, 1952.

53. Mayden, P.M., What Shall Psychiatric Patients Read? Am. J. Nursing, 52:192-193, 1952.

54. Mellow, J., An Exploratory Study of Nursing Therapy with Two Persons with Psychosis, Master Thesis, 1953.

55. Mereness, D., Meeting the Students' Emotional Needs, Am. J. Nursing, 52:336-338, 1952.

56. Montag, M.L., The Education of Nursing Technicians, New York, Putnam, 1951.

57. Morimoto, F.R., Favoritism in Personnel-Patient Interaction, accepted for publication by Nursing Research.

58. Morimoto, F.R., Greenblatt, M., Personnel Awareness of Patients' Socializing Capacity, Am. J. Psychiatry, Vol. 110, No. 6, 443-447, Dec. 1953.

59. Morimoto, F.R. and Kandler, H.M., A Comparison of Skills and Interests of Patients and Nursing Personnel in a Psychiatric Hospital, accepted for publication by Nursing World.

60. Morimoto, F.R., The Socializing Role of Psychiatric Ward Personnel, Am. J. Nursing, Jan. 1954.

61. Muller, T.G., The Nature and Direction of Psychiatric Nursing, Philadelphia, Lippincott, 1950.

62. National League for Nursing press release, 3/26/53.

63. National League for Nursing letter No. 34, 5/28/52.

64. Nielsen, J.C., Report of Second National Psychiatric Aide Programs Workshop, The National Association for Mental Health, Inc., Aug. 12, 1952.

65. Peffer, P.A. and Astryke, M., Extensive Use of Female Aides in Care of Male Mental Patient, Am. J. Psychiatry, 108:929-930, 1952.

66. Peplau, H., Interpersonal Relations in Nursing, New York, Putnam, 1952.

67. Psychiatric Aide Programs Workshop Newsletter, Aug. 15, 1952, The National Association for Mental Health, Inc., New York.

68. Render, Helena W., The Nurse-Patient Relationships in Psychiatry, 1st ed., New York, McGraw-Hill, 1947.

69. Report of Stockton Pilot Study, Calif. Dept. of Mental Hygiene, 7/1/50 to 11/1/51.

70. Research Reporter, Nursing Research, 1:40-42, 1952.

71. Rich, R. et al., Report on the Structure of Organized Nursing, Am. J. Nursing, 46:10, October, 1946.

72. Robinson, Alice, Psychiatric Aide, Lippincott, 1954.

73. Rosenberg, P., The Nurses Groups, personal communication.

74. Schwartz, C.G., Schwartz, M.S. and Stanton, A.H., A Study of Need-Fulfillment on a Mental Hospital Ward, Psychiatry (1951) 14:223-242.

75. Schwartz, M.S. and Stanton, A.H., A Social Study of Incontinence, Psychiatry, 13:399-416, Nov. 1950.

76. Semrad, E.V., Menzer, D., Mann, J. and Standish, C.T., A Study of the Doctor-Patient Relationship in Psychotherapy of Psychotic Patients, Psychiatry, Vol. 15, No. 4, Nov. 1952.

77. Semrad, E.V., The Psychiatrist Looks at Occupational Therapy, Am. J. Occ. Therapy, Vol. I, No. 5, Oct. 1947.

78. Shea, N., Klatskin, E.H. and Jackson, E.B., Home Adjustment of Rooming-In and Non-Rooming-In Mothers, Am. J. Nursing, 52:65-67, 1952.

79. Sleeper, F.H., Present Trends in Psychiatric Nursing, Am. J. Psychiatry, 109:203-207, 1952.

80. Smith, H., Sociological Study of Hospitals, unpublished Ph.D. dissertation, Dept. Sociology, Univ. of Chicago, 1949.

81. Solomon, H.C., "Psychiatric Nursing", read before the Michigan Society of Neurology and Psychiatry, Oct. 19, 1950.

82. Stanton, A.H. and Schwartz, M.S., The Management of a Type of Institutional Participation in Mental Illness, Psychiatry, Vol. 12, 13-16, Feb. 1949.

83. Stanton, A.H. and Schwartz, M.S., Observations on Dissociation as Social Participation, Psychiatry (1949) 12:399-354.

84. Study of Ward Patient Care in Hospitals for the Mentally Ill, Am. J. Nursing, 42:721, 1952.

85. Szurek, S.A., Dynamics of Staff Interaction in Hospital Psychiatric Treatment of Children, Amer. J. Orthopsychiatry (1947) 17:652-664.

86. Tudor, Gwen E., A Sociopsychiatric Nursing Approach to Intervention in a Problem of Mutual Withdrawal on a Mental Hospital Ward, Psychiatry, 15:193-217, May, 1952.

87. Vaccaro, J., Judging the Adequacy of Psychiatric Aides, Hospital Management, 73:46-48, 1952.

88. Wessen, A., The Social Structure of a Modern Hospital, unpublished Ph.D. dissertation, Dept. Sociology, Yale, 1951.

89. Whitehorn, J.C., "Emotional Responsiveness in Clinical Interview," Am. J. Psychiatry, 94:311-315, 1937.

90. Wilson, A.T.M., Hospital Nursing Auxiliaries, London, Tavistock Publications, 1950.

91. Woodward, J., Employment Relations in a Group of Hospitals, London Institute of Hospital Administrators, 1950.

92. Zetzel, E.R., The Dynamic Basis of Supervision, Social Casework, April, 1953.

93. Zilboorg, G., The Struggle of the Patient Against the Doctor, J. of the Michigan State Medical Society, Vol. 52, April, 1953.

Identifying Some Concepts Nursing Personnel Need to Understand in Relation to the Nature of Therapeutic Functions

Eleanor W. Lewis

Ms. Lewis is Associate Professor, School of Nursing and Associate Director of Nursing, Columbus Receiving Hospital and State Institute of Psychiatry, The Ohio State University.

This paper was an NLN Psychiatric Nursing Conference Project, Eastern Region, Washington, D.C., presented in April 1956.

This paper is directed toward the identification of some concepts nursing personnel need to understand in relation to the nature of therapeutic functions. Its special focus is on concepts and experiences related to therapy as a part of effective nursing in:

1. intensive treatment situations
2. supervisory and administrative processes

We should like to open our discussion with a consideration of what nursing is and can be. This will enable us to view nursing as a helping process based on knowledge, understanding and use of the natural, social and psychological sciences; it will also enable us to consider the levels of nursing care which are currently being provided. On the basis of our discussion of what nursing is and can be, we shall endeavor to identify concepts and experiences related to therapeutic functions which nursing personnel need in an intensive treatment situation. The supervisory and administrative processes needed to facilitate the therapeutic functions of nursing in an intensive treatment situation will then be discussed.

The Function of Nursing[1]

"Nursing is one of the services for the care of the sick, for the prevention of illness, and for the promotion of health which is carried on under medical authority. Its distinctive function is to give close and individualized service to the patient, performing for him what he cannot do for himself, giving supportive care, physical and emotional, to bring him through dependence to self-directive activity toward his own health.

"Professional nursing is always patient-centered, either through service given directly, or through instruction given the patient and his family, or through coordination of services given the patient or his family during the period of nursing care. It is based on an understanding of the total therapeutic plan and the concept of preventive medicine and community health, and on the physical, emotional, and intellectual state and capacity of the individual and his family.

"Its further function, in a society increasingly aware of the values of positive health, is to participate actively, or to assume a position of leadership, in community efforts to achieve physical, mental and social well-being of all the population."[1]

Culturally, nursing is seen as a helping process ministering to and helping people where they are not able to help themselves. Medically, nursing is seen as one of the many helping functions of a professional health team. Nursing as a process incorporates certain scientific knowledge, understandings, attitudes and skills which are used to promote both the physical and emotional well being of people. Because of its goal-directed and on-going nature, it necessitates serial steps and operations between nurse and patient. This makes of nursing a process which is interpersonal and one which may be both therapeutic and educative. While carried on under medical authority and based on an understanding of the total therapeutic plan, nursing has its own distinctive function, characterized as close, prolonged participation in the patient's living through experiences intimately involving the nurse in the patient's health problems.

One of the outstanding characteristics of a human being is his natural tendency toward growth and change unless he is in some way prevented from this. The nurse's interaction with the patient in the interests of his recovery can be effectively based on this concept of personality growth and development. The purpose in offering help to an individual undergoing health difficulties is to aid him in taking steps in the direction of productive action, growth and change. Within the framework of his relationship with the nurse, the patient can be seen to progress along a continuum from dependence through independence to interdependence. Nurses can help patients to direct action toward identifying and removing blocks which prevent their natural progress toward goals and thus, in terms of experience, lead to variations and changes in goals. This may be a matter of helping the patient to remember and better understand what is happening to him in the present situation, so that the experience can be integrated with, rather than cut off from, other experiences in life.

In the face of the rapidly increasing demand for nursing services, the professional nurse of today must be able to take leadership in making her distinctive contribution to the curative and preventive aspects of illness and to the creative aspects of health. She must be able to assume leadership in the improvement of those understandings and skills which nursing now has as well as in the development of new ones. She must be ready to assume responsibility for the teaching and supervision of other nurses and auxiliary nursing personnel. She must cooperate with other professions in planning for positive health in a creative and on-going health program.

Levels of Nursing Care

Nursing, like education, medicine, social work and other professions of social origin, aims to promote progress in meeting human needs. The needs which nurses attempt to meet through their behavior (actions, thoughts, attitudes and feelings) may be studied or analyzed in different ways. Nursing, for example, can be divided into three general types or levels of care which can then be studied or examined in relation to the satisfaction of the common human needs.

Because of its simplicity, we should like to refer to Maslow's system of classifying basic human needs. "This system arranges the totality of human needs from the most biologically basic to the most socially oriented:

1. Those needs which are essential to sustaining life itself: needs for food, water, air, warmth, sexual gratification, elimination of bodily wastes, etc.
2. Those needs which are related to maintaining the physical safety of the individual, such as the need for defense against attack.
3. The needs for love: the need to be loved, cherished, and aided by another individual or individuals.
4. The need for esteem: the needs to have worth and value as an individual, to respect and value oneself because one is respected and valued by others.
5. The need for self-realization: the needs to be creative and productive, to cope with life effectively, to work for and attain worthwhile objectives, etc."[2]

Three commonly recognized types or levels of nursing care are the custodial, the supportive and the rehabilitative. Custodial care is that type of care given "to" or given "for" a patient, probably most frequently done "for" a person to maintain his present level. It is intended to ease without necessarily curing or improving the condition, and it is basic and essential to all nursing. In terms of Maslow's system of classifying basic human needs, custodial care seems to satisfy those basic needs which are essential to life itself. It also seems to satisfy those needs which are related to maintaining the physical safety of the individual. Within the framework of the relationship with the nurse, this type of care tends to keep the patient dependent and to add nothing to his capacity to help himself.

Supportive care is that type of nursing care given "for" or "to" the patient; it is generally concerned with restoring physical health. It is more or less concerned with the carrying out of mechanical or technical skills based on varying degrees of application of scientific principles. At its higher levels it moves toward rehabilitation. In addition to the needs satisfied on the custodial level, the need for acceptance, which is experienced as support when one individual is aided by another individual or individuals, is now met. At its higher levels such supportive care moves toward the satisfaction of the need to respect and value oneself because one is respected and valued. In the nursing relationship a considerable degree of independence is experienced by patients receiving this type of care.

Rehabilitative care is that type which encourages the patient to participate in his own care. It not only improves health but also releases energies for continuing growth and self-realization. In terms of basic needs it enables the patient to become both creative and productive, to learn to cope with life effectively, to work for and attain worthwhile goals in living. In the nursing relationship, on this level, the patient experiences a high degree of interdependent participation with the nurse in the achievement of their common goals.

The Nature of Therapeutic Functions

As previously stated, nursing is an interpersonal process which may be both therapeutic and educative. For purposes of this paper, we shall confine ourselves to a discussion of the nature of therapeutic functions and from this point shall direct our attention toward nursing in a psychiatric setting.

The distinctive function of nursing is rooted in the nurse's round-the-clock participation in the patient's everyday affairs of living. This places her in close proximity to expressions of the patient's difficulties in living and in a position to give him continuous support and help in his use of the total therapeutic experience. Her participation with the patient is determined by his manifest expressions of behavior (actions, thoughts, attitudes, feelings) in the nursing situation.

In order to function therapeutically in the nursing situation, the nurse, like other professional practitioners (example, social case work), proceeds from a set of principles which constitute a logical base for her practice. Nursing began as a simple human service to sick people and has been in the process of evolving from that stage of practice. In order now to consolidate the professional character of nursing it is necessary to state and examine some of the basic principles under which it can function.

There is inherent worth and dignity in each human being.

Respect for the individual includes respect for and acceptance of individual and group differences compatible with democratic responsibility.

Cause and effect relationships exist.

Behavior, as well as other natural phenomena, is caused and does not just happen.

Scientific method is essential to the nursing process.

The scientific method of observation-interpretation-test is analogous to the process in nursing of impression-analysis-intervention.

The right to self-determination belongs inherently to man.

The professional nurse can constructively carry out her ethical commitment to the promotion of the patient's capacity for self-determination only on the basis of a correct appraisal both of the patient's capacities and the social realities.

In human beings there is a natural tendency toward growth and change.

One of the outstanding characteristics of human beings is their natural tendency toward growth and change unless they are in some way prevented from this.

With these principles as a frame of reference, we are now ready to identify three interlocking therapeutic functions inherent in the practice of nursing at the rehabilitative level:

1. To create and maintain a therapeutic milieu
2. To function as a participant observer
3. To engage in the therapeutic use of the self
   a. to use the self as a catalyst in interpersonal situations
   b. to participate in specific therapeutic experiences with patients

Concepts and Experiences

In view of the markedly interlocking nature of the above therapeutic functions it seems impossible to separate the concepts and experiences relating to them. There are, of course, certain concepts and experiences which are more closely related to one than to another of these therapeutic functions. There are, however, many concepts and experiences which appear to be closely related to each of these functions. Hence, for purposes of this paper, it seems desirable to state these concepts and experiences in general groupings.

Concepts

Every human personality has intrinsic worth and dignity.

Survival of the human organism depends on adaptations of internal and external stress.

Human nature is plastic and carries possibilities for numerous cultural modes of behavior.

Mental illness is a mode of participation with other people.

The purpose of hospitalization is to provide experiences in living which will enable the patient to establish relationships which are less anxiety provoking and more comfortable, thereby making the possibility of further relationships less threatening.

In the hospital, patients have the right to be as sick as they need to be in order to get well, although it may be necessary to prevent the rights of the one patient from interfering with the rights of another.

Behavior is meaningful.

Behavior includes moods, ideas and attitudes as well as motor activity.

Behavior can be modified.

Needs, both normal and neurotic, are like internal pressures which operate to produce behavior.

Present experience of a person is effected by all his past experience.

Behavior of a person is effected by, and effects, all persons and events in a situation.

A potential for growth toward maturity exists in all organisms.

A relationship is a two-way process.

Acceptance of a patient involves considering the meaning of behavior and recognizing the dignity of the patient, regardless of his behavior, without compromising one's own set of values.

The nurse's emotional needs and system of values are part of the patient's therapeutic environment.

In the hospital, all aspects of the patient's daily living, from admission to discharge, should be appropriate to the purposes they serve in the total treatment program.

The physical setting of the hospital should be appropriate to the purposes the hospital serves in the life of the patient.

To be therapeutic, the hospital environment must provide both for spontaneous and planned socialization of patients.

In a therapeutic environment there must be opportunities for motivating patients on each nursing unit.

The therapeutic milieu should provide opportunities for patients to participate in the planning program.

There are therapeutic indications and contraindications for the use of permissiveness and control.

The milieu in which patients live increases therapeutically as perceptions sharpen to expressed and unexpressed needs.

Needs, to be understood, must be communicated.

Communication becomes rational when it is understood.

When needs are met, new and more mature needs emerge.

The nurse plays an important role in identifying patients' problems and patterns of relationships and in planning useful methods of intervention.

Nurses, like other human beings, act on the basis of the meaning of events to them.

Observation, communication and recording are three interlocking functions in the nursing process.

Observation always precedes interpretation of the collected facts.

The nursing process of impression-analysis-intervention is analogous to the scientific method of observation-interpretation-test.

In order for the nurse to fulfill her role it is important for her to recognize the reciprocal nature of her experiences with patients by becoming aware of her own feelings, thoughts and actions.

As a participant observer the nurse must recognize and note cues from herself as well as cues from the patient.

Self-understanding by the nurse includes an understanding and acceptance of what her needs are and how they can be met.

When a nurse's needs are unmet they require attention in the situation and serve as barriers to the patient's goals.

The use of the self as a therapeutic tool involves continuous self-evaluation.

The psychiatric team needs to be mutually nourishing and supportive so that nurses can continue to find satisfaction in the day to day practice of nursing.

"The therapeutic milieu is a living, moving, changing atmosphere which breathes the air of people where the air is free enough for people to put their ideas on the table to see and question, where criticism is constructive and unfeared, where the job each one is doing is recognized for its worth and therefore people considered worthy."[3]

Experiences

Some experiences related to therapeutic functions which nurses need in an intensive treatment situation are:

Examination of one's own preconceptions, ideas, feelings, thoughts and actions in relation to the patient.

Acquisition and utilization of knowledge pertinent to the practice of nursing.

Orientation to the purpose of the intensive treatment situation.

Orientation to the policies and attitudes employed

in the specific intensive treatment situation.

Opportunities and time to study and get to know individual patients.

Guidance in learning to understand the situation from the patient's point of view.

Opportunities to become acquainted with the communication system in the intensive treatment situation.

Opportunities to study the role and function of the nurse in relation to the purpose of the hospital.

Guidance in developing awareness of oneself and what goes on in different nursing situations.

Opportunities to develop the abilities required of the individual nurse in the intensive treatment situation.

Observation, retention and the making of inferences about what goes on in the patient situation.

Recognition and the noting of cues in self as well as of cues coming from patients.

Analysis of data collected in the patient situation.

Evaluation and the testing of data.

Identification of needs and the setting of goals with patient.

Collaboration in planning for and with patients.

Participation in problem solving.

Practice in counseling (examples: initiating a contact, establishing rapport, listening meaningfully, utilizing silence, clarifying, etc.).

Provision for physical needs and safety of patients.

Practice in providing supportive care.

Sharing patient experiences with nursing, medical and other professional colleagues.

Helping patients to learn something about their present patterns as well as new patterns in living.

Communicating what is known, or what is not known, how one feels about patients, about what one thinks of policies, doctors' orders, treatment, etc.

Supervisory and Administrative Processes

It is our belief that the concept of nursing which we have been discussing can be translated into action only in those situations where the supervisory and administrative processes are committed to the same basic principles as those providing the basis for the therapeutic function of nursing. We here refer to those basic principles which support the professional character of nursing, namely, belief in the inherent worth and dignity of the individual, cause and effect relationship, the use of the scientific method, the right to self-determination and the natural tendency toward growth and change. Basic principles such as these provide the dynamic in supervisory and administrative processes and give rise to a strong, stable, vital situation within which people can live and work creatively together. Within such a situation communication is open, free, rich and full. Here, values are shared, differences respected and action is responsible. Within this situation people have a chance to experience growth freely and meaningfully. Here, collaborative effort is directed toward the solution of problems and the achievement of goals. Within this framework there is mutual trust and respect. Here, authority based on competence, skill, knowledge and understanding is directed toward its valid end, facilitating the common task.

In support of these convictions we should like to quote from a recent paper by Claire M. Fagin, who says, "I believe that the creation of any kind of environment from the nursing point of view is directly related to the kind of nursing administration which exists in a particular setting. To be more specific, I believe that the participation of staff and patients in a particular setting is directly related to the type of administration in that setting, and that the kinds of experience which patients have in a hospital will be similar to or related to the kinds of experiences which staff have.

"For example, a rigidly organized nursing service where the staff is limited by strong rules and regulations will often be mirrored in the work situation which will have strong limits and policies controlling the patient's daily living. One might take a look at a nursing service which has poor communication and see how often the nursing staff finds itself unable to understand the "irrational" communication of patients.

"I should like to repeat the hypothesis that 'the participation of staff and patients in a particular setting is directly related to the type of administration in that setting, and that the kind of experiences which patients have in a hospital will be similar to or related to the kinds of experiences which staff have.' "[3]

The usefulness of the supervisory and administrative program will also depend upon a strong, skillful, reliable communication system which is built on strong, close and reliable relationships. Possibilities for the development of such a communication system are limitless. Some tools which have been found useful in the implementation of this are: the study and improvement of reports and meetings between the nursing personnel scheduled on days, evenings and nights; provision for regular nursing team conferences which include doctors, nurses, social workers, psychologists and occupational therapists; provision for a weekly conference of all nurses in which there is collaborative participation in various kinds of problem solving; and continuing study of the use of various forms of written communication such as the nursing care cards and psychiatric nursing notes.

Individual and group growth may effectively be promoted and maintained through the supervisory process in which the individual or group has the opportunity to share experiences, feelings and attitudes centered around their roles. In such relationships there is the opportunity to identify and work through problems and so to develop new insights, abilities and skills for use in the therapeutic function of nursing.

References

1. Division of Nursing Education, Teachers College, Columbia University, *Work Conference on Regional Planning for Nursing and Nursing Education,* New York, Bureau of Publications, Teachers College, Columbia University, 1950, p. 8.

2. Lindgren, Henry Clay, *The Art of Human Relations,* New York, Hermitage House, Inc., 1953, p. 38.

3. Fagin, Claire M., *The Therapeutic Milieu,* Paper read at the 4th Annual Seminar, VA Hospital, Roanoke, Virginia.

Bibliography

Cockerill, Eleanor and Others, *A Conceptual Framework for Social Case Work,* Pittsburgh, University of Pittsburgh Press, 1952.

Fagin, Claire M., *The Therapeutic Milieu,* a paper read at the 4th Annual Seminar, VA Hospital, Roanoke, Va.

Kreuter, Frances Reiter, *The Establishment of Valid, Reliable, Objective and Usable Criteria For the Appraisal of the Quality of Medical Nursing Care that Selected Patients Receive in Hospital,* Teachers College, Columbia University, New York and U.S. Public Health Service (An Unpublished Report).

Lindgren, Henry Clay, *The Art of Human Relations,* New York, Hermitage House, Inc., 1953.

National League for Nursing, *Curriculum Suggestions For a Pre-service Psychiatric Aid Program,* 1955.

Peplau, Hildegard E., *A Beginning Checklist of Socio-Psychiatric Curriculum Content,* Rutgers University, School of Nursing, Newark, New Jersey (An Unpublished Paper).

Peplau, Hildegard E., *Interpersonal Relations In Nursing,* New York, J.P. Putnam's Sons, 1951.

Permission to reprint granted by the National League for Nursing.
Reprinted from *The League Exchange,* No. 26, Section A, 1957.

Aspects of Psychiatric Nursing: League Exchange No. 26*

Considered at the 1956 Regional Conferences of the National League for Nursing

The League Exchange

The League Exchange was instituted as one means of sharing ideas and opinions. Many other means are available, notably, biennial conventions, national and regional conferences, and meetings of state and local Leagues for Nursing. Further opportunities for the exchange of knowledge and information are afforded in *Nursing Outlook,* the official magazine of the National League for Nursing (NLN), and other professional periodicals.

It is recognized, however, that the time available at meetings and the pages of professional magazines are limited. Meanwhile, the projects in which NLN members are engaged and which they should be sharing with others are increasing in number and scope. Many of them should be reported in detail, yet such reporting would frequently exceed the limits of other communication media. The League Exchange has been instituted to provide a means for making useful materials on nursing, which cannot be published elsewhere, available.

It should be emphasized that the National League for Nursing is merely the *distributor* of materials selected for publication in the League Exchange series. The views expressed in League Exchange publications do not represent the official views of the organization. In fact, it is entirely possible that opposing opinions may be expressed in various articles in this series. Moreover, the League assumes responsibility only for minor editorial corrections.

It is hoped that NLN members will find the League Exchange useful in two ways: first, that they will benefit from the experience of others, as reported in this series, and, second, that they will find it a stimulus to the dissemination of their own ideas and information. There are undoubtedly many useful reports that are as yet unwritten because of the lack of suitable publication media. NLN members are urged to write these reports and submit them for publication consideration as a League Exchange item.

To the extent that all NLN members draw from, and contribute to, the well of nursing experience and knowledge, we will all move forward together toward our common goal — better nursing care for the public through the improvement of organized nursing services and nursing education.

Foreword

Improving the nursing care of patients by improving psychiatric nursing education is one of the important objectives of the National League for Nursing. Grants from the National Institute of Mental Health have assisted the NLN in its efforts to achieve this aim.

In line with this objective, the NLN sponsored a series of five regional conferences and one national conference on psychiatric nursing education in 1956. Nurses, psychiatrists, and social scientists were asked to participate. Prior to each of the regional conferences, papers on assigned topics were prepared by some of the participants and distributed to all the participants. The discussions at the five regional conferences, in turn, served as a basis for the deliberations at the national conference.

It is hoped, of course, that the conference series will stimulate further discussion about and explorations in psychiatric nursing education. For this reason, the NLN is publishing the report of the national conference and is making available, through the League Exchange, the majority of the papers from the regional conferences. A few of these papers have not been included at the request of their authors. Also omitted are two papers that are available from other sources. These are: Guideposts to Better Patient Care in Large Psychiatric Hospitals, by Milton Greenblatt, Richard H. York, and Esther Lucile Brown. Available in: *From Custodial to Therapeutic Patient Care in Mental Hospitals,* New York, Russell Sage Foundation, 1955, pp. 416-423, and Frontiers in Psychiatric Nursing, by Elvin V. Semrad and Theresa G. Muller. Available in: *Nursing World,* vol. 129, October 1955, pp. 12-16.

Since all papers cannot be published in one volume, they are being issued in four sections of League Exchange No. 26:

Section A: Concepts of Nursing Care
Section B: Therapeutic Concepts
Section C: Administration
Section D: Education

*Editor's note: Since it is not possible to reproduce the entire League Exchange No. 26, the Table of Contents is presented to give the reader an idea of the scope of the original series.

This arrangement may be of benefit to those who are particularly interested in one aspect of psychiatric nursing. Because of the interrelatedness of these subtopics, however, those concerned with the further development and improvement of psychiatric nursing education will undoubtedly wish to have access to all four sections.

Kathleen Black, Director
Mental Health and Psychiatric Nursing Advisory Service
National League for Nursing

CONTENTS

ASPECTS OF PSYCHIATRIC NURSING
(in four sections)

Therapeutic Concepts*

Hildegard E. Peplau, R.N.

Ms. Peplau is Assistant Professor in Nursing, Director, Program in Advanced Psychiatric Nursing, School of Nursing, Rutgers University.

This paper is Section B of League Exchange No. 26: *Aspects of Psychiatric Nursing*, 1957.

The planning committee has requested the author to prepare this paper on therapeutic functions. The questions raised by the committee were:

> What are the concepts nursing personnel need to understand in relation to the nature of therapeutic functions? What context of experiences are therapeutic for the patient?
>
> How are concepts and experiences related to therapy a part of effective nursing in:
> a. intensive treatment situations;
> b. supervisory and administrative processes; and
> c. community public health programs (prevention, intervention, treatment, and rehabilitation)?

This paper is a response to the stated questions. The ideas presented are offered as suggestive and provocative ones, rather than as a comprehensive system of the theory and practice of therapeutic functions in nursing. Such a theoretical system is evolving, but it is restricted by a paucity of findings in answer to the enormous and urgent need for clinical research in nursing situations. The lack of research findings and a time limit for the writing of this paper circumscribed this effort, which is largely a report based upon ideas selected from nursing literature and upon analysis of the author's experiences.

The author wishes to acknowledge the assistance of many interested, able, and available persons in the preparation of this work: Miss Ella V. Stonsby, Director, Rutgers School of Nursing, and Miss Florence Schorske, a member of the nursing faculty; Miss Jeanette White, Managing Editor, American Journal of Nursing Company; Miss Jane Schmahl, member of the faculty of the School of Nursing, Seton Hall University, Newark, N.J.; Miss Letitia Roe, Director of Nursing, Miss Margaret Larkin and Miss Betty Maloney, members of the education staff, New Jersey State Hospital, Greystone Park, N.J. While these persons have assisted significantly in the clarification and presentation of ideas offered in this paper, none bears the responsibility for this effort, which is primarily that of the author.

Introduction

All nursing practice is therapeutic when expertly performed. This assumption is particularly true when the term therapeutic is used to refer to the general helpfulness of nursing practices. The beneficial effects of devices used in treatment, and of rehabilitative procedures, are observable. A pill, a bath, a cool smooth pillow, a heel ring, a pleasant and interesting social conversation or diversion, all are practices of value in nursing. They may produce sleep, comfort, or relief from pain, or develop interest in living or a new outlook on life — all of which are, at times, beneficial. A tourniquet, a tracheotomy tube, or a properly operating oxygen or Wangensteen apparatus may be not only therapeutic but lifesaving, and therefore of inestimable value. The gestures, attitudes, verbal communications, and activities of the nurse in a situation where a person is undergoing panic, envy, despair, self-destruction, loneliness, or the effects of mutilating surgery or death can also be therapeutic, albeit in a different way. In general, the potential of the entire range of direct services to patients in nursing situations may be said to be therapeutic; the considered performances of nurses in relation to patients' recognized needs are or can be helpful.

In order to limit the length of this paper, it will be desirable to distinguish between general helpfulness and those therapeutic functions that are more specifically psychotherapeutic. For purposes of this paper, the phrase "psychotherapeutic nursing functions" implies general statements (of function), each of which refers to definable, purposive interventions (actions, practices, roles, techniques) used by a professional nurse. Such interventions are intended to meet needs formulated from observations made in nursing situations, i.e., a situation in which the nurse relates to another person in a professional capacity. These psychotherapeutic nursing functions occur in the context of the nursing situation and always in relation to one or more of the other helpful performances that are aspects of customary nursing practices. The differentiation of psycho-

*Editor's note: Appendix A, *A Beginning Checklist of Socio-Psychiatric Curriculum Content,* has been omitted.

therapeutic functions is merely intended to clarify them, rather than to show unusual importance. The significance of any performance of any nurse is determined by what is needed and by evaluating the consequences of what is offered in relation to what is needed. Recognition of the psychotherapeutic potential of nursing practice, however, is relatively new, and the exceedingly complex relation of these new functions to the customary, familiar ones will be the subject of nursing research yet to be done.

For purposes of this paper, the term "psychotherapeutic" implies facilitation of the development of learning products in another person, and providing an opportunity and a setting for experimentation in the use of new patterns of relating to people based upon such learning products at speeds and in directions that are easiest for the learner to follow. It is based upon an investigative approach utilized in connection with other customary aspects of nursing practice. Later in this paper, the concept of learning is defined. This concept suggests the competencies associated with the process of learning. Psychotherapeutic intervention seeks to enhance and/or develop these needed human competencies. Personal and social growth and favorable change in an individual's interpersonal relationships are outcomes of learning. Recognition and formulation of patterns of difficulty in living, which indicate growth and learning, may require psychotherapeutic intervention in order to secure these products.

All nurses have at least two psychotherapeutic functions: (1) the study of interpersonal relations between the nurse and any other person in the nursing situation, and responsible intervention by the nurse so as to promote changes favorable to the patient or persons concerned; and (2) the study of interpersonal relations among groups of patients, workers, or family members, and responsible intervention so as to promote changes favorable to all participants.

These two psychotherapeutic nursing functions are inherent in two definitions stated by nurses, which are pertinent here:

> *Psychiatric nursing* is "...a branch of the art and science of nursing, is concerned with the total nursing care of the psychiatric patient through the development and guidance of interpersonal relations, the creation of therapeutic situations and the application of other nursing skills in psychiatric treatment, and prevention of mental illness and the promotion of mental health."[1]

> A *psychiatric nurse* is "...a professional registered nurse 1) actively engaged in the care of mentally ill patients or in the prevention of mental illness; 2) engaged in the preparation of professional registered nurses to render such services; or 3) enrolled as a full-time student in an advanced psychiatric nursing program."[2]

Both of these definitions suggest situations that are primarily psychiatrically[3] oriented and modes of intervention that are psychotherapeutic, including those in which psychiatric problems may be prevented by early intervention.

Any situation can be or become, in whole or in part, a psychiatric situation — one which requires the use of psychiatric nursing theory and practices. See for example: Bowlby, J. *Maternal Care and Mental Health,* World Health Organization, Geneva, 1952, 194 pp., and Klein, D.B. *Mental Hygiene,* Henry Holt and Co., New York, 1956, 654 pp.

The Context of Psychotherapeutic Functions

The nurse's two psychotherapeutic functions — the study of interpersonal relations with both individuals and groups and nurse intervention — are one aspect of the total role of all staff nurses. These functions do or should go on in a variety of work situations, each of which may, at some time, develop into a so-called psychiatric situation. Professional staff nurses customarily work in general and psychiatric hospitals, schools and clinics, industrial plants, and homes, serving either as private practitioners or employees of public health agencies. In all of these work areas, the nursing practices needed will, at one time or another, require performances that are associated with the two psychotherapeutic nursing functions. Such situations can be called psychiatric situations inasmuch as the problems that arise call for the use of a body of knowledge and technique called psychiatric nursing theory. In psychiatric situations, the presenting needs that suggest the nursing problems have to do, primarily, with relationships among people.

It may be of interest to the reader to consider here needs listed by Peplau in June 1955 as one aspect of work on the NLN Demonstration Project in Methods of Integration in a School of Nursing. "Operational statements of needs of patients: a) suggest the report and command aspect of the need; b) therefore, suggest the possible meaning to the patient and the implications for nurse intervention; c) therefore, are more useful generalizations than broad subject-matter categories such as physical, social, emotional." Needs stated included: 1) Need for maintenance of conditions for optimal physiological functioning; 2) Need for bodily movement, to express self, to reduce tensions of bodily need and anxiety; 3) Need to count on others for help when needed; 4) Need for interpersonal intimacy — to feel close to, in touch with, at least one other person; 5) Need to experience and use rational control in relation to present and future situations; 6) Need to experience external events of one's own choosing, to express independence of others; 7) Need to feel belonging, participation, as a member of a group; 8) Need to struggle toward a working knowledge of emergent problems, an understanding of current contexts in which one is integrated; 9) Need to maintain status, position, prestige, and therefore to avoid the discomfort of anxiety; to identify self and to make changes in views of self in ways and at speeds that facilitate favorable improvements; and 10) Need to utilize capacities through functioning, in the service of learning, and in order to reduce the tensions of bodily need.

Such needs may arise incidental to or as a consequence of what a patient experiences during treatment for a physical defect or organ dysfunction of one or more kinds. For example:

> Mrs. B. has suffered a cerebral hemorrhage. Both of her right extremities are paralyzed. She is unable to move her arm or leg; she cries and appears completely helpless. The doctor has ordered that she be taken out of bed and put into a wheelchair twice each day. When moving her from the bed into the wheelchair, Mrs. B. sobs continuously. Physiotherapy is a part of her treatment and, on her own behalf, the patient is to exercise the paralyzed limbs. These orders distress her greatly as she very quickly comes to the conclusion that she will "never be right again," and that the whole procedure of treatment is useless.

In situations of this kind, the nurse will observe changes in the patient's behavior, determine the need, and use psychotherapeutic techniques. These latter activities, however, may account for only a small portion of the nurse's time and effort.

In other work situations, the presenting difficulties may be largely or entirely interpersonal in nature, i.e., having to do with feelings and thoughts and their bearing upon behavior and difficulties in relationships with people. An example given in a paper by a student nurse illustrates this point:

> I had a patient on the neurological floor, a girl who was 19 years old. She is a singer, or at least wanted to be, and she had had a few jobs with local bands but hadn't set the world on fire so to speak. Her chief complaint was a severe pain in both legs and she complained so much that the doctors decided to bring her into the hospital for tests. After extensive testing nothing explanatory was discovered but it was felt that traction might do some good. After about an hour of traction she seemed to feel better and after about a week she took the traction off or put it on whenever she felt like it. She would get out of bed and limp or use her crutches when she noticed others were watching her. I saw her walk across the hall without limping and without her crutches. She would spend hours setting her hair or 'putting on a face' and would do many things for other patients.

In situations of this kind, where the psychiatric emphasis can be easily recognized, the application of concepts, techniques, and modes of intervention derived from psychiatric nursing can encompass the total effort of the nurse.

In both of the foregoing examples, the observations of the nurse were required to determine that the emphasis in the nursing situation had shifted and the situation had become a psychiatrically oriented one. When this inference about the nursing situation is made, psychotherapeutic functions are authorized by the new needs that have emerged. In other words, the authority for much of the nursing service that is offered, and particularly for psychotherapeutic performances, is determined by and derived from the situation. A nurse must respond in one way or another where and when the needs of persons in the nursing situation emerge. When a need, demand, or problem arises, the nurse examines it in order to formulate the need so expressed. Such needs may be hidden or disguised in the form of a demand or problem. For example: A patient who is on a restricted fluid regime and has been so informed may continuously demand fluids. A patient who is lonely and anxious may complain of insomnia and demand medication, extra nursing care, and the like.

In both of these situations, the patients' needs must be inferred, either from the demands made or from further observation and study of the nursing situation. If the nurse in both of these nursing situations is discerning and competently educated for the workrole, she will respond psychotherapeutically, i.e., she will observe, study her observations and interactions with the patient, determine the presenting need, and structure her intervention accordingly. However, without the discipline of effective education, and the consequent inability to use the required intellectual operation, the nurse may fail to discern the need or to attempt to meet it psychotherapeutically. She may actually reinforce difficulties by failing to recognize a need, by deferring all action until someone grants her permission to act, or by labeling behavior as "demanding" and acting on this preconception. The authority of the situation may be heeded or it may be delayed, denied, or ignored, but few would disclaim that when a patient acts, a nurse must respond in one way or another. Because the behavior or symptoms seen in psychiatric situations are rarely explained simply, being outcomes of complex and often hidden dynamics, simple one-to-one equations of symptom or behavior *to* nurse response cannot be prescribed. Relief of a symptom — effecting change in behavior or attitude — requires sensitive observation and thoughtful inquiry as to multiple and alternative meanings of such behavior, which to the behavior is a mode of self expression. A psychotherapeutic response is based upon conscious use of intellectual operations rather than on an order or prescription coming from outside of the nursing situation.

Rational Control: a Psychotherapeutic Performance

The rational control of the structure of a nursing situation is one aspect of the nurse's psychotherapeutic function. The structure is made up of the formalized elements of the situation, such as the lines of authority, lines of communication, stated policies, etc. The structure also includes other elements that give form or shape to the psychotherapeutic context — the nurse-patient relationship in a nursing situation. These formal elements include, among others, such elements as the phases of the nurse-patient relationship, the roles taken by the nurse and patient,[6] the techniques used, the physical facilities,[7] and the like. These formalized and formal elements not only shape the context but may also influence the content, and the themes of feelings, thoughts, and actions of both the nurse and patient. The formal elements, therefore, have an important bearing upon psychotherapeutic functions and how they may best be carried out. Psychotherapeutic performances are conceptualized and go on in relation to all these elements in the nursing situation, as well as still others in the stated formal administrative structure of the institution in which the nursing situation develops.[8] However, within the scope of this paper, only discussion of roles taken by the nurse can be presented to illustrate the principle of rational control.[9]

Rational control occurs when the nurse is aware of her own affective reactions in the nursing situation, and when such awareness is coupled with consciousness of the role the nurse is taking in that situation. The principle of control is often misinterpreted to mean "bossiness" or rigid manipulation of the nursing situation to suit immediately perceived ends that occur to the nurse. The principle appears most clearly when the absence of rational control is observed. In such situations the nurse may become increasingly anxious without knowing it, communicate this anxiety to a patient already burdened with anxiety, and, later on, convert her own mounting anxiety to anger, punitiveness, etc. Such actions are then justified in terms of the safety of other patients. A physician's orders for patient sedation and seclusion may then be used to further reduce the nurse's anxiety. In such situations, the interaction between nurse and patient involves dissociated components of the experience of each, with neither one being aware of what is going on.

An example of an occurence in a nursing situation where a student was involved may clarify this point:

> The patient had been talking about her husband. I suddenly began to feel very hot all over and I noticed that I was trembling. I looked at my watch and knew it was time to leave in five minutes. So I excused myself and left. When I got outside I felt chilly and I was actually shaking. I don't know what precipitated this. The patient knew that I was married because I have 'Mrs. ____' on my pin and I wear a wedding ring. But I had never said anything to her about my husband. I never mentioned him in any way.

In this situation, the interaction was largely between dissociated components of the nurse and patient's experience. The anxiety felt by the nurse was very great, and the patient did not recognize connections among experiences to which her statements about her husband referred.

A similar interaction of dissociated nurse and patient needs can also occur. A nurse who has an extensive but dissociated need to help others may work best with patients who are actually helpless, and in situations where patients wish to and are able to express self-help, this nurse may become anxious. Her exclusive need to help may require that the other persons in the situation have exclusive needs to be helped. Similarly, it is sometimes observable that the nurse, being unaware of the needs behind the demands the patient makes, meets those demands, thereby reinforcing the pathology of the patient by participating in it.

Rational control by the nurse also requires the nurse to use concepts that explain what is observed. Such concepts explain either the structure or the function (dynamics) of the situation. The concept of *frustration* offers, perhaps, the simplest illustration.

The concept of frustration is applied to explain the structure of an experience when the observable behavior or inferences made from such observations include: 1) evidence that a goal has been set, 2) evidence that movement toward that goal has begun, 3) evidence that an obstacle has intervened to prevent movement toward the goal, and 4) expression of aggression in direct or indirect form. These operations of the frustration concept also suggest that further information is needed to ascertain the intrapersonal dynamics of the individual's experience of frustration. Questions that can be investigated: What was the goal? How important was it? What steps were taken to achieve it? What was the investment in such movement? What were the barriers to achieving the goal? Further, the operations of the concept also suggest aspects of nurse intervention. For example: Was the goal one that is compatible with the present situation of the patient? Did the nurse, by her behavior, block the patient in his movement toward a reasonable goal? This explanatory concept, among many others, is useful to the nurse in estimating the significance of the behavior that is observed and in structuring the workrole in a way that meets patients' needs.

Workrole of Staff Nurse

Psychotherapeutic functions can be understood most easily if taken in relation to *the total workrole of the staff nurse.* Taken in its entirety, this workrole is a very complex one, perhaps moreso than most other professional workroles. It is made up of several distinct subroles of which the psychotherapeutic is but one. Each subrole has its corresponding role-actions or activities. Different emphases in nursing situations at different periods in time call for different subroles. A choice must be made among such subroles as: 1) mother-surrogate, 2) technical, 3) managerial, 4) teacher, 5) socializing agent, and 6) counselor or nurse psychotherapist. A brief discussion of each subrole follows.

The earliest use of the nurses' workrole was in terms of *mother-surrogate* activities. Today, the professional nurse still performs such "mothering" acts as bathing, feeding, dressing, warning, protecting, disciplining, supporting, persuading, reassuring, and comforting a patient. When a sick person is hungry, perspiring, or unable to manage dressing himself, a nurse can be helpful by offering the food, bath, or assistance in dressing that is needed. The nursing profession has studied these necessary activities in relation to health promotion. It has accumulated a body of knowledge about how to perform these activities with minimum strain to both the patient and nurse. It has refined these skills, which are native to the mother role, and returned such knowledge to the community by teaching health hygiene and child rearing practices, particularly through mothers' classes and Red Cross home-nursing classes. What nurses taught mothers about child care 20 years ago became, in part, an aspect of the social experience of students now entering nursing schools. Whatever refinements have occurred in the professional understanding of activities related to the mother-surrogate subrole would, for these students, constitute new knowledge to be examined in light of the preconceptions of the mother role held by the student entering nursing school.

Although these activities in the mother-surrogate subrole are often helpful, they are not psychotherapeutic in and of themselves. At best, they are devices or vehicles that influence the nurse-patient relationship. They can be used to establish and promote a working psychotherapeutic relationship. They may also serve as standpoints for observing the behavior of a patient — the maneuvers used to get or avoid approval or disapproval, the expression of feelings through symptoms or actions toward the nurse, responses to tenderness, and interest and other expressions of the nurse that touch upon the patient's values or self-concept. For example:

> A 19-year-old boy was admitted for surgery and, the following day, an operation for pilonidal cyst was performed. Several hours after the operation, the nurse offered the patient evening care. When the nurse asked the patient to turn so that his back could be bathed, the patient appeared agitated and angry, offering many reasons why this could not be done. Later that night, the patient continuously made demands and complained to the nurse that he could not sleep. By morning, the patient complained of severe abdominal pain, which subsequently led to a laporotomy. This investigation, which uncovered nothing definitive, led to the referral of this patient to a psychiatrist.

In the situation just described, the mother-surrogate subrole offered ample opportunity for observing direct and indirect expressions of need arising from surgery in the rectal area and subsequent performances of the nurse; such observations apparently were not made. If they had been noted, referral to the psychiatrist might have been made earlier based upon evidences of need secured by the nurse, or the nurse might have intervened psychotherapeutically.

In some psychiatric nursing situations, the activities in the mother-surrogate role may have very great therapeutic value, affording the nurse an opportunity to provide a mothering experience and affording the patient a richly rewarding therapeutic experience. Such experience might lead the way to psychotherapy. It might offset longings or needs for such a relationship based upon trauma in earlier child-rearing experiences. On the other hand, the nurse needs an almost canny shrewdness at the outset of some nurse-patient relationships in order to hunch the probable value of a particular mother-surrogate activity with a particular patient at a specific time. For example:

> A private practitioner was sent by a nurse's registry to the home of an individual who had been drinking for several weeks. Upon the practitioner's arrival, and immediately following introductions, the patient said, "I want you to sit here on the bed and hold my hand. I am afraid." The nurse, being a stranger to the patient, did not know the intent of the request, the patient's preconceptions of nurse, and the needs that governed this demand. The nurse said, "I will be glad to hold your hand when I see how this will help you. Perhaps we could talk about it first." This response, in the form of an investigative approach, was new to the patient and subsequently led to a working relationship. On the other hand, several less well-prepared nurses who later entered the situation met the demand without examining the need, only to find themselves unwittingly caught up in the patient's seductive maneuvers.

Transforming the role-actions of mother-surrogate into vehicles for psychotherapeutic intervention requires sensitive observation and awareness disciplined by the use of concepts that help explain what is observed. It is this product of professional education that marks one principal difference between the quality of work done by professional and nonprofessional nursing personnel — the ability to observe and evaluate demands made by patients in terms of underlying needs. In this connection, the following quotation is pertinent: "...the schizophrenic's dependency needs and his anxiety about them are greater than are those of the neurotic; the schizophrenic has, usually, very strong identifications with the early mother. These identifications become manifest in therapy as strong maternal qualities which tend to call forth infantile-dependency feelings in the therapist....the schizophrenic has such an inability to make distinctions among thinking-feeling-and-acting that he tends to express his dependency needs in seeking physical contact. This is much more likely to stir up anxiety...than is the neurotic's verbalized wish... and because the therapy of a schizophrenic usually requires a very considerably longer time than does the analysis of a neurotic, the therapist is faced with a relationship in which the patient's dependency will be not only more intense but a lot longer-lasting."[10]

In this connection, Adland comments: "It is clear that in the face of these kinds of pressures the dependency needs of all the personnel will be acute and ever present."[11] Activities in the mother-surrogate subrole tend to activate dependency needs in the patient and at the same time provide an opportunity for the nurse to meet such needs in a helpful or therapeutic way. However, favorable change in the patient depends upon recognition of such needs and the development of ability to express independence and interdependence. To foster recognition and formulation is a psychotherapeutic performance.

The second subrole in the workrole of staff nurse developed as the practice of medicine enlarged in scope, as the profession of nursing evolved further, and as more and more "treatments" or procedures were brought within the customary purview of nursing practice. The *technical subrole*[12] of the nurse, therefore, developed side-by-side with the evolving technology of medical men. The general staff nurse practitioner in all institutions and agencies must know how to perform technical procedures competently, efficiently, and correctly. If a pedestrian is hemorrhaging from a severed artery, the nurse who passes by is expected to know how to apply a tourniquet correctly. If a lumbar puncture is to be performed by a physician, the nurse is expected to secure and prepare all of the proper equipment and to assist the physician in using it in a way that is safe for the patient. If insulin coma or subcoma treatment is ordered, the nurse is expected to administer the treatment correctly throughout all its phases, from injection of insulin to termination of the coma, by gavage or an intravenous injection if necessary. If a patient is choking with asphyxia, the nurse, in the absence of a physician, may be expected to perform a tracheotomy. These technical activities are of the utmost significance, depending upon the authority of the situation. They require the observation and judgment of the nurse. But the day-to-day practices of nurses contain many more customary technical procedures prescribed by the physician but carried out by the nurse — accuracy, safety, efficiency, and economy are principles governing their use, which, for the most part, is determined by the physician who prescribed them.

While these technical procedures may be life-saving and helpful, they are not psychotherapeutic. To speak of psychotherapy for a comatose patient is nonsense. These technical procedures may be vehicles that the nurse uses to promote a trusting, working relationship with a patient. They may be a basis for teaching the patient something of value in understanding his bodily functioning. But they may also coerce the patient's view of the nurse as a person who "has all the answers," "knows what to do," "disciplines," and "reports you to the doctor." It is these very coercions, and still others to be determined by nursing research, that may well interfere with a relationship that could be psychotherapeutic. The discerning nurse will intervene to bring these coercions to light, so as not to sacrifice the core of the workrole, which is a working relationship between nurse and patient that promotes growth and learning for both. The nursing situation is a special instance of living from which both nurse and patient can derive greater understanding about themselves and their patterns of behavior.

In the course of the evolution of nursing practice, a *managerial* subrole was acquired, particularly in relation to sick patients. In view of the limited time the physician spends with each patient, and the round-the-clock ministrations of the private duty or hospital nurse, management of the patient's environment by the nurse was inevitable. In earlier days, nurses frequently bought food for patients, cooked meals, cleaned patients' rooms, and even washed sheets as a part of private practice. These performances by the nurse were needed for the well-being of the patient. In hospitals, quite within the memory of the author's practice, nurses have washed walls, arranged furniture, determined who may visit and for how long, and even dashed to the hospital laundry for fresh sheets. Hopefully, today, many of the housekeeping activities associated with this subrole are rapidly being shifted to nonprofessional and/or non-nursing personnel. Nonetheless, the nurse still has a managerial role, and it is even more complicated.

The managerial subrole is primarily concerned with overseeing the achievement of purposes of nursing care through the manipulation of the context or situation. The term "manipulation," as it is used here, refers to abilities to put to use, for example: ability to conceive outcomes, to develop plans toward their gradual achievement, and to utilize necessary techniques as and when needed. Manipulation of the physical and material aspects of a situation implies rearranging them; with reference to the interpersonal situation, the term implies that the nurse can structure her relationship to the patient, to some extent, so as to produce investigation by the patient through which he can rearrange his life situation in terms of his greater understanding of himself and the situation in which he finds himself — in this instance, the nursing situation. The context includes both the physical and material aspects as well as the interpersonal factors surrounding the patient. The way in which these factors bear upon and facilitate or hinder the working nurse-patient relationship, so that purposes are or are not achieved, is the subject of inquiry and focus in the managerial subrole. In this connection, Stainbrook's comments are worthy of note:

> "...it is the physical space which determines a good deal of the possibilities of interaction in the life space...we mustn't forget that although there is a great deal of corrective communication in participant interaction with others, there is also a great deal of necessity in everyone, and particularly in the person who has become disturbed in his living, to have also considerable self-communication or privacy. How one provides in the psychiatric hospital for the time to be alone as well as for the time to be together is not only an administrative problem, it is also an architectural problem."[13]

Although the material aspects of the environment — the furniture, flowers, food — are important, the focus in the managerial subrole has shifted to concern with the social situation, the human context in which persons get sick or recover, in which they grow or fail to grow as persons. This focus requires the nurse to perform such new activities as the following:

> Observation and collection of data for study regarding the acculturation[14] of patients to and within the ward setting, sampling the interpersonal atmosphere in a ward or family situation in order to identify the principal themes and patterns that are operating,[15] identifying the central figures among patients as a group and

devices they use to maintain their position,[16] identifying the purposes of patterns which serve to link patients together as a group, promoting patient government and constructive self-help interaction among dormitory groups of patients, assisting patients to have a needed group experience despite isolating techniques which they use persistently. These new activities associated with this subrole can and should be psychotherapeutic. They are pertinent to all nursing situations. They require all nurses to use concepts, principles, and methods drawn from the social sciences, principally from the findings of workers who recently have concerned themselves with studies of psychiatric situations.[17]

Nurses function psychotherapeutically when they study and intervene constructively in the social environment that is the context of the nursing situation — a hospital,[18] a home and family situation,[19] an industrial situation,[20] a school,[21] and any overlap of these social environments. One vehicle for collecting data needed for the study of social contexts in hospitals is developing in the form of "nursing teams."[22]

Psychopathology has been identified, initially at least, as a social phenomenon, an adaptive pattern that is demanded by and/or rewarded in a social context. The person who becomes ill, and is in need of professional help that is based upon psychiatric knowledge, is at least in part acting upon coercions initiated by others in his life situation. The patient who acts out helplessness has experienced situations in which the needs of others to have him feel or act helpless have operated. Moreover, the patient, in part, has agreed with this view of himself, i.e., he tends more and more to see himself as helpless and to become more helpless in his actions. Moreover, anxiety arises in such a social context in which such patterns are communicated and acted upon unwittingly by all parties in the situation. In the managerial subrole, such interaction of patterns is identified and nurse intervention is developed so as to favor learning for all parties. Management through study will also form the basis for preventive practices, which largely have to do with interventions based upon the next subrole.

The *teaching* subrole has developed considerably since World War I, but there is still great need for textbooks on how teaching is used in the staff nurse workrole in nursing situations. In general, the teaching that is or should be done can be categorized in one or the other of the two forms discussed below.

Instructional teaching has to do with organized or planned teaching and consists largely of giving information, facts, or needed know-how to the patient or family members through telling, showing, reading, and the like. This form is explained extensively in educational literature. It is based on the assumption that the teacher has information or skill that another person needs, that this knowledge can be actively taught through known methods, and that the acquisition of such information by the other person can be measured or tested in one of several ways. Such teaching is based upon a plan that outlines the organization of the information to be "gotten across" to the person who is in the student role. Building such plans occurs before the teacher and student begin to work together; most teacher training institutions suggest that a "good" plan will include such elements as purpose, objectives, overview, units of instruction, tests to be used, and the like. See for example: Burton, W. *Guiding Learning Activities,* Appleton-Century-Crofts, New York, 1944. Mittler, A. "The Procedure Breakdown: A Teaching Tool," *Nursing Outlook,* Apr. 1955. Mursell, J. *Developmental Teaching,* McGraw-Hill Book Co., New York, 1949. Muse, M. *Guiding Learning Experiences,* Macmillan Co., New York, 1950.

Nurses use this form of teaching in nursing situations when noticeable gaps in information, on the part of the patient or members of the family, are observed and when such information must be relayed quickly or in an economical way for many reasons — duration of nursing services, numbers of patients, and the like.

Experiential teaching is a relatively new form of teaching. It has to do with using the experience of the learner as a basis from which learning products are developed. Neither the teacher nor the learner knows in advance what the learning products will be. The learning products are formulated as nurse and patient together evaluate the experience of a patient.

When experiential teaching is used, a current life situation or problem is analyzed, learning products are abstracted, gaps in information are located and closed, and shifts in the focus of teaching are initiated by the learner. The instructor focuses on helping the learner to develop learning products — generalizations about experiences and techniques for appraising experiences. This form of teaching requires an understanding and use of counseling techniques and other still-to-be-defined methods[23] that encourage the development and use of the abilities described in some detail below under the concept of learning. This subrole overlaps with the nurse psychotherapist role described below, but the similarities and differences in role-actions are still to be defined by nurses.

The overlap of experiential teaching and psychotherapeutic counseling can be understood in terms of the common elements in the processes of education and psychotherapy.[24]

The goals of education and psychotherapy are the same — the improvement of persons and their ability to live and work productively and creatively with people. The phases and steps undergone in each process show similarities; effort is shared in promoting movement from dependence to independence to interdependence and in the development and use of human capacities for feeling and reasoning. Both education and psychotherapy are concerned with developing awareness and understanding of experience; i.e., effort is shared in aiding individuals to move from the autistic or the highly personal interpretation of events toward the consensually validated ones, the shared experience of developing meanings upon which several or many individuals are in agreement. Both are interested in bringing to the notice of individuals those selectively unattended portions of experience, i.e., those observations and impressions that have been made but are not formulated or even noticed within the awareness of an individual. Both are concerned with examining currently operating frames of reference, and the bases from which perceptions are selectively made. And they are concerned with fostering improvements in these bases from which observations and inferences are made. This is to say that both are concerned with helping individuals to become aware of the widest range of possibilities from which future choices, that will be self-evolving rather than self-limiting, can be made. These possibilities would include views about people, events, courses of action, and the like. However, one *notable difference* needs to be pointed out — only psychotherapists are specifically trained to attempt aiding in the release and formulation in awareness of dissociated perceptions of experience, i.e., with unconscious materials. Yet, in the nursing situation, these emerge sometimes spontaneously — even in general nursing situations.

Both educators and psychotherapists are concerned with the identification of conditions that will improve situations or contexts in which an individual can improve himself. The particular situational circumstances, however, i.e., the milieu in which different psychotherapists or educators work, are different. Likewise, there are differences in focus, in vehicles used to promote learning, in the roles as seen by the professional worker concerned, among other colleagues in different professions, and among the citizens in society. Moreover, training for different work situations, or contexts in which the psychotherapist works, stems from different standpoints with different emphases.

The nurse in her customary workrole must determine, on the basis of observation and circumstances, which form of teaching will help the patient to secure and use the learning products he needs. She must be familiar with both forms and, at this point in the development of the nursing profession, she can perform a real service by helping to develop the latter form more fully. Such development will require study of the overlap of the role of teacher, the experiential form of teaching, and the role of counselor or nurse psychotherapist.

A fifth subrole exists in a variety of activities in which the nurse participates as a *socializing agent*. These activities include conversing with a patient about current events, taking walks with patients, watching television, playing cards, and the like. Such activities are widely used in psychiatric situations and are thought to be beneficial, giving the patient an opportunity to test out social skills in a relationship with the nurse, who is presumed to be a mature person. These activities have been studied in part through research projects and are often actively taught to student nurses as a part of certain clinical experiences such as pediatric and psychiatric nursing. See for example: Boyd, Richard, et al. "Ward Social Behavior: An Analysis of Patient Interaction at Highest and Lowest Extremes," *Nursing Research*, October 1954. Galioni, E.F. et al. "Group Techniques in Rehabilitation of Backward Patients," *American Journal of Nursing*, August 1954. Greenblatt, Milton, York, Richard H., and Brown, Esther Lucile. *From Custodial to Therapeutic Care in Mental Hospitals*, Russell Sage Foundation, New York, 1955, 497 pp.

In the subrole of socializing agent, the professional nurse should be aware of her intentions and expectations as these govern her behavior toward a patient, and she must also observe to find out how her behavior is received and interpreted by the patient. Moreover, the nurse should conceptualize in advance the extent of her role as a socializing agent, i.e., to have a mental picture of the ramifications and consequences so that the limits of the role are clear to her.[25] This is particularly useful since the patient may wish to convert the nurse-patient relationship into a peer or chum relationship, and there are some substantial differences in the expectations that may operate in each of these relationships. For example, in the professional relationship, which emphasizes psychotherapy, the needs of the patient are the focus while the needs of the professional person are met in social situations other than the work situation. In a peer or chum relationship, the needs of both parties are given some consideration. Moreover, in the latter relationship, the beliefs, values, and feelings of both parties are open to examination and the patient may fully expect that the nurse will discuss her family as much as the patient will refer to hers as the chum relationship develops. This is the way peers and chums tend to relate in society in general. See for example: Jones, Maxwell. "The Concept of a Therapeutic Community," *Am. J. Psychiat.*, Vol 112, Feb. 1956, pp 647-650. See differences in "Community Meetings" and "Group Meetings." Sullivan, H.S. *The Interpersonal Theory of Psychiatry*, W.W. Norton & Co., New York, 1953. See chapter 16, pp 245-262.

The reality factor is that the nurse is not a chum, nor is this the reason people come to nurses or hospitals — to secure chums. However, it is quite possible that the patient has missed this valuable experience in the course of his development and that the nurse can supply what is needed. The problem, then, is not whether the nurse is or is not a chum, nor whether she should or should not function in a chum relationship. The question is whether the nurse has conceptualized what is involved in being a chum and how this relates to possible expectations that the nurse and patient may generate about each other when a chum relationship is used. It also requires awareness of how the role of chum, when taken by the nurse, will influence the possibility of the nurse taking still other roles. The patient may properly come to wonder what the actual role of nurse is. Or the patient may come to use the nurse's readiness to step out of the professional role as a way of avoiding facing his own difficulties. For example:

> A very attractive student nurse walked into the room of a patient and observed that the patient looked worried. She commented, "Are you upset about something?" The patient quickly replied, "No. My, what lovely hair you have. How do you keep it looking so nice?" The nurse then proceeded to describe how she went about caring for her hair. Meanwhile, the patient prompted the nurse to continue by asking questions to which the nurse responded. Afterward, the instructor asked the student, "What happened to the worries of the patient?" The student replied, "Oh, my goodness, I forgot all about that!"

Many of the problems connected with the use of the socializing agent subrole can be classified as the problem of role reversal in which the patient may take on the customary activities of nurse and the nurse soon finds herself largely in the role of patient, in the sense of being taken care of by someone other than herself. Role reversal also occurs among patients, i.e., when nurses withdraw from roles that are useful to patients, these needed roles are taken. Nurses tend to act them out in ways that often reinforce pathology, their own and that of patients whom they nurse. In the exchange of social information, the nurse may actually burden the patient with information the patient doesn't need or cannot use wisely, which may lead to competition, envy, and other difficulties. If the patient has a need for a favorable mothering experience, or to formulate that this is what he is seeking in the nursing situation, the patient may act this out in the form of offering to take care of the nurse. He may do this by getting a chair for her, by getting the playing cards the nurse wants, by turning the television to her favorite program, etc. In home situations, a psychiatric patient may actually cook for the nurse — and this is beneficial in many ways. Or, nurse and patient may do the cooking together. It is up to the nurse to be aware of the role she is actually taking, to help the patient to recognize the limits she imposes on her participation in socializing events, and also to see the relation of the subrole of socializing agent and still other roles that may be needed.

The overlap of two or more subroles that a nurse might take is often crucial when the nurse has to rapidly shift from being a socializing agent to the subrole of *counselor or nurse psychotherapist*, or when the situation requires a merging of the two roles. It is recognized by the author that staff nurses are currently unprepared for this role, which is one used by psychiatric nursing specialists, but this subrole is potentially a part of the workrole of staff nurse. Greater social distance must be taken by the nurse who is observing and listening closely for latent content in communications than is possible when the nurse is partly engaged in work or play activities with a patient or a group. These activities tend to absorb some of the nurse's interest which, to some degree, tends to distract her from exclusively focusing on observation of intrapersonal and interpersonal relations, i.e., connections between events that concern the patient or go on in the nurse-patient situation.

There are two forms that nurses use in the subrole of nurse psychotherapist: spot investigations and intensive counseling. *Spot investigations* of commonplace events that the nurse observes or that a patient, in passing, tells the nurse about, require a marginal type of counseling intended to promote the use of capacities for learning. In such situations, the nurse works with a patient, using investigative techniques, to assess with the patient what the patient describes as a current difficulty. For example:

A patient in a psychiatric ward approached a graduate nurse, saying, in a quiet voice, "It is not fair having your mail read by people belonging to this hospital." The nurse looked at her watch and said, "I have five minutes. Shall we sit down and talk about this?" Both sat down on a bench in the ward and the patient continued, "The patients hit each other; some are so sick they don't know it." The nurse commented, "Is there more to this that you want to discuss?" The patient answered, "The patients kick and scream but they are sick; I am a very quiet person." The nurse commented, "You have noticed this difference in the behavior of other patients and your own." The patient said, "I am really afraid to scream." "What would happen if you did?" the nurse asked. "I am not that sick," the patient replied emphatically. The connection which the nurse observed was that screaming implied illness in severe degree and that this patient was questioning his pattern of behavior, namely, being quiet. The nurse's time was up, which she pointed out to the patient, and on leaving said, "If you want to discuss this further with me, let me know and I'll arrange some time for another conference."

There are several points about "spot investigations" that are illustrated in the example given. The nurse set a time limit and adhered to it. She let the patient know she was in the role of counselor by specifying "talk about this" by sitting down, by exclusive attention focused upon the patient, and by concluding with the word "conference." Recognizing that there was not sufficient time to extensively investigate the problem, and realizing that the nurse was not able, at that time, to support the patient through a prolonged investigation, the nurse did not interpret or attempt to get the patient to formulate possible connections between what was said.

The nurse might also initiate spot investigations. For example: A physician made his rounds in a psychiatric ward for the first time in one week. The staff nurse observed the responses of several patients. One patient immediately sat down on the floor, as if to assume a subordinate position and certainly to make it more difficult for the physician to talk with her. Another patient immediately approached the nurse saying, "It is about time he got here;" apparently she could not say this to the physician directly. Another patient commented to another nurse, "He is a nice man, but the patients chase after him too much." Another patient nearby joined in saying, "Oh, he is handsome enough, but I wonder if he is sincere." Another patient, who had been speaking to a student nurse, immediately jumped up, ran down the hall to greet the doctor, and brought him to the student to whom she formally introduced the doctor saying, "I've been talking to the nurse and telling her why I am here." The doctor commented briefly, then turned to the nurse and asked several questions while the patient looked on somewhat enviously.

After the physician left, the graduate nurse made it a point to spend some time with each group of patients to discuss the doctor's visit, and to help patients express their feelings and yet realistically view the doctor's time schedule.

Intensive counseling may be used by nurses, particularly in private practice or in home visits by a public health nurse, but also in ward situations. Intensive counseling obligates the person who offers it to finish what is started, i.e., the consequences for the patient must be taken into account at the outset. When the nurse encourages lengthy ventilation on the part of a patient, suggests interpretations from limited data, and then discontinues the relationship, the patient will interpret the nurse's performance on the basis of past experience; it is highly likely that feelings of mistrust, abandonment and the like will be reinforced. However, when a nurse has any continuing relationship with a patient in home or ward situations, with a specific time made available each day, over a long period of time, for investigation of difficulties on a regular basis, intensive counseling may be used.[26]

The activities and techniques used in this subrole need to be described by nurses with particular reference to nursing situations.[27] The nurse psychotherapist functions in somewhat the same way as other psychotherapists, albeit in a different situation — the nursing situation. The fact that the psychotherapist's role is merely one among several subroles is one principal difference between the practice of psychoanalysis and the practice of nursing. Moreover, the nurse psychotherapist uses this role primarily in relation to a wide range of "nursing problems" or difficulties that the patient acts out in the nursing situations; the behavior observed is the starting point in the use of role actions connected with this subrole. Furthermore, the primary purpose, particularly in nonpsychiatric situations, for which the patient seeks nursing services is not strictly psychotherapeutic. The patient who comes to the hospital for surgical removal of a pilonidal cyst does not come with anticipations of the need for psychotherapeutic assistance; the need emerges in the nursing situation. The work situation, the starting point of therapy, and the goals of the patient at the outset are all different in different work situations. In this paper, the concern is with the beginning description of the potential workrole of nurse in nursing situations.

The nurse also needs explanatory concepts and directional principles which aid her in interpreting what is observed, and in guiding interventions. Three central concepts are discussed below. All of these concepts pertain to areas of knowledge pertinent to the entire workrole of staff nurse in a psychiatric situation.

Areas of Knowledge and Concepts Relevant to the Workrole of Staff Nurse

- *Theory of personality development:* The nurse needs to explore prevailing theories concerning development of human personality in terms of observations of growing children, the nurse's own child-rearing experiences, and the observation of unfinished developmental tasks that can be observed in adult behavior.
- *Theories of human behavior:* The nurse needs to explore prevailing concepts and theories that offer explanations of the genetic, structural, and dynamic meanings of behavior, and to use these prevailing explanations cited in literature as one basis for comparison with generalizations made from observations of behavior in clinical nursing situations.[28]
- *Unconscious motivation:* The nurse needs to explore existing theories and to generalize from her own experiences and observations of unwitting behavior. An understanding of the concepts of awareness and unawareness, attention and inattention, especially with regard to relations between feelings, thoughts, and actions, is needed to grasp the hidden meaning of symptoms and other forms of communication used by patients diagnosed as having psychiatric and/or psychosomatic disorders.
- *Sociological theory:* The nurse needs to explore the findings and methods of social sciences, particularly to understand social interaction, the nature of social contexts, and such social phenomena as values, customs, mores, roles, status positions, uses of mass media of communication, and the like. The findings relate directly to the content of behavior of persons whose living is disturbed; the methods relate to development of the workrole of staff nurse in psychiatric facilities.
- *Theories of therapy:* The nurse needs to explore the stated concepts, principles, and procedures used in psychotherapy as described in professional literature. The relevance of these findings for improvement of the workrole of nurse in nursing situations should be the emphasis of such exploration.

There are two closely connected concepts that render the purpose and nature of psychotherapeutic functions more intelligible. These two concepts are *learning* and *adaptation*. In this connection, Maier says:

> "Changes in an individual imply learning, and in this sense therapy becomes closely associated with learning. Problems of learning, however, are very complex and many variables influence learning progress, hence the association of therapy with learning does not simplify views on therapy. Rather, confusion may be created because various learning theories have given clinical theory as well as clinical practice different types of emphasis."[29]

The term or concept "adaptation" is often very loosely and vaguely defined in textbooks and dictionaries. It is frequently considered to be synonymous with the concept of learning, either in whole or in part. For purposes of this paper, there are advantages in separating these two concepts and showing the operational meaning of each in its significance to nurses. These concepts will be operationally defined after a consideration of what is meant by the term "operational definition."

To operationally define a concept is to specify the behaviors or performances associated with the concept. Conversely, when such behaviors are observed, they can be identified as being parts of a concept. The constellation of such related behaviors can be referred to by using the name of the concept. "An operational definition states a rule that relates some term to some publicly observable processes, objects, or events."[30]

In very simple form, an operational definition of frustration as a concept has already been given (see page 95). A second example would be the concept of conflict. The behaviors that comprise the constellation of operations referred to in this concept are: 1) observed behavior relates to two opposing and incompatible goals that are held; 2) movement toward both goals has started, but at least one of the goals is to be avoided; 3) hesitation, vacillation, blocking, and fatigue are observable behaviors; and 4) finally, one goal becomes dominant. As in the previously shown concept, the concept or conflict refers to the structure of the experience, but the operations stated can be used to secure the dynamics or meaning of the experience to the person involved. For example, the nurse may observe only hesitation, vacillation, blocking, or fatigue. On the other hand, the patient may comment in a way that suggests peripheral aspects of a core conflict. For example, a patient commented, "It isn't what Jesus wanted, but people say I am fast." Further discussion revealed evidence of conflict between the goal of behavior guided by Christian beliefs and a goal related to behavior actually engaged in by the patient prior to admission to the hospital. In order to secure data regarding the dynamics of the conflict, questions such as the following must be answered: What were the incompatible goals — the peripheral aspects shown in the patient's behavior on the ward and perhaps the goals in the core conflict revealed in intensive psychotherapy? Which goal is the patient avoiding, or are both goals being avoided? What is the strength of each goal? What steps have been taken toward goal achievement?

Application of concepts in nursing practice, particularly to explain what has been observed by the nurse, is an important aspect of professional nursing practice. The concept *application* requires the following operations, or behaviors, on the part of the nurse: 1) observation of behavior in a situation; 2) sorting and clustering of what is seen or interpreted from observation; 3) naming the cluster by using the concept appropriate to both the behavior observed and the actions to which the concept refers; and 4) further inquiry as to the dynamics or meaning of behavior, using the structural aspects of the concept(s) that were used to interpret behavior. When used in this way, operational concepts serve as guides to the recognition of behavior and the determination of its meaning.

Defined in terms of observations of a person's behavior, or the interpretation of varieties of such behavior, the term *adaptation* is a concept that refers to: 1) feeling a need or observing a difficulty in oneself; 2) using a pattern of behavior automatically (without further intervention of thought about the difficulty); and 3) experiencing a feeling of relief from the initial tension or anxiety connected with the felt difficulty, without understanding what happened or developing foresight, which would enable the person to meet similar situations in the future without anxiety or with less tension.

One of the simplest examples of the foregoing sequence occurs when an individual: 1) feels uncomfortable about the possibility of disapproval from another person for an aspect of behavior; 2) says "I'm sorry;" and 3) feels relief from the initial tension.

In contrast, *learning* is a concept that refers to observable behaviors of the learner such as the following:

1. Feeling a need or observing a difficulty, or indications of the anxiety or tension associated with it;
2. Making an effort to locate the difficulty (e.g., describing what was experienced by recalling associated, though dimly perceived, details, facts, occurrences, ideas, or feelings);
3. Analyzing the data collected;
4. Formulating the meanings and relations (connections) seen in the data available and clarifying such relations by stating them;
5. Validating with others the correctness of inferences made, or the usefulness of relations drawn from the data; and
6. Acting upon validated formulations (which are the learning products) so as to produce observable and favorable changes in one's behavior in the present context, and foresights that will influence behavior in the future.[31]

Learning can be said to be in process when any one of these behaviors is observed; a learning product derives from the serial completion of all steps indicated in the definition.

The Nature and Purpose of Psychotherapeutic Functions

It can be observed, in the definitions given above, that *adaptation* and *learning* share only the first operation of observable behavior. This points to an important difference between adaptation and learning, and it suggests the nature of psychotherapeutic functions.

The purpose of such functions is to promote the development of behavior that is new to the learner, and to refine the meaning of the experience of the learner through the use of capacities for reason. It can be speculated that psychiatric problems are primarily problems in learning that arise in and as a result of interpersonal situations. In the course of growing up, a person experiences many feelings, thinks many thoughts, and draws many conclusions about the behavior of others as well as about one's own behavior; many interpersonal situations arise in the home, neighborhood, school, church, and the like, where it is noticed to be inappropriate to examine, and therefore to formulate, what these experiences mean to the individual. In many of these situations, what is being said to the person may be the direct opposite of what is felt by that person. In the face of such pressure, dissociation, or failure to notice what goes on and the automatic use of approved behavior may be necessary in order to restore feelings of comfort. In this sense, the difference between the concept of adaptation and the concept of learning becomes self-evident.

Psychiatric nursing problems can be conceptualized in terms of the two foregoing concepts as a basis for designing and stating a useful and workable theory of psychotherapeutic counseling in nursing practice. Patients in psychiatric hospitals very quickly adapt to the ward routines. Such adaptation is often merely reinforcement of patterns of behavior that, in situations before hospital admission, brought relief from anxiety and tension. The nurse has the task of encouraging learning, which, in the sense of the definition given, requires the nurse to use an investigative approach in patient care and to promote interest and skill among patients in utilizing their capacities toward development of each operation of the learning process.

This task may be further conceptualized when the total learning of a person is seen as an integrated, interconnected system of beliefs, values, feelings, and patterns of behavior, each of which bears some relation to the other. Moreover, these relations or connections between events, perceptions, and formulations of meanings of experiences can be stated by the person who has learned what they are. On the other hand, adaptive patterns are more or less additive; they are more like accretions that form a kind of superstructure or facade. Such patterns are built upon and often hide the person's actual learning, the formulated beliefs, feelings, and patterns, which are products of situations that have been observed, analyzed, formulated, and validated. In a sense, it can be said that the use of the latter learned behavior implies a person who "knows what he is doing, feeling, thinking," in contrast to a person who just acts, feels, or ruminates without considering further what goes on.

In situations of extreme stress, of which there are many in present-day society, the ability to learn, to use all of the operations of the concept of learning stated above, is perhaps the only guarantee against the quick development of anxiety into panic. It is when anxiety increases that further observation is particularly difficult to pursue, and with greater degrees of anxiety, the formerly useful adaptive patterns are no longer effective; they fail to work to relieve or ward off anxiety. As these accretions fall apart, having been held together by the singular purpose of bringing relief, the individual is revealed at the point where his learning has been seriously interrupted. He is revealed at the point where description, analysis, formulation, and validation of experience, or effort in these directions, has failed to produce learning products based upon the use of capacities for reason. And he has failed, therefore, to build and refine skills in learning that are dependent on the present situation.

For many persons, the interruption of learning occurs within the early years, between the emergence of speech and the beginning of school; for others, the learning process may be slowed down during the school years. The present system of public education is largely built on more mechanical theories of learning,[32] and very little attention is given to the experiential teaching suggested in this paper. The implications for education and psychotherapeutic work in clinical situations seem abundantly clear. Everyone has the need, beginning with the emergence of speech, to develop powers of reasoning into abilities to learn and to derive learning products that are consciously formulated from and revised with experience. This is a major focus for all preventive work in the mental health field, and it is also a suggestion for what is needed in psychotherapeutic functions. To help growing children, students, and patients alike to describe, analyze, formulate, and validate their experiences in living and to feel comfortable in the process of so doing, those persons who are mothers teachers, or nurses must see themselves as models of these behaviors. Such a view of self is necessary to promote learning products and develop learning abilities in others, but is also necessary for continuously extending the learning and the formulated foresights of these mothers, teachers, and nurses. A test of the general need for such a focus on experiential learning can be made with any random sampling of high school students, nursing students, adults in the general population, and patients in psychiatric facilities. It is indeed easily noticeable that patients in mental hospitals have considerable difficulty in describing their participation in any experience, particularly their feelings and thoughts, and the sicker the patient is, the less well developed are these abilities. But the same limited development of those most significantly human functions, can be seen, albeit in different degree, in any sampling of the general and nursing population.

The purpose of the two psychotherapeutic functions of staff nurses is to promote learning. These two functions are: 1) the study of interpersonal relations of nurse and patient prior to responsible intervention to promote changes favorable to the patient and 2) the study of interpersonal relations among groups of patients, family members, and nursing personnel, with responsible intervention to promote learning. These functions have several principal characteristics that may be utilized, in part, in relation to any of the subroles cited above, or that may be the sole emphasis, as in the subrole of nurse psychotherapist. These characteristics are as follows: 1) facilitation of the patient's communication; 2) facilitation of the patient's social participation; 3) interpreting the needs of the patient or group and assisting in their formulation and/or fulfillment; 4) identifying learning inabilities and assisting the patient in developing the needed skills; and 5) identifying gaps in factual information and promoting the understanding and use of concepts and principles.[33]

These psychotherapeutic functions of the nurse require a theoretical framework that includes concepts and principles such as those listed in the appendix. These concepts are learned when the clinical experience of the student nurse is examined in detail, with sufficient time for the student to utilize, for herself and with the student group, the operational steps in the concept of learning cited above.[34]

Effective Nursing in Intensive Treatment Situations

The phrase "intensive treatment situations" refers to hospital and home situations in which the emphasis in the total psychiatric care of the patient utilizes all available resources within, or that can be brought into, that situation. In such situations, sensitive observation by the nurse is of utmost importance. In the early stages of need for psychiatric nursing care, the amount of anxiety experienced by the patient fluctuates considerably, and the nurse who is in that work situation must be able to notice and interpret changes in the degree of anxiety so as to forestall panic reactions where possible, or to sit through such reactions in the most helpful way known to nurses. The nurse must have a working, theoretical knowledge and be able to use explanatory concepts as well as techniques of intervention that will tend to see the patient through such periods of anxiety in a growth-provoking way.

Admissions or reception units in psychiatric hospitals often serve as intensive treatment units. In such units, the emphasis in nursing care should also include a concerted effort by nursing personnel to establish, in the awareness of each patient, the importance of an investigative approach as an aspect of the role of patient in a psychiatric unit or hospital. The role of psychiatric patient is not clearly stereotyped in the mind of the public. Mass media communications such as radio, television, newspapers, and periodicals for laymen have promoted and expanded upon the parts to be played when a layman gets into the sickrole, as in a general hospital. However, the sickrole of mental hospital patient, i.e., the part he is expected to play in order to recover, has not yet been widely popularized. On first admission to a hospital, psychiatric patients discover and very quickly act upon the role they must play either to "get out" or to "stay up front," but neither of these goals is synonymous with "getting well." The information about how to behave in order to get out or to avoid the "back wards" is relayed from one patient to another, and nursing personnel, often unwittingly, contribute by indicating behavior that nurses approve. The approved behavior should emphasize an investigative approach, i.e., the patient making every effort to locate and understand his difficulties that led to hospital admission, the part the nurse can play in this effort the patient is to make, and the ways open to the patient to use the resources of the entire hospital in behalf of his own learning.

A second emphasis should be on the idea that psychiatric hospitals are specialized educational institutions set up by the community to assist the patient in learning about living — learning that did not occur sufficiently prior to hospital admission. The patient needs to develop his abilities to use reason to describe, analyze, formulate, and validate the meaning of experience with other persons. The patient may also need to learn social and vocational skills essential for productive living. All of these learnings are primarily the responsibility of other existing social institutions — the family, school, church, community centers, and the like. But when these institutions have failed and the individual has therefore not succeeded in securing the competencies he needs for living comfortably and productively with people, the psychiatric hospital, as a special educational institution, offers specialized techniques for promoting such learning later in the person's life.

A third point that seems pertinent is the nurse-patient ratio in relation to the patterns of care offered by nursing service, and the selection of nursing hours that are ample for each nurse to show interest and establish working relationships in the ward setting with individual patients and with small groups of patients. The selection of nursing personnel should be based upon ability and educational preparation for this task. Moreover, both personality factors and intellectual ability should be taken into account; nurses who are able to express warmth and acceptance of patients experiencing serious difficulties in living and who, at the same time, can conceptualize the nature of those difficulties from available data are greatly needed. A concentration of able nurses in intensive treatment units should do much to reduce the backlog of patients who do not show progress toward community living. The hours and nurse-patient contact should probably not exceed a total of six hours, with an interval of two hours interposed between continuing contacts, during which recording of data and conferences among personnel should be arranged. This consideration of hours of contact with the patient is based upon the double strain imposed upon nurses when they are in contact with anxious patients and, at the same time, are observing and conceptualizing what is going on. Similar strains are not felt by nursing personnel who do not conceptualize the problems, inasmuch as they are not constantly putting forth effort to solve problems — problems which they cannot conceptualize. Such members of the nursing staff can comfortably function in other ways for longer periods of time.

Effective Nursing in Relation to Supervisory and Administrative Processes

There are nurses, other than the author, who are better qualified to clarify this question. However, two points can be suggested here.

The values held by and the techniques used by the supervisor or administrator tend to influence nursing personnel. If these values are recognized as worthy, and the techniques experienced as "democratic," nursing personnel will tend to emulate and utilize them in their own relationships with patients. However, if the values and techniques of the administrator run counter to the integrity of the "idealists" among the nursing staff, they will become a source of dissention and unrest that may undermine the nursing service program.

The various units of the hospital often operate more or less independently of each other; sometimes each is a private hierarchy with lines of communication only to the "front office." In order to develop nursing service as a whole, some provision must be made for open discussion among various segments of the total services. This discussion should ultimately lead to the examination of the structure for decision making, with some explicit statement of policy, regarding matters that are dealt with by nursing service as a whole and those matters that can be decided locally.

Nursing service, however, does not function apart from other services that comprise the "health team." All of the services offered to the patient represent a complex system of alliances through which patients are served, a system so complex that some regularized, interdisciplinary deliberations are urgently needed in order to clarify goals and procedures for achieving them. Such deliberations might lead to the development of mutual goals and/or to the explicit statement of differences, either in goals or in modes of achieving them.

Community Health Programs

The various mass media are informing the public so rapidly about the nature of psychiatric difficulties that laymen are beginning to expect understanding and help from nurses who work closest to the community. The focal points of such demands are maternity, child health and school nursing. All of the available knowledge about the prevention of difficulties — and prevention implies primarily the development of ability to learn and to be aware of difficulty when it arises — should be actively put to use by nurses in every contact with the public.

With the advent of tranquilizing drugs, more persons are remaining in the community despite difficulties that previously would have required hospitalization. Moreover, patients are being discharged earlier from psychiatric hospitals and many are returning to work, continuing their activities with the aid of these new drugs. This trend means that public health nurses, industrial nurses, and private practitioners need to understand what is known about these drugs and need to be able to utilize customary contacts with people to observe when the drugs are not sufficient for the problem for which they have been prescribed. The referral system between hospital and community agency nurses, as well as interagency conferences, are needed in order to prepare for what may be a groundswell in this direction. Moreover, the development of day-care centers for psychiatric patients will also increase the number of now-entirely-recovered psychiatric patients in the community — and the protection previously afforded through hospitalization of such patients will not be available to the public. This constitutes a problem on which much thought is needed.

Education of Nurses for Work in Psychiatric Situations

This paper suggests a number of problems in the education of nurses. What is a concept? How are concepts taught? How should they be taught so that the student perceives connections between the concepts that are available in psychiatric theory and the observations she makes in a clinical situation? Is there a minimum number of concepts that all nurses must have for effective practice in the workrole of staff nurse? Can these be identified apart from facts, principles, generalizations, and current opinions? Can some of the concepts be integrated in the basic curriculum? At what points in the curriculum is it best to introduce which concepts? Must concepts be repeatedly reviewed in different clinical situations in order to help students see their relevance in all nursing practices?

References

1. *Conference on Advanced Psychiatric Nursing and Mental Hygiene Programs,* University of Minnesota Center for Continuation Study, Minneapolis, 1950, p 32. (not available for distribution).

2. National League of Nursing Education. *Criteria Suggested as a Basis for Approving Post Graduate Programs and Courses in Nursing,* 1945. (out of print).

3. The definition of psychiatry given by Sullivan, H.S. *Interpersonal Theory of Psychiatry* p 368. "...scientific psychiatry has to be defined as the study of interpersonal relations...That which is studied is the pattern of processes which characterize the interaction of personalities in particular recurrent situations or fields which include the observer."

4. For a full statement of the meaning of the concept of "authority of the situation" see: Metcalf, Henry C., and Urwick, L., eds. *Dynamic Administration: the Collected Papers of Mary Parker Follett,* Harper & Bros., New York, 1940, p 59.

5. Peplau, Hildegard E. *Interpersonal Relations in Nursing,* G.P. Putnam's Sons, New York, 1952, p 54.

6. For discussion of illness as a social role see: Henderson, L.J. "The Patient and Physician as a Social System," *New England Journal of Medicine,* Vol. 212, 1935, pp 819-823. Parsons, Talcott. *The Social System,* Free Press, Glencoe, Ill., 1951, chapter 10, "Social Structure and Dynamic Process: The Case of Modern Medical Practice."

7. Stainbrook, Edward. "The Hospital as a Therapeutic Community," *Neuropsychiatry* (A Quarterly Report of the Department of Neurology and Psychiatry of the University of Virginia), Vol 3, No. 3, Fall 1955, pp 69-87.

8. For references on administrative structure see: Barrabee, Paul. "A Study of a Mental Hospital: The Effect of its Social Structure on its Function," unpublished Ph.D. dissertation, Harvard University, 1951. Caudill, W., Redlich, F.C., Gilmore, H.R., and Brody, E.B. "Social Structure and Interaction Processes on a Psychiatric Ward," *American Journal of Orthopsychiatry,* Vol 26, 1952, pp 314-334. Dembo, T., and Haugmann, E. "The Patient's Psychological Situation upon Admission to a Mental Hospital," *American Journal of Psychology,* Vol 47, 1935, pp 381-408. Devereux, George. "The Social Structure of a Schizophrenic Ward and its Therapeutic Fitness," *Journal of Clinical Psychopathology,* Vol 6, 1944, pp 231-65. ______. "The Social Structure of the Hospital as a Factor in Total Therapy," *American Journal of Orthopsychiatry,* Vol 19, 1949, pp 492-500. Fromm-Reichmann, F. "Problems of Therapeutic Management in a Psychoanalytic Hospital," *Psychoanalytic Quarterly,* Vol 16, 1947, pp 325-356. Hall, Oswald. "The Informal Organization of the Medical Profession," *Canadian Journal of Economics and Political Science,* Vol 12, 1946, pp 30-44. ______. "Sociological Research in the Field of Medicine: Progress and Prospects," *American Sociological Review,* Vol 16, 1951, pp 639-44. Lentz, Edith. "Morale in a Hospital Business Office," *Human Organization,* Vol 9, 1950, pp 17-21. Schneider, David M. "The Social Dynamics of Physical Disability in Army Basic Training," *Psychiatry,* Vol 10, 1947, pp 323-333. Stanton, Alfred H., and Schwartz, Morris S. *The Mental Hospital,* Basic Books, New York, 1954, 484 pp. See especially Appendix B, pp 414-425.

9. For further discussion of professional roles, including nurse roles, see: Devereaux, George, and Weiner, F.R. "The Occupational Status of Nurses," *American Sociological Review,* Vol 15, 1950, pp 628-634. Lee, A.M. "The Social Dynamics of the Physician's Status," *Psychiatry,* Vol 7, 1944, pp 371-377. Parsons, Talcott. "Illness and the Role of the Physician: A Sociological Perspective," *American Journal of Orthopsychiatry,* Vol 21, 1951, pp 452-60. Schwartz, Charlotte G., Schwartz, Morris M., and Stanton, Alfred H. "A Study of Need-fulfillment on a Mental Hospital Ward," *Psychiatry,* Vol 14, 1951, pp 223-42. Schwartz, Morris M., and Stanton, Alfred H. "A Social Psychological Study of Incontinence," *Psychiatry,* Vol 13, 1950, pp 399-416. Tudor, Gwen E. "A Sociopsychiatric Nursing Approach to Intervention in a Problem of Mutual Withdrawal on a Mental Hospital Ward," *Psychiatry,* Vol 15, 1952, pp 193-217.

10. Searles, Harold F. "Dependency Processes in the Psychotherapy of Schizophrenia," *J. Am. Psychoan. Assoc.,* Vol 3, Jan. 1955.

11. Adland, Marvin L. "Personnel — Effect on Patients," *Neuropsychiatry,* Vol 3, No 3, Fall 1955, p 130.

12. For an extensive listing of activities that are related to the technical subrole, from the standpoint of staff nurse in psychiatric facilities, see study by: Fagin, Claire Mintzer. *A Study of Desirable Functions and Qualifications for Psychiatric Nurses,* National League for Nursing, 1953, pp 44-48.

13. Stainbrook, Edward. "The Hospital as a Therapeutic Community," *Neuropsychiatry* (A Quarterly Report of the Department of Neurology and Psychiatry of the University of Virginia), Vol 3, Fall 1955, p 73.

14. For a definition see: Kroeber, A.L., ed. *Anthropology Today,*

University of Chicago Press, Chicago, Ill., 1953. See chapter on "Acculturation" by Ralph Beals, pp 621-641.

15. For example see: Foote, Nelson N., and Cottrell, Leonard S. *Identity and Interpersonal Competence: A New Direction in Family Research*, University of Chicago Press, Chicago, Ill., 1955, 305 pp.

16. For example, patients often use devices which are generic to the juvenile era. For a discussion of the juvenile era see: Sullivan, H.S. *The Interpersonal Theory of Psychiatry*, W.W. Norton & Co., New York, pp 217-244.

17. See references given in footnotes 7 and 8. Also see: Bettelheim, Bruno, and Sylvester, Emmy. "A Therapeutic Milieu," *American Journal of Orthopsychiatry*, Vol 18, 1948, pp 191-206. Jahoda, Marie, Deutsch, Morton, and Cook, Stuart. *Research Methods in Social Relations*, Vol 1 and 2, Dryden Press, New York. Rioch, D. McK., and Stanton, A.H. "Milieu Therapy," *Psychiatry*, Vol 16, 1953, pp 65-75. Rowland, H. "Interaction Processes in a State Mental Hospital," *Psychiatry*, Vol 1, 1938, pp 323-337. Stanton, A.H., and Schwartz, M.S. "The Management of a Type of Institutional Participation in Mental Illness," *Psychiatry*, Vol 12, 1949, pp 13-26. Sullivan, H.S. "Socio-psychiatric Research: Its Implication for the Schizophrenia Problem and for Mental Hygiene," *American Journal of Psychiatry*, Vol 10, 1931, pp 977-991.

18. Ackerman, Nathan. "Interpersonal Disturbances in the Family," *Psychiatry*, November 1953, p 359. Hyde, R.W., and Solomon, H.C. "Patient Government: A New Form of Group Therapy," *Digest of Neurology and Psychiatry*, Vol 18, 1950, pp 207-18. Jones, Maxwell. *The Therapeutic Community*, Basic Books, New York, 1953. Main, T.F. "The Hospital as a Therapeutic Institution," *Bulletin Menninger Clinic*, Vol 10, 1946, pp 66-70. Rowland, H. "Friendship Patterns in a State Mental Hospital," *Psychiatry*, Vol 2, 1939, pp 363-73. Szurek, S.A. "Dynamics of Staff Interaction in Hospital Psychiatric Treatment of Children," *American Journal of Orthopsychiatry*, Vol 17, 1947, pp 652-64.

19. Henry, Jules. "The Inner Experience of Culture," *Psychiatry*, Vol 14, 1951, pp 87-103. ______. "Family Structure and the Transmission of Neurotic Behavior," *American Journal of Orthopsychiatry*, Vol 21, 1951, pp 800-818. Naegele, K.D. "Some Problems in the Study of Hostility and Aggression in Middle-Class American Families," *Canadian Journal of Economics and Political Science*, Vol 17, 1951, pp 65-75. Szurek, S.A. "The Family and the Staff in Hospital Psychiatric Therapy of Children," *American Journal of Orthopsychiatry*, Vol 21, 1951, pp 597-611. Thomas, J.L. *The American Catholic Family*, Prentice Hall, 1956.

20. King, Pearl H.M. "Task Perception and Interpersonal Relations in Industrial Training, Part II," *Human Relations*, Vol 1, pp 373-412. "Occupational Health," *Chronicle of the World Health Organization*, Vol 10, No 1, 1956, pp 14-20.

21. El-Koussey, A.A.H. "Education for Mental Health in a Changing World," *The Educational Forum*, Vol 20, No 2, 1956, pp 191-197. Trager, Helen G., and Yarrow, M.R. *They Learn What They Live*, Harper & Bros., New York, 1952. Van Til, W.A., and Denemark, G.W. "Intercultural Education," *Review of Educational Research*, Vol 20, October 1950, pp 274-86. Wedge, R., Pittinger, R., and Whitman, R. "Spontaneous Neurotic Clique Formation in University Students," *Psychiatric Quarterly Supplement*, Vol 25, 1951.

22. Lambertson, Eleanor. *The Nursing Team*, Bureau of Publications, Teachers College, Columbia University, New York, 1953.

23. Follett, Mary Parker. *Creative Education*, Longmans Green & Co., New York, 1943. Fuerst, Elinor. "Dramatic Representation: A Teaching Method," *American Journal of Nursing*, May 1955. Jersild, Arthur T. *When Teachers Face Themselves*, Bureau of Publications, Teachers College, Columbia University, New York, 1956. Kelley, Earl, and Rasey, Marie. *Education and the Nature of Man*, Harper and Bros., New York, 1953. ______. *This Is Teaching*, Harper and Bros., New York, 1954. Orage, A.E. *The Active Mind: Adventures in Awareness*, Hermitage House, New York. Tatum, Julien R. "Changing Role of Professional Personnel in the Field of Medical Care," *Nursing Outlook*, Dec. 1953. Thelan, H.A. *Dynamics of Groups at Work*, University of Chicago Press, Chicago, Ill., 1954. Ubbink, Mary R. "Patients for a Day," *Nursing Outlook*, Apr. 1954. Wandelt, Mabel A. "Planned versus Incidental Instruction for Patients in Tuberculosis Therapy," *Nursing Research*, Oct. 1954.

24. Peplau, Hildegard E. "An Exploration of Some Process Elements Which Restrict or Facilitate Instructor-Student Interaction in a Classroom," unpublished Ed.D. thesis, Teachers College, Columbia University, 1953, pp 55-60.

25. For some excellent reasons why limits are necessary see: Kelly, George A. *The Psychology of Personal Constructs*, Vol 1 and 2, W.W. Norton & Co., New York, 1956, 1218 pp. See Especially pp 96-97.

26. For a paper by a nurse of historical interest here see: Olsen, Marie. "Mental Nursing a Privilege," *American Journal of Nursing*, Vol 29, Sept. 1929, pp 1080-1084.

27. Sullivan, H.S. *The Psychiatric Interview*, W.W. Norton & Co., New York, 1954, 246 pp.

28. Such subject matter areas as anatomy, physiology, etc., would be included in this area. An extensive research project, which unfortunately did not define the term "concept" or discriminate between concept and generalization, has been done. See: Fedder, Helma Julia. "Basic Science Concepts Essential in Planning Nursing Care," *Nursing Research*, Vol 4, No 3, pp 100-124.

29. Maier, Norman R.F. *Frustration*, McGraw-Hill Book Co., New York, 1949.

30. Schmidt, Paul F. "Some Merits and Misinterpretations of Scientific Method," *Scientific Monthly*, Vol 82, No 1, Jan. 1956, pp 20-24.

31. The concept of learning presented here presupposes the use of language; for forms of "learning" used earlier in personal development see: Sullivan, H.S. *The Interpersonal Theory of Psychiatry*, W.W. Norton & Co., New York, 1953. See chapter 9, pp 150-157.

32. See critiques by: Hildegard, Ernest R. *Theories of Learning*, Appleton-Century-Crofts, New York, 1948. Kramer, Samuel A. "Are Theories of Learning Helpful?" *The Educational Forum*, Vol 19, No 2, Jan. 1955, pp 227-235. Tuttle, Harold S. "Ambiguous Is the Word for 'Transfer,'" *The Educational Forum*, Vol 19, No 2, Jan 1955, pp 159-164.

33. Characteristics 1-3 have been paraphrased from the work of Tudor, Gwen E. "A Sociopsychiatric Nursing Approach to Intervention in a Problem of Mutual Withdrawal on a Mental Hospital Ward," *Psychiatry: Journal for the Study of Interpersonal Processes*, Vol 15, No 2, May 1952, p 193.

34. Peplau, Hildegard, "An Undergraduate Program in Psychiatric Nursing," *Nursing Outlook*, July 1956.

Permission to reprint granted by the National League for Nursing.
Reprinted from *The League Exchange*, No. 26, Section B, 1957.

Identifying the Needs of Emotionally Ill Patients and the Extent to Which the Needs Can be Met Through Nursing

Madeleine Leininger, R.N.

Ms. Leininger is Director, Advanced Psychiatric Program University of Cincinnati, College of Nursing and Health.

This paper was considered at the 1956 Regional Conferences of the National League for Nursing.

In the more progressive centers of psychiatry, the psychiatric nurse is moving quite rapidly in the changing area of functioning as a therapeutic person in constructive relationships with patients. Our educators in nursing and our more progressive medical colleagues are continuing to recognize the significant part the prepared nurse has in all the various forms of therapy for patients. They have recognized that the nurses' relationship with patients and team members have a profound influence on the total recovery processes of the patients' illness. With the close support of the psychiatric team, the nurse is finding that her work offers professional and intellectual stimulation with increasing worth and professional esteem.

There still remain, however, other psychiatric centers where considerable focus is needed to orient the psychiatric nurse and other members of the team to new concepts related to her role. This orientation means a transition from the past concepts of the nurse functioning as a relatively impersonal custodial agent carrying out written medical recommendations and procedures, to the present concept of the nurse functioning in therapeutic relationships with individuals and groups of patients. It implies that the nurse use herself and the social environment in assisting patients with their underlying difficulties.

Considerable direction for helping the nurse to move into her role has come through the improvement of psychiatric nursing educational programs. In achieving future direction and growth in professional programs, a significant area to be considered is identifying the needs of patients with emotional and non-emotional illnesses. The topic which I have been asked to discuss with you, or to provide an impetus for discussion at this conference, is: How the needs of emotionally ill patients differ from the needs of other patients and the extent to which these needs can be met through nursing.

The first part of the topic indicates a difference to be made between the needs of the emotionally ill patient and those of other patients. In attempting to make this point of differentiation, I was concerned with finding a useable and acceptable definition of emotional and mental illness. After considerable searching, Ginsberg's statement seemed to be the point of view expressed by several authors regarding emotional or mental illness; "...Even statistical norms are lacking to help us in our search for a definition."[1]

The term "emotional illness" has a broad connotation both in the description and use of the words. The meaning of the term ranges from minor illnesses, including certain personality disorders and transient neurotic disturbances, to the major types of emotional illnesses, including the more severe neuroses and psychoses. The terms emotional illness, mental illness, and psychiatric illness are frequently used interchangeably without definition of the words. One finds several general descriptive phrases to describe emotional and mental illness. These descriptive phrases include: increased deviation in the modes of the individual patient's behavior related to change in the patterns of thinking, feeling, acting, and productive activity; changes in the patterns of eating, sleeping, and other basic living activities; disturbances in the interpersonal relationships with other people; decrease in the integrative capacity of the personality; loss of accurate awareness of reality testing and the environment; and a lack of adjustment in society.[1,2]

In attempting to compare the needs of emotionally ill patients with other patients, it would seem well to identify the latter group. "Other patients" apparently refers to all patients who do not present obvious clinical evidence of a psychiatric or emotional illness. These patients may be generally considered to be on clinical services other than a psychiatric service. Recently, there has been impressive evidence that this group of patients has a high incidence of emotional illness and that there is a need to place equal significance on the emotional conflicts of patients with somatic disturbances. The importance of emotional disturbances and the manner in which they affect different patients with different types of illness is under close study with systematic research findings accumulating in an impressive amount. The reports from these studies are somewhat startling, yet indicate the extent and the relationship of emotional disorders in a significant portion of these other, apparently nonpsychiatric, patients. A recent study at the University of Cincinnati, in the departments of surgery and psychiatry, reports that of 200 randomly selected patients with surgical illness, there was a diagnosable mental disorder in 86 percent of the patients.[3] The 86 percent included patients with psychosomatic disorders, severe neuroses, psychoses, and asocial behavior patterns. The study also showed that emotional factors operated with other cases. Delirium was brought on partly by emotional factors and was often the first sign of serious complications to surgical treatment, and 71 percent of the patients' illness was aggravated by delays in seeking treatment due to complex emotional attitudes of fear and anxiety. It was found that ignorance, lack of intelligence, or poor education were seldom causes of delay. As indicated in the report, the investigating group was extremely conservative in the boundaries of indicating that emotional illness was present. Elsewhere, it has been estimated that about 50 percent of all patients seen by general practitioners of medicine have a significant emotional or mental illness, whether associated with physical illness or not.[4]

With due allowance for statistical inexactness of such data, there is still an impressive picture of the significant part emotional factors have in initiating, aggravating, and perpetuating somatic illnesses. It could perhaps be concluded that other patients have needs similar to those of the emotionally ill patient and that further research is indicated to identify the specific needs for these patients. Modern medicine has recognized many of the general psychodynamic patterns and needs of patients with psychophysiological disorders such as peptic ulcer, asthma, and dermatitis whose illness has been greatly precipitated or conditioned by emotional factors of a chronic nature. However, it is essential to identify the particular needs related to the nursing care of these patients.

Returning to the consideration of identifying the needs of emotionally ill patients and other patients, one could conclude that the majority of "other patients" have some degree of emotional illness.[5] Also, any patient with a physical illness has varying degrees of emotional regression associated with the illness. The degree and severity of the emotional illness seems to have a wide range, varying from minor to major types of emotional illnesses. It would seem that perhaps one might best attempt to make the differentiation of emotional illness between the minor and the major types of personality disorganization and identify some apparent needs of each group.

Before identifying the needs of patients with minor types of emotional illness, a description of the general characteristics of the group might provide a frame of reference for the discussion. Patients with minor emotional illness have maintained most of the integrative capacities of their personality structure, have some capacity to relate generally in a socially acceptable way, have occasional inappropriate judgment and behavior in social situations when under pressure, have a reservoir of fears and anxiety that breaks through frequently, and have lost considerable spontaneity in the real feeling for living.[2,6] This would include the range of patients considered to have a "non-emotional" illness — from patients with minor character and trait disturbances to patients with minor psychiatric disturbances.

The *kinds* of needs seem to be more readily identified and specified than the *degree* or quality of the need. Many of the kinds of needs could be identified by interdiscipline conferences related to understanding the intrapsychic and environmental conflicts influencing the patient's illness, analysis of the quality of personnel-patient relationships, and understanding the kind of patient illness. Cues for the degree of each need would seem less tangible and would thus be more difficult to specify. What may have seemed an adequate degree of a need for one patient might be quite different from the degree of need for another patient with a similar psychopathological illness. The extent of meeting the degree of patients' needs would therefore be highly individual both for the patient and the personnel providing the need. The variable factors, to the degree of the need, would also be related to the kind of patient illness, the patient's ego strengths and integrative capacities, the quality of the patient-personnel relationship, and the type of social rehabilitative environment for the patient.

The needs of the patient with minor emotional illnesses would concern not only nurses in the clinical area of psychiatric nursing but nurses in all other clinical areas and public health agencies. The last two groups have close opportunities to meet the need of this large group of patients. Some of the general needs of patients with minor emotional illnesses might be identified as the following:[6,7,8]

1. The patient needs recognition of his individual adjustment patterns with consideration of the social practices and mores that are consistent with the patient's cultural and economic status.

2. The patient needs to be understood in terms of his anxious and fearful feelings concerning seeking medical or psychiatric assistance, the

reasons for postponing seeking help, being ill and hospitalized, and the kind of care and treatment he expects to receive during hospitalization.

3. The patient needs to have a reconstructed hospital environment comparable to his home environment.
4. The patient needs to be understood in terms of the patient's own concepts of his illness, the circumstances leading to his illness, and the "why" of his behavior.
5. The patient has a need to be accepted and understood in his varying phases of regression and dependency needs.
6. The patient needs a supportive communicant (not only verbal but also nonverbal) who understands him as a person and who provides for opportunities of emotional growth during his illness.
7. The patient often needs to be supported in his physical and psychological defenses that he may be using in his illness, or the support may indicate that the defenses need to be modified or withdrawn. This would include supporting the expression of anxiety and utilizing anxiety so it will be a constructive learning experience to the patient.
8. The patient needs to be relieved of the stresses and pressures that are closely related to his illness or that affect the patient's equilibrium of emotional health to the extent that they determine whether he will remain ill or recover.
9. The patient needs to have the environment and psychological factors assessed which aggravated or perpetuated the existing illness.
10. The patient needs to have his somatic complaints correctly interpreted and supportively managed.
11. The patient needs a therapeutic atmosphere and climate and relationships that assist him in the expression of his behavior, in gratifying his needs, in facilitating his communication, and in enhancing his social participation.
12. The patient needs to have the meaning of his expressed needs interpreted and a plan of action made together with other members of the team.
13. The patient needs to have assistance from others in providing security, in setting limits, and in protection of the patient when he is unable to do so in an acceptable way.
14. The patient needs to have a continuity in the total rehabilitative care that extends from the hospital to the home and into the community.
15. The patient needs to have a degree of consistency in therapeutic attitudes of personnel.
16. The patient needs to have his personal values respected with the therapeutic plan of care continuously centered on him as a person.
17. The patient needs to have his illness understood by his family, his social home environment, and persons in his work situation.

The patient with a major type of emotional or psychiatric illness might be identified as one of a group who is acting out his behavior in a more diffuse and socially inappropriate way, so there is an impending danger to the patient and to others in his environment. He is unable to handle in a socially acceptable way the freedoms to which he was entitled, has lost considerable ego strengths and integrative capacities, has marked decreased capacity for object relationships, and has severe disturbances in reality testing.[5,6]

The patients in this group would be considered those patients with the major psychiatric illnesses including the more severe neuroses and psychoses. Nurses who have achieved a degree of skill in meeting the majority of the needs of patients with minor emotional illnesses and who have had an advanced educational program in psychiatric nursing would be concerned with this group. The needs listed for the minor emotionally ill patients would be basic to this group, and these needs would have qualitative and quantitative degrees of difference. The basic need would be further considered in terms of the social context in which the need is provided and the degree of professional skill to which the need is being met.

Other needs of this group with major emotional illness could be perhaps identified as follows:

1. The patient needs to be relieved of the more prominent shame and embarrassment still associated with the more severe emotional disorders.
2. The patient needs to have the more pathological forms of defenses carefully understood and evaluated; in addition he needs to have the defenses either supported, modified, redirected, or suppressed according to the goals of psychiatric therapy for the patient.

3. The patient may need to be provided with more protective and close therapeutic relationships during the acute phase of the illness and with a progression in the type and degree of support as the patient is reconstituted.
4. The patient needs an environment which supports degrees of flexibility for the expression of behavior, yet retains a consistency in maintenance of therapeutic attitudes.
5. The patient needs help in re-establishing his grasp for reality.
6. The patient needs supportive relationships over an extended period of time to meet the more severe regressed patterns of behavior.
7. The patient needs assistance in re-establishing his basic needs and the more acceptable living patterns.
8. The patient needs protection of his democratic and natural rights of freedom.
9. The patient needs assistance in re-establishing himself in his community.

The extent to which the needs of patients with major emotional illness can be met through the various types of therapies might be considered under four principal categories or a combination of any of the four categories for psychiatric disorders:

Psychotherapy......including group therapy, individual therapy, and social milieu therapy

Somatic therapy......including electric therapy, insulin therapy, lobotomy, and hydrotherapy

Chemotherapy......including the tranquilizing therapies (thorazine and serapsil therapy), narcotherapy, and other medical therapies

Adjunctive therapy......including occupational therapy, recreational therapy, music therapy, art therapy, bibliotherapy, diet therapy, and educational therapy

The extent and degree of success to which the needs of the patient could be met through these various forms of therapy would depend on a number of related factors: the extent to which the goals of the therapy were understood and communicated effectively, the degree of personal skills in administering or participating in the therapies (interpersonal skills, physical dexterity, communicative skills, etc.), the extent of background of knowledge and understanding of the therapy, the resourcefulness of the person in modifying the method and techniques of the therapy to meet individual needs of the patient, the type of attitude maintained in the therapy, the type of environment (physical and psychological) in which the patient is receiving the therapy, and the extent of consistency with which the patient's needs are viewed and met by the personnel.

The last factor, consistency, would seem to be a most significant consideration in the therapy plans and goals for the patient. If true therapy is in practice, every contact of the patient by the personnel would have an influence on the patient's recovery. This consistency would depend on collaborative conferences with the psychiatrist and all personnel concerned with the therapy. It would imply effective communication, continuous therapy planning, progress evaluation conferences, and close experiences with the patient. An attitude of continuous and cooperative sharing of information, with an understanding that no one person is the sole purveyor of therapy, would contribute to the assurance of consistency and success of therapy for the patient. The way the doctors, nurses, and aides view the patient's needs are frequently different from the way the patient views his needs. A delusional patient may say, "I need ten FBI men to protect me so they won't steal my money in this room." This need for ten men expressed by the patient would be interpreted not in the literal connotation but according to the dynamic processes of the patient's illness. This does not imply that we are less concerned with what the patient expresses as his need, but that the patient's needs often must be reinterpreted and evaluated according to the most therapeutic need for him. This is one of the basic reasons for a patient who requires psychiatric or medical assistance to say, "I need care." It gives us a natural entree to help the patient in identifying his needs.

The question to be raised is: To what extent can these needs and the differences in the needs of emotionally ill patients be met through nursing? It would seem that this is one of our greatest problems yet to be solved. There is a paucity of literature which reports research studies regarding the extent to which the patient's needs are being met by professional nurses and nurses with advanced psychiatric nursing education. We need to examine closely the problems related to emotional needs of patients and the specific areas in which students in the various levels of undergraduate and graduate education need support in the case of patients in all areas of nursing. We need to identify, clarify, and define with our professional colleagues the extent to which emotional need of patients are now being met and can be met through nursing, as well as the extent to which the various needs are being met by other members of the therapeutic team. We would also be concerned with an analysis of the full implication of the general concepts related to patient needs.

The differences in the extent to which the emotional needs of patients could be met through nursing would depend on some of the factors which are listed below and which still need to be discussed and clarified:

1. The kinds and degree of emotional needs of patients with various types of emotional disorders
2. The degree of the nurse's self-knowledge and self-understanding
3. The degree of finely attuned judgments the nurse is capable of making based on rich, diversified, professional and nonprofessional life experiences
4. The degree of natural sensivity the nurse has to the individual patient's problems and needs
5. The depth of knowledge of dynamic processes of normal behavior and the processes of deviant behavior
6. The quality of communication and interrelatedness between the nurse and other members of the therapeutic team

A candidate for graduate education in psychiatric nursing should have achieved a basic understanding, knowledge, and some abilities in the majority of needs listed for patients with minor emotional illnesses. The needs for patients with minor emotional illness could be correlated in all areas of nursing in the basic professional program. The student in a graduate program in psychiatric nursing would then have content and related field experience to increase and strengthen her skills to meet the needs of patients with both minor and major emotional illnesses. The goal in graduate psychiatric nursing programs would be a degree of expertness in functioning as a clinical specialist with emotionally ill patients. A clinical psychiatric nursing specialist would have competence in working with individual patients and groups of patients. This goal would enable her to function effectively as a therapeutic person in constructive relationships with a patient and give her a better assurance of a close collaborative relationship with other members of the professional team.

The implications for graduate educational programs in psychiatric nursing which are based on the needs identified in this paper for emotionally ill patients would include:

1. Depth of knowledge and understanding of the nurse's own self, attitudes, limitations, and strengths
2. Skill in utilizing the creative aspects of the nurse's own personality
3. Skill in developing, maintaining, and terminating a close supportive relationship with patients
4. Skill in identifying and analyzing the common grounds for meaningful and natural interpersonal interactions between nurse and patients
5. Skill in working with a variety of behaviors of patients who express feelings of dependency, independency, rejection, hostility, depression, and withdrawal
6. Skill in dealing with expression of emotional content which is delusional, accusatory, or laden with much emotional feeling and which is centered around daily living experiences such as eating, sleeping, interactions with others, etc.
7. Skill in modifying and reconstructing the social milieu that is most therapeutic to the patient, including:
   a. Modifying administrative policies for the needs of patients
   b. Modifying nursing procedures to individual patient needs
   c. Allowing patients freedom of choice in the details of daily living when possible
   d. Consideration of the legal aspects related to a patient's illness
8. Increased knowledge and skill of the various methods and types of therapies for nonpsychiatric and psychiatric patients, including the group of patients with psychophysiological disturbances (peptic ulcer, asthma, etc.)
9. Knowledge of factors which may be barriers to the nurse's effective participation in the therapy of patients and skill in working through some of the barriers
10. Some ability in working with groups of patients who are in a structured or nonstructured group
11. Increased leadership and relationship abilities in working with and guiding professional and nonprofessional workers
12. Increased understanding of the dynamic foundations of human behavior and the psychopathological influences in types of emotional illnesses

13. Knowledge of cultural and social influences on emotional illnesses with an orientation to some sociological theories of psychopathology
14. Knowledge of the various philosophical schools of thought in psychiatry

In summary, I have attempted to identify some of the needs of patients with minor and major emotional illness and discuss some varying factors which would influence the extent to which needs could be met through nursing. It would seem timely to discuss these needs with other nurses both in education and service to determine if these needs can be met by graduates of the basic professional program and graduates of an advanced program in psychiatric nursing. An interdisciplinary conference with representation by psychiatrists, psychologists, social workers, physicians in medicine and surgery, and other professional colleagues would seem highly desirable to obtain their suggestions and thoughts of how they feel the needs can be met through nursing.

In closing, I would like to raise these questions for consideration and discussion by the group:

1. To what extent do you feel the needs listed for patients with minor emotional illness can be met in the basic professional programs in nursing?
2. To what extent do you feel the needs listed for patients with major emotional illness can be met in the graduate program in psychiatric nursing?
3. What are the present emotional problems that confront students in the undergraduate and graduate psychiatric nursing program in their relationships with patients?
4. What kind of educational guidance for students in the clinical areas could best provide assurance for students in meeting the minor and major emotional needs of patients?
5. How can the student in nursing be brought closer to other members of the health team to help in identifying the needs of patients and to participate closer in the therapy plans and goals for patients?
6. What extent of theoretical knowledge in dynamic psychopathology is necessary for the nurse to function effectively with minor and major emotional illnesses?
7. To what extent can the needs listed for minor and major emotional illnesses be met by others?

References

1. Ginsburg, Solomon Weiner. The neuroses. *Annals of the American Academy of Political and Social Science*, 286:55-64, March 1953.

2. Fromm, Eric. Do we live in a sane society? Speech delivered at Hebrew Union College, Cincinnati, Ohio, February 28, 1956.

3. Zwerling, Israel, et al. Personality disorder and the relationships of emotion to surgical illness in 200 surgical patients. *American Journal of Psychiatry*, 112:270-277, October 1955.

4. National Association for Mental Health. *Facts and Figures about Mental Illness*. New York, The Association, 1952. p. 14.

5. Noyes, Arthur. *Modern Clinical Psychiatry*. W.B. Saunders Co., Philadelphia, 1954. p. 84-87.

6. Group for the Advancement of Psychiatry, Committee on Psychiatric Nursing. *Therapeutic Use of the Self*. (G.A.P. Report No. 33). The Group, Topeka, Kansas, June 1955.

7. Black, Kathleen. Appraising the psychiatric patient's nursing needs. *American Journal of Nursing*, 52:718-721, June 1952.

8. Greenblatt, Milton, York, Richard H., and Brown, Esther Lucile. *From Custodial to Therapeutic Patient Care in Mental Hospitals*. Russell Sage Foundation, New York, 1955.

Recommended Reading

Black, Kathleen. Nursing in psychiatric hospitals. *Mental Hygiene*, 39:533-544, October 1955.

Lohr, Mary. Interpersonal relations — in an advanced program. *American Journal of Nursing*, 55:1088-1091, September 1955.

Semrad, Elvin, and Muller, Theresa. Frontiers in psychiatric nursing. *Nursing World*, 12:12-16, October 1955.

Titchner, James L., et al. Psychosis in surgical patients. *Surgery, Gynecology and Obstetrics*, 102:59-65, January 1956.

Weiss, Olga. The skills of psychiatric nursing. *American Journal of Nursing*, 47:174-176, March 1947.

Permission to reprint granted by the National League for Nursing.
Reprinted from *The League Exchange*, No. 26, Section D, 1957.

Individual Supervision: A Method of Teaching Psychiatric Concepts in Nursing Education

D.E. Gregg, E.A. Bregg, and F.E. Spring

Ms. Gregg is Chairman, Training Specialist, Psychiatric Nursing, Training Branch, National Institute of Mental Health, National Institutes of Health, Public Health Service, United States Department of Health, Education, and Welfare. Ms. Bregg is Assistant Professor, Psychiatric Nursing, Western Reserve University. Ms. Spring is Assistant Professor, Psychiatric Nursing, Duke University.

This paper was reprinted from *Psychiatric Nursing Concepts and Basic Nursing Education*, National League for Nursing, 1960.

Introduction

Throughout clinical nursing there is a need for goal-directed professional relationships with patients in which the nurse has an awareness of how her own behavior influences a patient's progress and his use of health services. Education that deepens the student's understanding of human behavior, that develops her perception of how her own behavior affects others, and that fosters her personal growth toward a mature, integrated personality contributes to her ability to develop useful interpersonal relationships.

To teach the student to use her nursing relationship in a therapeutic way requires some modification of teaching methods, particularly those used in clinical teaching. Psychiatric nursing has become concerned with this teaching problem, because the development of dynamic psychiatry has emphasized the importance of the patient's interactions with others. This paper focuses on one method of clinical teaching, individual supervision, which is particularly useful in teaching psychiatric concepts and principles of therapeutic interpersonal relationships. The term "supervision," as commonly employed in nursing, has a meaning that is different from the supervisory process described in this paper.

In traditional administrative nursing supervision, the primary responsibility is to see that good care is given to patients. The supervisor usually has some system of making rounds to see patients and to evaluate the quality of the care given them. She discusses patient care and ward-management problems with the head nurse and other nursing personnel, assists with personnel and interdisciplinary problems and issues, and coordinates the services of one unit into the total structure of the institution. In traditional nursing education supervision, the primary responsibility is the education of the student. Usually the teaching in this type of supervision encompasses some form of demonstration of nursing care to the student and return demonstration by the student to the supervisor. The supervisor observes and guides the student's clinical work and evaluates the student's learning and the quality of care she gives patients.

These traditional supervisory methods do not adequately meet the demands of either administrative or educational supervision in psychiatric nursing. A more comprehensive supervision of the therapeutic relationships with patients and the complicated interrelationships in the clinical setting is needed. Out of this need, new supervisory processes have been developed. Both administrative and educational nursing supervisors have done some very creative work along these lines.

Psychiatric nursing is the clinical context for the discussion, in this paper, of individual supervision as the authors use it in clinical teaching. This does not imply that individual supervision applies only to this field. Individual supervisory process will be discussed with no attempt to cover other aspects of a supervisor's work with students or to discuss the individual variations in the process used by various teachers.

Definition of Individual Supervision

Individual supervision is defined as a working relationship developed between a teacher and a student in planned individual conferences for the purpose of guiding the student's learning of therapeutic nursing intervention in the patient's behavior and disease process. The teacher's objective is to create an understanding, helpful relationship in which the student can learn. The process used is the examination of a student's work with a patient in which the teacher helps the student to interpret what is going on in her nurse-patient relationship and to plan further nursing intervention. The supervisory relationship is one in which the student obtains assistance when she needs it, feels secure enough to express her reaction to any clinical experience, experiments with new ideas and new skills, and assumes responsibility for her own growth. (It will be noted that the teacher is a supervisor, and the terms are used interchangeably in this paper.)

Need for Individual Supervision

Clinical Experience

The need in psychiatric nursing education for the type of supervision that is described in the preceding paragraph arises out of several circumstances. It is well documented in the literature and the teaching experiences of the psychiatric professions that the early clinical experiences and the introduction to certain psychiatric concepts have an emotional impact upon the student. The process of the nurturing role, the behavior of a patient, and the concepts that identify the meaning of behavior bring to mind the student's own early experiences and often exacerbate old conflicts.[1,2,3] Elizabeth Zetzel, in a discussion of supervision in social work, points out that these experiences are potentially maturing ones for students, but students have to deal with them without much time for assimilation.[3] This situation calls for a kind of supervision that provides the student with the security and freedom she needs to develop as a compassionate, flexible, and thinking person. A permissive, democratic supervisory structure has been found to promote this kind of growth more effectively than an autocratic, authoritarian structure in which the student is given directives and has less opportunity to reason through the problems for herself.

Age of Student

Undergraduate education in psychiatric nursing presents some unique problems when compared with education in other psychiatric professions. Nursing is the only one of these professions that offers clinical instruction in the psychiatric area on the baccalaureate level. The nursing student is therefore younger in chronological age and in emotional maturity than are students in the other psychiatric disciplines. She has less experience in dealing with the concepts from the various sciences and humanities, for she is in the process of obtaining this instruction as an undergraduate student. The impact of the emotional experiences in the clinical situation may, in some instances, be greater on this younger age group. Also, in comparison with other students in the psychiatric setting, the nursing student's psychiatric clinical experience is very brief. This means that the nursing student will not have time to adequately work through and understand certain situations to which she has an emotional response. It is therefore quite possible that she will develop a need to use unconscious defenses against stress situations in ways that are not constructive. Such defenses may damage her perception and sensitivity in later nursing situations. This places a responsibility on the psychiatric nursing teacher to develop means for assisting the student to attain at least a beginning acceptance and understanding of the emotionally disturbing experiences she encounters in the clinical setting.

Milieu of Nursing

Another unique aspect of the nursing student's experience is that, in the clinical nursing setting, she is always surrounded with a complicated social situation. She has to be concerned with individual patients within a group-living situation. This is quite in contrast with working with one patient by appointment in the privacy of an office. In addition, the nurse is in the work setting and in contact with patients for longer periods of time than are other professional workers. The nurse in an institutional setting works with individuals and with groups in an almost constantly changing social structure. If her work setting is in a patient's home, she is concerned with the patient and his family group. The potential for emotionally disturbing experiences is probably greater in either of these situations than in contacts with individual patients.

Clinical Patterns

Certain patterns in the clinical settings affect the student. For example, the adequacy or inadequacy of nursing and psychiatric staffs and the character of the interdisciplinary relationships greatly affect the student's learning experiences. Attitudes toward students, toward patients, and toward those who give the patient care influence the learning experience.

These are some of the factors that point up the need for individual supervision throughout the clinical learning experiences of nursing students in the psychiatric setting.

Philosophy of Undergraduate Education

Although this discussion deals only with supervision in psychiatric nursing, the method described is applicable in other areas of nursing education. The widening interest, in all clinical nursing, in developing meaningful interpersonal relationships with patients indicates that an individual supervisory process may be increasingly useful in other clinical areas.

This discussion of individual supervision in psychiatric nursing is related to the undergraduate student. The authors concur with the philosophy that the undergraduate collegiate student is educated to assume beginning (staff) nursing positions in psychiatric agencies. She is expected to attain a baccalaureate level of professional competence, which means she can give quality patient care under the *guidance and direction of a qualified supervisor.* A wide individual variation among students is expected in their development beyond the minimum course requirements in this work, for each student differs from others in her experience, her level of emotional and intellectual maturity, and her creative ability.

The authors believe that the essence of professional nursing is the meaningful, understanding, and scientific use of the interpersonal relationship with a patient. It is only through the full understanding of the therapeutic use of this relationship that the nurse can give expert nursing care and can assign duties to nonprofessional personnel and supervise them in carrying out the tasks. *The physical and emotional components in any procedure or contact with a patient are inseparable in a therapeutic relationship.* The meaningful nursing relationship will become increasingly important as medical procedures continue to become more complicated and as research activities are extended to involve more patients. The sympathetic, compassionate, "mothering" roles are a natural part of nursing. The student enters nursing education with a natural endowment in certain of these roles and needs help to develop and use this endowment and bring it into harmony with the scientific discipline of nursing so that the ability to understand and help others becomes an integral part of her behavior.

The Supervisory Process

The individual supervisory process can be considered in three phases. The first phase is one of orientation in which the preparations for supervision are made. Next is the phase in which the actual working relationship between teacher and student is in progress. A termination phase follows in which the final evaluation and summarization of the student's work are made and the clinical work and supervision are terminated.

Orientation Phase

The Teacher's Work Within the Clinical Setting

The teacher's work within the clinical setting in which the student has her experience can be considered a part of the preparation for supervision; however, the work is on-going and not just a "preparatory procedure."

Preferably, psychiatric nursing is taught in settings where the student is associated with talented staff nurses, head nurses, and clinical supervisors. These people are very important in the student's learning as models and individual teachers, since one of the first steps in learning is identification with people who are significant to the learner.[4,5,6] In only a few institutions for psychiatric patient care are we so fortunate as to have a complete staff of professional nurses. Often the supervisor is the only one or one of the few skilled professional psychiatric nurses with whom the student comes in contact. This increases the importance of having the supervisor in the clinical setting with the student. She demonstrates to the student and nursing staff the use of particularly perplexing concepts and interprets and intercedes in situations in which misconceptions might be learned. The teaching supervisor's role is different from that of the staff nurse, head nurse, and administrative supervisor. Therefore, without these models, a student cannot get a true appreciation of the significance of these positions to the care of patients and of the special talents each position requires, nor can she become aware of the pressures involved in each of the roles. In addition, the teacher's work with the personnel in the clinical setting is complicated if a professional staff does not exist.

It is important that a cooperative and constructive working relationship between the teacher and the nursing personnel be maintained so that the student may use the learning opportunities in the clinical setting constructively. Such a relationship enables the nursing service staff and teacher to share ideas, work out problem situations together, and introduce new concepts to both nursing personnel and students in ways that will be beneficial to both groups and useful in the care of patients.

A similar working relationship is necessary between the teacher and the members of other disciplines in the clinical setting. The staff and the teacher need to have a mutual understanding of each other's responsibilities and roles and of the student's participation in the clinical setting. Both formal and informal means of communication between the nursing staff, medical staff, teacher, and student are required for the maintenance of useful working relationships.

Differentiation Between Therapy and Supervision*

One of the goals of individual supervision is to provide a secure supervisory relationship in which the student is given the freedom and responsibility to learn. The unique teaching opportunity in supervision is to help the student further the development of her personal endowment, correlate her learning from various areas and experiences, and integrate it into her professional behavior.

A distinction between therapeutic process and supervisory process is always a concern in a discussion of individual supervision.[7,8] In each of the disciplines where a similar kind of supervision is employed, there are controversies in relation to this problem. The goal in supervision is to teach the student, and this is to be distinguished from the goal in therapy which is to promote a basic behavioral change in the patient. There are important similarities and differences in these two processes.

One of the similarities is that both are learning processes. Behavioral changes may occur in both situations, but one difference lies in the goal of each process. The student is in a learning situation in which she is expected to increase her knowledge and skill. In other words, the emphasis is on gaining new information. In the process of learning, some of the educational experiences foster emotional growth and the development of certain insights that may change some aspects of her behavior. In contrast, the patient is in a therapeutic situation in which the goal is a behavioral change rather than the acquisition of information.

An understanding of the differences between therapeutic process and supervisory process is essential and is one of the various ways that the supervisory relationship can develop into a therapeutically oriented one. The supervisor intervenes in a student's conscious or unconscious attempts to use the supervisor as a therapist. She is aware of the ways she may stumble into meeting a student's therapeutic needs. For example, when a student's reaction to a situation includes the expression of a personal problem, the extent to which the problem is explored may determine the difference between a supervisory process and a therapeutic one. The supervisor should also be clear about what kinds of remarks constitute a probe into the student's personal emotional life.

In the supervisory relationship, the supervisor does not respond to the therapeutic needs expressed by a student or demonstrated in her handling of the nurse-patient situation. It is assumed that the student, without therapeutic intervention, can work through her emotional conflicts, whether these are a recapitulation of early emotional problems precipitated by work with psychiatric patients or reactions to new concepts.[9] If a problem seems to be a serious one which the student cannot resolve alone, the supervisor must be able to recognize the student's need for therapeutic help and refer her to the available resources. Occasionally, if the student is too handicapped to work, the teacher is confronted with the decision to discontinue, temporarily or permanently, the student's educational experience.

Another similarity in the therapeutic and supervisory relationships is that each is a permissive, understanding, helpful relationship that provides freedom for growth. The differences lie in the extent of freedom and the responsibilities and techniques of the helping role. The student, for example, is at liberty to express what she thinks and feels about her work, including those thoughts and feelings that do not fit the stereotypes of her professional role. The patient is allowed full expression of his thoughts, feelings, and actions, including his neurotic or psychotic behavior, with unconditional acceptance from the therapist. In the student-teacher relationship, expression of extensive neurotic or psychotic behavior would be an indication that another kind of help than supervision is needed, and in this sense, the teacher cannot continue to "accept" the acting out of personal conflict that interferes with the teaching process. In therapy, the patient is free to work at his own pace. In the learning situation, the student also has this liberty, but it is altered by the time limitation of the program or course in which the learning must be accomplished. She is also required to meet certain minimum standards.

There are marked differences between the student and the patient in the extent of the need for help and the realization and expression of such need. There are also many differences in the procedures of offering assistance and the utilization of the help offered. The student is assumed to be a well person who can recognize a need for assistance and who is motivated and self-directed in taking action to solve a problem or to get new information in order to learn. Blocking in her learning process will more

*Many points in this section are developed from the discussions on supervision in the second Chicago Conference of the NLN Basic Psychiatric Nursing Education Project, October 1958.

often be due to lack of information and experience than to emotional conflict. The patient, on the other hand, is troubled by emotional conflicts which may interfere with his recognition of his needs, his ability to request assistance, his ability to use help, and his capacity for problem solving.

The basic dynamics of a good supervisory relationship and a therapeutic relationship are essentially the same, although the functions are different. In psychiatry, those who supervise students are prepared as psychiatrists and psychoanalysts, and a discussion of the differentiation between therapy and supervision is colored by this fact. In psychiatric nursing, the nurse works with a patient's emotional problems and conflicts along with the psychiatrist but usually does not participate in the interpretations of unconsciously motivated behavior and the examination of the early life experiences that are done by the psychiatrist. In this respect the teacher-student and nurse-patient relationships contain some similarities that may not be present in the psychiatrist's therapy and supervisory relationships. For example, when a patient is immobilized by conflict which requires intensive work with the psychiatrist in which the nurse does not necessarily participate, the nurse waits, accepts the patient's inability to move in the nursing relationship, and offers support as indicated until the problem can be worked through in therapy. In supervision, the teacher may have a similar period of supportive waiting until the student can resolve a conflict on her own in order to proceed with her learning.

The intensive study of a student's interpersonal relationship with a patient which takes place in individual supervision entails an understanding of the dynamics of both the supervisory relationship and the therapeutic nurse-patient relationship.

Differentiation Between Student and Supervisor Roles

A differentiation between the role of the supervisor and that of the student is essential to the supervisory process. One point of differentiation is in the authority role. The supervisor needs to be able to use rationally the authority vested in her, to be reasonably comfortable with the responsibility involved, and to perceive the student's concept of authority. She has to be willing to examine supervisor-student interaction in order that she may behave in a way that will allow the student to continue to work effectively. Her ability to give the student an experience in the constructive use of authority will influence the student's learning.[10] The supervisory relationship can be a prototype for the student's handling of authority in the nurse-patient relationship.

In relation to the authority role in supervision, the student is in a dependent position in the teacher-student relationship. The supervisor needs to understand the dynamics of dependency and to be able to accept the student's normal dependence upon her. She also has to be aware of the ways she can interfere in a student's development by misuse of this element of the relationship. There is a continually shifting quality in the student's dependence as she progresses. The supervisor needs to be able to perceive when a student is ready for more independence and to support her growth in this direction. This is one of the significant decision-making areas for the supervisor. It requires a supervisor's willingness to recognize the student's growth and an ability to relinquish certain responsibilities to the student. It sometimes involves taking calculable clinical risks in the student's work with a patient. The supervisor's ability to develop a secure working relationship with the clinical staff influences the risks that can be taken in allowing the student the freedom to act independently.

In addition to the teacher's skill in observing and judging a student's readiness to move, the degree to which she is free from a need to keep a student dependent will determine whether or not a constructive experience can be provided. An important point in role differentiation is that the student has the responsibility for giving the nursing care and the supervisor guides the student in this work.

The handling of dependence that takes place in the supervisory process is also a model for the student in her own work with the normal dependence of a patient. The skill with which the supervisor works in this area of her relationship with the student will be one of the determinants in the student's ability to be accepting of the patient's dependence and useful in working with problems of overdependence. There are many aspects of the dependency-independency interaction and the dynamics of dependency and related hostility that would be worthy of exploration in a further discussion of supervision. One certainly must be concerned about an understanding of this area in considering the question about who shall give supervision.

Role differentiation between supervisor and student is also demonstrated in the teacher's use of certain limit-setting areas. Inherent in the teacher's role are decisions regarding the minimum competence required of the basic student, clinical decisions involved in the student's work with patients and personnel, and evaluation of the student's progress (including grading). She is also responsible for establishing the structure for the supervisory relationship (including the interpretation of how the supervisory conference will be used) and for demonstrating its usefulness. Her advanced knowledge and skill are brought to bear in the choices of learning assignments and the clinical decisions involved in guiding the student's nurse-patient relationship.

A well-worked-out supervisory relationship offers stimulating learning for both the teacher and the student. As the supervisor works with a variety of students, she has the opportunity to grow in teaching skills and to extend her understanding of human behavior. In the process of helping students grow she realizes the endless individual variations that can be constructively used by different personalities in therapeutic nursing relationships with patients. The student, in turn, has the rewarding experience of personal creativity and growth in her work with patients within a supervisory process that offers just enough control to allow the security that makes possible a real freedom in learning.

Preparation of the Student for Individual Supervision

Orientation to Therapeutic Nursing. Prior to her orientation to the supervisory relationship, the student needs to have some understanding of the philosophy of therapeutic psychiatric nursing. Most of this philosophy is learned in her nursing classes in which principles and techniques of patient care are discussed. The philosophy of psychiatric nursing, the concepts used in psychiatric nursing, and the process of the therapeutic nurse-patient relationship are discussed in other papers in this conference. As a point of reference for this paper, the authors agree with the philosophy that psychiatric nursing offers a patient therapeutic learning experiences in interpersonal relationships that enable him to test out and change his concepts about himself and his relationships with others and thus further his work toward health. In the nursing contacts with patients who are not in need of a therapeutic experience, the nurse has the responsibility for creating a relationship in which growth and learning can take place.

Nursing meets a need for care which is different in many ways from that met by psychiatry. A patient may be in psychotherapy and remain in his usual environment and carry on most of his usual activities. Nursing is employed when he can no longer deal with his environment by himself. Nursing's task, then, is to provide an interpersonal experience that is differnt from any the patient can get otherwise. This therapeutic experience is developed through the collaboration of the psychiatrist and the nurse, and it can take place in an institutional setting or in the patient's home.

The student, in her academic classes, will increasingly expand her knowledge of therapeutic intervention in a patient's behavior. She is assisted in learning to use this knowledge in nursing practice through individual supervision of her clinical work.

Orientation to the Supervisory Procedure. A student's orientation to individual supervision will include a discussion of the expectations of both student and teacher and a clarification of the supervisory process. The planning of appointments for the supervisory conference, the manner of recording nurse-patient relationship material, and the utilization of this material in the supervisory conference will be covered in the preparatory discussions.

Various ways of planning appointments for supervision are used by different teachers. The authors believe a student should be given individual supervision throughout her work with a patient and, therefore, supervisory conferences should be required rather than appointments that may be used at the discretion of the student. The authors have found the most useful arrangement to be a standing appointment which the student keeps throughout the time she is under supervision.

The student brings a written process record of the nurse-patient interaction to the supervisory conference. This record is an interpersonal relationship study with one patient which is recorded throughout the student's work with the patient. After each nursing contact the student records as much as she can recall of what took place, the patient's actions and the thoughts and feelings he expressed, and what the student said, did, and felt in her responses to the patient. The study also includes a notation of the student's impressions and an evaluation of what is taking place in the relationship. In compiling this study, the student gives considerable thought to her interaction with the patient before she comes to the supervisory conference. This is a useful preparation for supervision, and it helps her learn to study her own work.

The examination of the nurse-patient relationship in the supervisory conference can be done in a variety of ways, and more than one approach may be employed in any one supervisory relationship. The authors, in their conferences, review the entire interpersonal relationship study presented by the student. In some instances, the supervisor studies the written material before discussing it with the student in the conference; in others, the student brings the study to the conference and the supervisor and the student review and discuss it. These discussions constitute the main work of the supervisory process.

Working Phase

Review of the Nurse-Patient Relationship Data

Purpose of the Review. In the process of examining the interpersonal relationship study together, the teacher helps the student interpret what is going on in the relationship. The intent of this interpretation is to help the student learn to study behavior in order to understand its meaning, and to use her own behavior as a means of therapeutic nursing intervention. In the search for the meaning of behavior, principles from psychiatry, psychology, sociology, and anthropology may be employed as the nurse-patient interaction is studied. The nursing intervention is based on these interpretations, and principles from psychiatry and psychiatric nursing direct the nurse's approaches.

The teacher and student may discuss the intervention measure step-by-step so the student will understand how a principle applies in the various aspects of the nurse's work, including what she says, what feelings she conveys, and what she does as she carries out the nursing measure.

The attitude of examining nurse-patient behavior in order to learn from it has to be well ingrained in the behavior of the supervisor. This is quite different from reviewing the nurse-patient relationship to detect errors. Errors will be discussed, however, in the process of studying the relationship. It is important for the supervisor to convey to the student that errors will be defined and discussed in order to work out solutions, not to blame the student for making them. The student will be expected to develop increasing ability to examine critically and to evaluate her own nurse-patient relationship, and the teacher will help her to appreciate the steps that indicate progress in her growth.

Student's Use of the Review. Since this type of supervision takes place in a permissive rather than a directive supervisory relationship, this structure is explained to the student in the orientation to the supervisory process. The real meaning of this structure is felt only as student and teacher work together. It is relatively easy for a teacher to convey to the student that she is interested in her and intends to help her learn. It is also a simple procedure to indicate that the student is free to express her feelings and thoughts in relation to her work without any expectation of censure. If some of the student's previous experiences with supervision have been unfortunate, she will have doubts about this supervisory process until she has an opportunity to test it out and verify that the supervisor means what she says.

The student's doubts may be demonstrated in various ways. For example, she may be reluctant to keep the appointment, may fail to bring in the interpersonal data for discussion, or may bring in only small portions of it. She may use various avoidance maneuvers to keep from discussing it when she comes to the conference. In these instances, the supervisor may listen to her expression of feelings about it and try to understand the factors that interfere with her work. She may recognize with the student that it is an anxiety-provoking experience to record nurse-patient interaction and have it examined by a supervisor, yet reinforce the fact that these requirements are made in order that the work may proceed. As the student meets with help and understanding from the supervisor, some of her anxiety is reduced. When the student becomes more secure in the supervisory relationship, she is able to report the nurse-patient interaction more fully and can examine it more freely and eventually develop flexibility and creativity in her work. It is usually reassuring to the student to find that many of the things she has done in the past in interpersonal relationships with patients, as well as those she intuitively employs in her present work, are therapeutically useful.

The student's security in the supervisory relationship also develops from experiences with the kind of supervisory intervention that encourages her to reconsider an approach that is leading toward an error or that assists her to reason through a knotty problem. The confidence that comes from successful problem solving in which she becomes aware of the strength in her own intellectual abilities is one of the factors that make it possible for her to develop the flexibility and inventiveness that are valued.

At first the student may identify with the supervisor or with other nurses in the setting and use the words and behavior of these models without much discrimination. When she passes beyond this phase of identification in her learning and becomes more aware of how her behavior affects the patient and more insightful in recognizing her own mistakes, she may, for a period, be increasingly sensitive to the critical examination of her relationship. In this instance (as well as in the examination of any part of the nurse-patient interaction), the supervisor needs to be quite adept at assessing the student's readiness for each step in the learning process. When the supervisor opens a particular area of interaction for discussion, the timing, manner of approach, and extent to which it is explored are important; otherwise, she may bombard the student with an examination of various aspects of an interpersonal situation that the student is not ready to handle. An understanding handling of the student's increased sensitiveness at this time, plus continuity in assisting her to work with the problems without blaming her, will make it possible for her to become more comfortable with the fact that certain errors will be made and can be resolved.

Confidential Nature of Supervisory Material. The integrity of the supervisor in handling the supervisory material is important to the security of the student. A certain privacy about the work that takes place in the supervisory hour is needed, and the supervisor's policy regarding this is conveyed to the student. Some of the things discussed in the conferences and some of the student's responses to clinical experiences cannot be shared with others if the student is to have the freedom to talk about the things that concern her in her work.

Nursing and Learning Goals. When the student first starts to work with a patient, some discussion of the reasons for selecting the particular patient for study is useful. The student's goals for the patient's care and for her own learning are reviewed. The supervisor helps the student develop goals that will be realistic for the patient and attainable for the student. The student learns how to relate the psychiatrist's therapeutic plan, the patient's proposed length of stay in the treatment situation, and the available clinical resources to her development of nursing goals. Her primary task, however, is to observe the patient's behavior to determine what he needs to learn that can be offered in a nursing relationship. When this is decided, she is ready to develop, within her relationship with the patient, the initial learning experiences, which are directed toward the ultimate therapeutic goal and which are provided through the use of her own behavior. The supervisor's assistance with this assessment of the goals and direction of the nursing relationship begins with the student's first contact with the patient and continues throughout her work with him.

In the classroom and in supervisory conferences, the student learns to develop her goals for nursing care in relation to the therapeutic procedure designed by the psychiatrist. For example, the nursing relationship with a patient who is receiving anaclitic therapy may be quite different from the relationship with one who is not. The student also learns that there are times when anxiety-reducing measures are desirable in relation to a patient's therapy and times when they are not. The nurse may function essentially in a supportive role in some instances, and in others she may function as the main therapeutic agent. In this second role she works with a psychiatrist, but she does not function as a replacement or substitute for the psychiatrist. Instead, her role is a therapeutic nursing one. The undergraduate student learns about the elements of this latter role, but graduate study is required to learn to function in it.

As the student and supervisor review the student's relationship with a patient, it is the patient's behavior that is studied for its meaning. His patterns of responses to situations and his verbal and nonverbal expressions of thoughts and feelings, as well as all of his behavioral responses, are examined. The purpose of this process is to help the student try to understand how the patient thinks and feels, what things are concerning him, how he is using the nursing relationship, and what he needs as a learning experience in the interpersonal relationship with the nurse. The student learns how to examine a patient's unconsciously motivated behavior in order to understand him better. She learns to respond to cues in his behavior in order to try new approaches of intervention in behavior patterns.

The student's behavior is not the focus of such examination. The supervisor directs her comments to what the patient seems to be doing, and she suggests interpretations of what his behavior may mean.[11] The student's behavior is discussed only in relation to how the patient seems to be responding to her and the alternative nursing responses that she might use as a means of intervention.

Communication Techniques

Throughout the examination of the nurse-patient relationship, various communication techniques are used by the supervisor. She may use direct or indirect questions in a variety of ways which indicate a desire for clarification, elaboration, or explanation of further information about a particular incident. The aim of such questioning may be to help the student to think through a situation, to explore the facets of it more fully, and to become more aware and more critical in her observations. On the other hand, the supervisor may use this technique to help the student learn to describe what she is doing and to evaluate more clearly what she can do.

Occasional comments or statements that pick up an idea or feeling are useful in accomplishing the same aims, or in emphasizing a point, raising doubt about a statement, or adding material for discussion.

The supervisor may also interject new information when it seems to be needed, make suggestions regarding further study, or introduce alternate methods of nursing intervention. By her comments she may indicate affirmation and encouragement when these reactions seem to be indicated.

A request that the student contrast and compare two incidents is used to help her identify themes and cues in the interaction and discover discrepancies and errors in her observations and formulations. Through the comparison of related incidents, she also can plan for continuity in the relationship and apply the principles learned in one situation to other ones.

Nonverbal communication is also important. The teacher needs to be aware of the many ways she may inadvertently communicate feelings that interfere with the student's work. The important role of nonverbal communication in listening and in expressing interest, respect, and support makes it obvious that the supervisor needs to be aware of how she uses nonverbal communication.

All of these techniques of communication are useful in the supervisory process in assisting the student to work with nursing problems and patient problems.

Problem Solving

The student needs to learn to employ a problem-solving approach to her work with patients. There are two areas of problem solving; one is the nursing-problem area which indirectly affects the patient, and the other is the patient-problem area in which the patient needs the nurse's help in working on a problem. The nursing problem is detected by the nurse through observation of the nursing situation. The work on this kind of problem need not be shared with the patient; however, he is usually involved in the process.

Nursing Problem. The nursing-problem group includes how to approach patients in the initial stage of establishing a relationship, how to withstand and handle the many kinds of testing behavior that patients may use, how to accomplish the necessary health measures such as rest and feeding, how to work with the many situations related to the patient's psychopathology or disease process, and how to work through problems related to terminating the treatment and nursing relationship. Also within the category of nursing problems are those related to the patient's interaction with others in his living situation, including other patients and staff or family and friends. Nursing intervention is sometimes necessary in the patient's behavior toward others and in their behavior toward him.

Process of Problem Solving. In the problem-solving process, the supervisor assists the student to: (1) gather information in order to identify a problem, (2) separate the significant factors from the insignificant, (3) select a solution, (4) explore the possible outcomes of the solution, (5) take action upon the selection, (6) evaluate the results, and (7) work with the outcome (either success or failure). In this work it is important that the student be allowed to do the work of the problem solving and to make the choices. The supervisor assists only when the student needs help. She detects this need either by direct verbal requests from the student or through her observations of the student in which she detects errors in the problem-solving process that require the supervisor's intervention.

Patient Problem. In the other problem-solving situation, the patient works on a problem of his own and indicates a need for help which the nurse perceives either through her observations of his behavior or by a direct verbal request from the patient. Many kinds of problems are presented to the nurse. She must determine whether the patient really needs and wants help or is simply talking about a problem which he is capable of solving alone. If help is needed, she has to judge whether she can give it or will have to refer the patient to another person for the kind of help he needs. The student is therefore concerned with learning how to assist a patient in problem solving and how to help him move toward other resources for assistance.

Supervisory Activity. In the supervisory process, the supervisor helps the student stay clear about the assisting role in problem solving with a patient. The steps of problem solving are the same in nursing problems and in patient problems, but in the latter the student learns the importance of allowing the patient to do his own work and to wait and support him as he struggles with each facet at his own pace. She also learns to help him work through the frustration, conflict, and anxiety that may be aroused.

When the student becomes blocked in the problem-solving process because of a lack of information or experience, the supervisor either offers the information or refers the student to resources where she can obtain it. If her block is due to an emotional response or conflict, the teacher waits until the student can work through or resolve her emotional problem, and she may reduce some of the pressures at this time.[12,13] She offers support by maintaining the security of the supervisory relationship through continuing interest and acceptance of the student. The supervisor has to evaluate the degree of the student's anxiety and estimate her anxiety tolerance in order to plan learning experiences in ways that will make it possible for her to work through her anxiety. The methods used to help the student deal with an anxiety-provoking experience and the timing of teacher intervention are important supervisory skills. There are many incidents in the student's work with a patient that may generate anxiety. Under ordinary circumstances the student resolves these in her own way.

As the supervisor studies the nurse-patient interaction, she continually assesses the learning needs of the student. She observes how the student utilizes an educational experience, how she approaches and works with a problem, and how she thinks, feels, and behaves in a nursing situation. The supervisor uses these observations to plan the student's learning experiences. In the process of this work with the student, the teacher has an interest in and concern for the patient's progress as well as for the student's development. The depth of the student's learning experience will be partly determined by how skillful the teacher is in evaluating the patient's therapeutic needs in the nursing relationship.

The student will also extend her own learning by asking questions, requesting additional experience, and seeking other resources. Occasionally a teacher has to intervene in a student's inappropriate or premature use of resources or clinical experiences.

As was mentioned before, the student's whole process record of her work with the patient is examined. This does not mean, however, that every facet of each incident is discussed. The supervisor and student select specific incidents for this step-by-step kind of examination and discussion. These incidents are usually in areas that seem to be a particular problem to the student. A series of incidents that show repeated patterns in the patient's behavior and that acquire new meaning when studied in sequence may be selected for close examination. In the same way, another series of incidents may be selected in order that the student may become aware of a pattern in her responses to the patient. Incidents may be selected by the supervisor to reinforce a previous learning, or to have the student examine the factors which led her to an inference or decision, in order that she may better understand how she reached the decision or in order that she may change an erroneous inference. The teacher is used throughout the supervisory process as a person with whom the student can test the realities, discrepancies, and distortions in her perceptions and inferences in the nurse-patient interaction. A step-by-step examination of the interpersonal process between the student and the patient may also be used when the student is unable to realize her own progress and the supervisor wants her to become more aware of the actual learning steps she has accomplished. Such an examination may be used when the student has made an unrealistic evaluation of her participation in a particular experience with a patient.

Supervisory Problems. There are several problem areas for the supervisor in working with a student in individual supervision. Because of the close association between teacher and student in this type of supervision, the supervisor has a greater opportunity than that offered in the traditional supervisory roles to make it possible for the student to think for herself. She has to be able to differentiate between a student's creative thinking and her simple identification with the opinions of the supervisor. She also needs to be able to detect when a student is functioning intuitively without really increasing her understanding. In working with a highly intuitive student, one can easily miss the cues that indicate that she is not learning some of the concepts and principles that she will need at a later time. On the other hand, it is also important for the student to be free to operate intuitively.

The supervisor needs to understand the dynamics of competition, the patterns of competitiveness in the clinical situation, and the hazards of unconscious competition between teacher and student. The supervisor, for instance, may behave as if she is the one who is giving the patient care and may compete with the student. As a result, she bombards the student with the way she would give the nursing care and does not allow her the freedom to develop her own approaches to nursing problems. This can cause the student to feel so incompetent and inadequate, or so angry, that her learning is blocked. A related problem is one in which the supervisor may perceive the student only as an extension of herself and cause the student to feel "used." She can become so concerned about how she is represented that she is severe in her criticism and can allow no errors. Role confusion is only one of the factors involved in such situations and is an outward demonstration of several problems.

A young, insecure supervisor may believe that the student will be able to accept the authority role of the supervisor better if she is "like the student." To create this impression, she attempts to reduce her authority, overemphasize her mistakes, and underrate her advanced preparation. This behavior creates role diffusion which precipitates anxiety in the student. Clearly defined roles in the teacher-student relationship, a clear interpretation of the necessary limits, and the supervisor's willingness to study her behavior so that she may become aware of her own errors and work out the problems precipitated by them are essential to good supervisory practice. This examination of the supervisory process is not shared with the student, except in instances when an error has directly affected the student and has to be discussed in order to be corrected.

Termination Phase

Termination of the Student-Patient Relationship

The supervisory relationship ends when the student's clinical work is completed, after she has terminated her therapeutic nursing relationship with the patient. As a part of supervision the teacher helps the student understand the principles of the termination process in her work with her patient and assists her in planning the conclusion of the nursing relationship.

Frequently, a student is confronted with the problem of prematurely discontinuing a nursing relationship that has barely begun to be significant to the patient. The student then has the problem of handling the termination process constructively and planning for continuity of the patient's care. The student also learns to work with the more natural termination process in which the patient progresses toward recovery; his needs for nursing care change, and he emancipates himself from and finally terminates the nurse-patient relationship. The supervisor helps the student perceive these needs, accept the changes in the patient, and function in a useful closure of the relationship.

Consideration of Further Learning

The undergraduate student usually moves into another supervised clinical experience upon completion of the course or courses in psychiatric nursing. Since clinical assignments are brief and students often do not adequately complete an adjustment to certain problems in the learning situation before having to leave the course work, the student can often profit by some discussion of the next steps needed in her educational experiences.

Cooperative Evaluation

The individual supervisory process includes an on-going evaluation of the student's work through the examination of the nurse-patient relationship in which the student assumes an increasingly responsible role. In keeping with this educational orientation, the traditional evaluation that is reported at the end of a student's clinical experience should also be a cooperative arrangement between the student and the teacher. Progress toward the teaching goals that the student become increasingly competent in examining her own work and increasingly responsible for assessing her own learning needs and that she develop a clear concept of her abilities is furthered by the evaluation summary as well as the total clinical experience.

Summary and Questions

Individual supervision, as it is used by the authors in teaching psychiatric nursing, has been presented. An attempt has been made to outline briefly the process of this supervision that takes place in a series of individual conferences in which there is an intensive study of a student's work with a patient. Some of the educational framework within which the supervisor and student work is touched upon as are some points in philosophy. Although the clinical focus in this discussion is psychiatric nursing, the supervisory process is applicable in teaching in other clinical areas.

There are many questions to consider in planning individual supervision for students:

1. What experience and academic background should one have to prepare for this kind of supervision?
2. How does a teacher in any field develop the understanding of the dynamics and interpersonal skills necessary to this kind of supervision?
3. Should an individually supervised interpersonal study with a patient be a part of each clinical experience of the undergraduate student?
4. Should this kind of individual supervision be a

part of the student's experience throughout the clinical courses?

   a. If so, how could faculty coordinate the supervisory experiences of the student, or would such coordination be necessary?

   b. How would the focus of the supervisory process differ in the various clinical areas?

5. What are the "hazards" in the individual supervisory process? How do they compare with those in traditional supervision?

6. How does a supervisor handle her own anxiety in this type of supervision?

7. What are the similarities and differences in the process in individual and group methods of supervision?

References

1. Coleman, Jules. "The Teaching of Basic Psychotherapy," *American Journal of Orthopsychiatry*, 17:622-627, Oct. 1947.

2. Feldman, Yonta, Spotnitz, Hyman, and Nagelberg, Leo. "One Aspect of Casework Training through Supervision," *Social Casework*, 34:150-155, Apr. 1953.

3. Zetzel, Elizabeth. "The Dynamic Basis of Supervision," *Social Casework*, 34:143-149, Apr. 1953.

4. Fleming, Joan. "The Role of Supervision in Psychiatric Training," *Bulletin of the Menninger Clinic*, 17:157-169, Sept. 1953.

5. Grotjahn, Martin. "The Role of Identification in Psychiatric and Psychoanalytic Training," *Psychiatry*, 12:141-151, May 1949.

6. Kelman, Herbert. *Compliance, Identification, Internalization.* Unpublished Monograph.

7. Coleman. *Op. cit.*

8. Zetzel. *Op. cit.*

9. Reynolds, Bertha. *Learning and Teaching in the Practice of Social Work.* New York, Farrar & Rinehart, 1942.

10. Murase, Kenneth. "A Problem in Supervision in an Authoritarian Setting," *Social Casework*, 35:117-122, Mar. 1954.

11. Searles, Harold. "The Informational Value of the Supervisor's Emotional Experiences," *Psychiatry*, 18:135-146, May 1955.

12. Zetzel. *Op. cit.*

13. Reynolds. *Op. cit.*

Bibliography

Allen, David W., Houston, Marietta, and McCarley, Tracey H., Jr. "Resistances to Learning," *Journal of Medical Education*, 33:373-379, Apr. 1958.

Austin, Lucile N. "Basic Principles of Supervision," *Social Casework*, 33:411-419, Dec. 1952.

Blake, Florence. "The Supervisor's Task," *Nursing Outlook*, 4:641-643, Nov. 1956.

Bregg, Elizabeth A. "How Can We Help Students Learn?", *American Journal of Nursing*, 58:1120-1122, Aug. 1958.

Cantor, Nathaniel. *Dynamics of Learning.* Buffalo, Foster and Stewart, 1946.

Cruser, Robert W., *et al.* "Opinion on Supervision: A Chapter Study," *Social Work*, 3:18-25, Jan. 1958.

Ebaugh, Franklin. "Graduate Teaching of Psychiatry through Individual Supervision," *American Journal of Psychiatry*, 107:274-278, Oct. 1950.

Ekstein, Rudolf and Wallerstein, Robert. *The Teaching and Learning of Psychotherapy.* New York, Basic Books, 1958.

Grossbard, Hyman. "Methodology for Developing Self-Awareness," *Social Casework*, 35:380-386, Nov. 1954.

Grotjahn, Martin. "Problems and Techniques of Supervision," *Psychiatry*, 18:9-15, Feb. 1955.

Heider, Fritz. *The Psychology of Interpersonal Relations.* New York, John Wiley, 1958.

Henry, Nelson B., ed. *The Integration of Educational Experiences.* The Fifty-seventh Year Book of the National Society for the Study of Education. Part 3. Chicago, University of Chicago Press, 1958.

Ingmire, Alice E. "Student and Teacher Share the Evaluation Process," *Nursing Outlook*, 3:155-158, Mar. 1955.

Lehnert, Bettina. "The Use of Case Material in Supervision," *American Journal of Orthopsychiatry*, 21:54-58, Jan. 1951.

Meerloo, J.A.M. "Some Psychological Processes in Supervision of Therapists," *American Journal of Psychotherapy*, 6:467-470, July 1952.

Mowrer, O. Hobart. *Learning Theory and Personality Dynamics.* New York, Ronald Press, 1950.

Norris, Catherine M. "A Structure for Learning," *Nursing Outlook*, 6:379-381, July 1958.

Peplau, Hildegard E. "What Is Experiential Teaching?", *American Journal of Nursing*, 57:884-886, June 1957.

Robinson, Virginia C. *The Dynamics of Supervision under Functional Controls.* Philadelphia, University of Pennsylvania Press 1949.

Rosenbaum, Milton. "Problems in Supervision of Psychiatric Residents in Psychotherapy," *Archives of Neurology and Psychiatry*, 69:43-48, Jan. 1953.

Skinner, B.F. "The Science of Learning and the Art of Teaching," *Harvard Educational Review*, 24(No. 2):86-97, 1954.

Smith, Dorothy. "Let's Help Students Learn and Grow," *Nursing Outlook*, 5:16-19, Jan. 1957.

Stainbrook, Edward. "On the Structure and Dynamics of Supervision in Psychiatric Training," *Psychiatric Quarterly*, 23:35-40, Jan. 1949.

Symonds, Percival. "Evaluation in Professional Education," *Nursing Outlook*, 5:166-168, Mar. 1957.

Towle, Charlotte. *Common Human Needs.* Washington, D.C., U.S. Government Printing Office, 1945, Chap. 7, "Supervision," p. 95-122.

______. *The Learner in Education for the Professions, As Seen in Education for Social Work.* Chicago, University of Chicago Press, 1954.

Von Bergen, Ruth and Cline, Nora. "Some Aspects of Learning How to Supervise," *Nursing Outlook*, 4:152-154, Mar. 1956.

Warson, Samuel. "Affective Learning and the Student-Teacher Relationship," *American Journal of Psychiatry*, 106:53-58, July 1949.

Will, Gwen. "Psychiatric Nursing Administration and Its Implications for Patient Care." Greenblatt, Levison, and Williams, *The Patient and the Mental Hospital.* Glencoe, Ill., Free Press, 1957, p. 237-247.

Williamson, Margaret. *Supervision: Principles and Methods.* New York, Women's Press, 1950.

Winokur, George. "Brainwashing — A Social Phenomenon of Our Time," *Human Organization*, 13:16-18, Winter 1955.
Wright, Elizabeth. "Creative Leadership," *American Journal of Nursing*, 53:720-722, June 1953.

Discussion

Robert L. Stubblefield

The paper on individual supervision by Miss Bregg, Miss Gregg, and Miss Spring is a stimulating presentation of many aspects of the problems in supervision. They have explored the various writings in nursing and in related fields of psychiatry, social work, and clinical psychology and have presented a review of our current understanding of some of the working processes in supervision. In the introduction they have stressed the value, importance, and limitations of individual supervision as a teaching method and have clarified the various uses of the term within the field of nursing. They have given a satisfactory definition of individual supervision and have discussed the various indications and needs for supervision in a clear manner. In my opinion, they have given an excellent description of the unique aspects of the nursing student's experience in a clinical setting and have emphasized the considerable differences that exist between nursing in a group living situation and psychotherapy as it is practiced in a ward or office.

My only quarrel with them in the early part of their paper centers around their statement that the impact of the emotional experience in the clinical nursing situation in psychiatry is very intense and their apparent implication that this impact is not felt with such intensity in other areas of nursing practice. In my opinion, it is quite likely that the nursing student may have the same kind of intense emotional experience in surgery, in pediatrics, or in medicine, depending on her own psychological experiences during the earlier years in her life.

In their definition of a philosophy of undergraduate education, the authors make some general statements about the goals of an undergraduate collegiate program in psychiatric nursing and relate these goals to the goals of professional nursing in their statement, "...the essence of professional nursing is the meaningful, understanding, and scientific use of the interpersonal relationship with a patient." They add, "It is only through the full understanding of the therapeutic use of this relationship that the nurse can give expert nursing care and can assign duties to nonprofessional personnel and supervise them in carrying out the tasks." Are the authors referring only to psychiatric nursing? What about knowledge of current nursing techniques as an added essential, especially in nonpsychiatric areas?

In one area I would like to take issue with the authors. They state, "The sympathetic, compassionate, 'mothering' roles are a natural part of nursing. The student enters nursing education with a natural endowment in certain of these roles." In my opinion, the second statement should be prefaced by a phrase like "ideally" or a similar qualifying term, since I believe that some nurses enter the field, not as a natural mothering type of person, but to defend themselves against feelings of being unloved and unwanted, with a need to resolve or minimize these past experiences by devoted service to patients and vicarious enjoyment of the nursing situation.

In regard to the authors' descriptions of the supervisory process, including the orientation phase, and their very careful attempt to differentiate between therapy and supervision, I feel that they have made a number of excellent observations and have given us a good understanding of the similarities and differences between therapy and supervision. For those of us who are not involved in actual supervision of nurses, however, and perhaps for others, I think that the paper would be strengthened materially by some examples of the specific things that are done in the supervisory processes in nursing itself. In addition, I would add that there should be an interest in other factors besides the understanding of the supervisory relationship and the therapeutic nurse-patient relationship.

Rudolf Eckstein has captured this very adequately in his recent book *The Teaching and Learning of Psychotherapy*, in which he describes in some detail four phases of the supervision process. As I interpret Eckstein's remarks, the student of psychotherapy may fail to understand the therapeutic process because of a sickness within himself, in which case therapy is indicated for him; or because of ignorance, in which case direct suggestion and education are indicated; or because of complex counter-transference feelings toward the patient, in which case the supervisor attempts to explore some of these underlying emotional feelings directed toward the patient; or because of problems in the supervisor-supervisee relationship, in which case the supervisor is obligated to make some specific efforts to interpret and clarify the problem within this relationship. In other words, I think you should be looking for the factors in the transactions in more specific areas than you defined.

I found the discussion of differentiation of student-supervisor roles diffuse and not too clear. For example, I did not understand what guidelines are used to help the supervisor decide when to recognize the student's growth and ability to accept additional responsibilities in work with patients. I am in complete agreement with the suggestion that the handling of dependence that takes place in the supervisory process serves as a model for the student in her own work in the normal dependency problems with patients.

In regard to the section on preparation of the students for individual supervision, I should like to make two general observations. I agree that the nurse attempts to offer a therapeutic learning experience to the patient in interpersonal relationships that "enable him to test out and change his concepts about himself and his relationships with others." It seems to me that the basic contribution of the nurse is to reduce the tendency toward regression; in this context it seems to me that even those patients who do not want a therapeutic experience need the support of the nurse in order to avoid regression in the course of ordinary nonpsychiatric medical and surgical conditions of various kinds.

I find it difficult to understand how one can discuss a philosophy of supervision in psychiatric nursing without some attempt to tie it to some particular therapeutic and psychological theory about behavior. In simple terms, one can assume that the individual's personality is part biologic, part psychological, and part social and that he has basic drives, including a drive to relationships with other individuals, and learned drives. When these objects are unavailable or are rejected, he retreats from them and has feelings of loneliness. In essence then, the nursing process is an attempt to prevent or minimize the effects of the regressive phenomena that are introduced when the memory of the previous stimulus, namely the loss of a significant figure in fact or fantasy, is reactivated within the hospital therapeutic experience.

As an illustration, a patient is conscious of the fact that his resident physician is leaving the ward service. One can predict his regression with some knowledge of his past history and personality diagnosis and can adopt some nursing techniques that theoretically will reduce or minimize the extent of his regression. For example, one can treat him in a more infantile supporting manner; one can give him opportunity to bring out aggressions without criticism or moralizing; or one can be more inclined to interpret rather than simply react to and support him in this period.

Is it the verbal interaction or the emotional experience of acceptance of regressive impulses that works? This is the old argument about what is effective in a psychotherapeutic experience, and it seems appropriate to mention that this is a problem in nursing as well as in the field of psychotherapy. In my own opinion, it is likely to be the experience of acceptance and understanding and clarification, rather than the dramatic effect of the interpretation, that makes the difference in the patient's behavior, understanding, and eventual maturation. Basically, infants begin their experiences by tactile impressions of their environment, and remnants of these events persist in our language ("I feel," "I was touched," "I am moved"). The infant gradually substitutes signals, signs, and eventually symbols to deal with his environment. Thus, any discussion of goals of nursing should be concerned with the level of the nurse's role (oral-tactile, anal-signal, oedipal-symbolic). Perhaps nursing does itself and medicine a disservice in focusing its supervision on efforts to develop highly skilled verbal symbolic communication with patients, thus, abandoning its earlier historical interest on tactile, kinetic, nonverbal communication (maternal roles) with sick patients.

In the details of the description of the working phase of a supervisory process, I found myself interested but full of many questions about what actually goes on. This section would have been strengthened a great deal by some examples at several points. I disagree with the statement, "The student's behavior is not the focus of [the] examination. The supervisor directs her comments to what the patient seems to be doing, and she suggests interpretations of what his behavior may mean." In my opinion, this places too many limits on the supervisory process, in that the nursing student is reporting a transaction and her own behavior should be subject to some examination, too. Theoretically, the patient's behavior is determined in part by identification with the mother, the identification with the father, the identification with other significant figures in the early environment, and the identification with the perceptions of the interaction between these various figures. Accordingly, I think the process of supervision should pay some attention to these various elements in the patient's behavior as they emerge in several interactions (patient-patient, patient-relative, patient-staff), in the patient's memories of past experiences, and in the patient-nurse interaction. Also, in this section I felt that the authors recommended too formal a relationship with the student.

I am in essential agreement with the section on

communication techniques in the supervisory process and the description of problem solving in the supervisory process. Again, however, I feel that my understanding of it is limited by the lack of examples. Since behavior operates at so many different dynamic levels, it is difficult for me to understand what the nurses mean when they talk about gathering information in order to identify a problem or separating the significant factors from the insignificant.

For example, if a woman patient states that her mother constantly belittles and scorns men and that she basically agrees with her mother's observations, the nurse has several choices in this situation. She may listen without comment; she may reflect anxiety in the current relationship; she may attempt to clarify the patient's underlying conflict about the mother's attitudes and the patient's own natural heterosexual feelings; or she may use many other responses. However, there are many possible sources of this behavior. The patient may be saying, "Shall we hate men together?", "Will you encourage me to rebel against my mother and carry out my heterosexual impulses despite her opposition?", "Will you permit me to grow up and be independent of you and of the hospital as my mother did not permit me to do as a child?"

As another example, an adult woman patient has been visited by her mother and is crying quietly in her room. On inquiry from the nurse, the patient states that her mother had talked about the time when the patient lived with her maternal grandmother from age one to seven, while the mother worked. These memories included a memory that the grandmother had said that she was "the meanest white girl alive." Later the patient spontaneously recalled pleasant memories about the late latency and early adolescent years in her life, when her mother had given up her work and returned to the home. Should the nurse concentrate on the patient's hostility toward the mother for refusing to take her home; or on the pleasant memories in the latency and adolescent period of her life; or on the guilt in the relationship with the grandmother, who was the most significant mother figure in her life; or on the deeper hostilities the patient feels toward her mother, whom she feels does not want her, did not mother her in the past, and is not interested in protecting and mothering her in the present? In my opinion, it is not enough to answer that the nurse should deal with this in terms of her spontaneous reaction. I believe that one should establish some theoretical goal in nursing therapy that would relate to the total goal in therapy of the particular patient, and then in this situation be prepared to deal with a specific area and to avoid discussions in other areas of the patient's life situation.

It is precisely in these areas that I think a great deal of competition develops between the nurse and the therapist. This creates many of our communication problems and results in lack of clarity about therapeutic goals. The search for dramatic information from the historic past may block us from a consistent individual and group cohesiveness, which is essential for the patient's new learning. You recognize my bias immediately; I am interested in having nurses deal with the reality types of conflict as they are experienced in the day-to-day living situation with the aid of an ever expanding knowledge about the patient's past and present personality. Thus, I believe that we should attempt to define the patient's behavior in simple, operational terms and require that our nurses attempt to respond in a warm, humane, and spontaneous manner that will enhance feelings of security and acceptance, and reduce feelings of loneliness.

I would prefer to see a supervision process concentrated on a very few episodes in an attempt to establish the common factors in human experience that are involved in emotional illnesses. I feel that it is the emotional experience within the transaction between nurse and patient that is meaningful and therapeutic for the patient, and not what is said in the magic of the interpretation. It is my opinion that the experience can be best understood by a detailed discussion of a small number of nurse-patient transactions, rather than by an attempt to review the details of several episodes in a particular supervisory session.

The author's review of the termination phase of a supervisory process is brief and concise. It is clear that they are aware of the fact that a number of people, especially in the field of social work, have found that a careful review of the results of supervision is of considerable value in rounding out the educational experience for the student. Unfortunately, the psychiatrists, by and large, have not been able to do this effectively.

In regard to the questions, I have a number of reactions to them, but will limit my remarks to two areas. Specifically, I feel that a teacher in any field develops the understanding of the skills in supervision by a detailed study of the process of supervision itself. Ideally, I think that some supervision should be recorded, so that the person who is learning supervision will have an opportunity to experience the process of being supervised, to observe supervision, and to study the actual processes involved in it. I feel that individual supervision should be a part of the student's experience throughout the clinical courses in pediatric nursing and other areas as well as in psychiatric nursing.

Finally, the authors have given us an excellent bibliography, which reviews much of the current literature in the field of education pertaining to the value and limitations of individual supervision.

Robert E. Switzer

I should like to congratulate the three authors of this paper on their ability and willingness to accept the commitment to prepare this paper, and on their ability to live up to their commitment so well in the face of many difficulties. The difficulties came from having to produce, within a given length of time while working on their regular jobs at great distances apart, a publishable paper on an area that I know each of the authors considers to be one of the most important and crucial areas in present-day psychiatric nursing education.

One of the big pressures came from the fact that, from the very beginning of this project, the non-nurse participants have been pushing the nurses to commit themselves to paper for their own benefit, as well as for the benefit of the non-nurse members, so that they may be better able to ascertain how their own particular discipline might add to the achievement of the goals of the project. Another pressure came from the fact that, in every regional conference, psychiatric nursing was repeatedly and threateningly told that psychiatric nursing had better find ways of integrating mental health and psychiatric principles into nursing school curriculums and into nursing, in general, or it would be done for them by the behavioral sciences. The spotlight was the interest in this project that must have already been engendered throughout nursing education and the anticipation with which the whole field of nursing education must be waiting for the final published report of this project.

For purposes of discussion, I prefer to think of this paper as divided into two parts. The first half I would call the theoretical and philosophical approach to individual supervision as a method of teaching in psychiatric nursing, and the second half I would call the operational consideration of this teaching technique. In the first half, I find many areas in which to offer constructive criticism. I think this is as might be anticipated. Psychiatric nursing, with great conviction and rightly so, has observed the efficacy of this teaching technique in psychiatry and psychiatric social work and is attempting to apply this technique in its own area. It is only to be expected that there will be misunderstandings, misconceptions, disagreements, and misapplications until the borrowed theories and concepts are restudied and reformulated to fit the particular needs of nursing education, which are in many ways vastly different from those of individual supervision in psychiatry or in psychiatric social work.

In the first part of the paper, there are many phrases such as: "goal-directed professional relationships," "useful interpersonal relationships," "therapeutic interpersonal relationships," "therapeutic nursing intervention," and "therapeutic use of self," but I could find no statement that was to me a clear, concise expression of the meanings of these terms, or, in other words, we are discussing supervision toward what?

I quarrel with the lack of a positive stand in the section that discusses the need for individual supervision. For the most part, the expressed indications have to do with preventive psychiatry, in terms of the impact of psychiatric patients on the relatively young and immature nursing student and the protection afforded her in a complicated social situation, in terms of her relatively short time on a service, compared with other professional workers, and in terms of concerns about protecting her from the "interdisciplinitis" that may be present. I believe that we should start from a positive statement.

I may be stuck on definition of words, but I would hope that the small group discussions this afternoon would take a very long and careful look at the following quotation from the section of the paper "Philosophy of Undergraduate Education": "The authors believe that the essence of professional nursing is a meaningful, understanding, and scientific use of the interpersonal relationship with a patient." I do not believe that this statement can stand alone. If this statement is true, then nursing had no essence for a long, long time. I believe that mothering care is the essence of all nursing, and that the meaningful understanding and scientific use of the interpersonal relationship with the patient is a refinement of that essence. I do not mean to quibble; I simply believe that nursing students should not be taught the concept I have just quoted. Such teaching could tend to "interpersonalize" and specialize the nursing student right out of her identity with nursing.

I have particular difficulties with the sections of the paper on the similarities of, and differences between, therapy and supervision. There are statements that seem to say to me that there is no difference between therapy and supervision. There are statements that make it difficult for me to convince myself that the supervision described is not psychotherapy. There are statements that make it difficult for me to convince myself that the student is being taught any distinction between being therapeutic and being an individual psychotherapist. When the discussion shifts to the area of the differences between the student and the patient, I have even greater difficulty convincing myself.

The dilemma I find myself in, in this portion of the paper, is exemplified by the following quotation: "The basic dynamics of a good supervisory relationship and a therapeutic relationship are essentially the same, although the functions are different." The sentence following this quotation is: "In psychiatry, those who supervise students are prepared as psychiatrists and psychoanalysts, and a discussion of the differentiation between therapy and supervision is colored by this fact." I would show my coloring by voicing an opinion that this comparison of the basic dynamics of a good supervisory relationship and a therapeutic relationship is unclear and incomplete. The operational dynamics in a good supervisory relationship and the operational dynamics in a good therapeutic relationship are very different, if we are going to hold to an opinion that supervision and therapy are not synonymous. This is the position, I think, that we must hold to in this discussion. In a supervisory relationship, the operational area is the conscious level. In a therapeutic relationship, the operational area is to a large extent the conscious level, although the person taking the therapeutic role may very well be in possession of considerable information about the unconscious of the individual to whom he is being therapeutic. In therapy, some of the area of operation is the conscious level, but the real areas of operation are the preconscious and the unconscious, through the active utilization of interpretation, the transference, material from early life experiences, dreams, and so forth. The goal of supervision is to help a nursing student to be a better nurse. The goal of therapy is to bring about a more successful handling of internal conflict.

Throughout the paper, there is an inconsistency to which I can find no resolution. At many points, great emphasis is placed on the fact that in the supervisory relationship the student finds permissiveness, freedom, and complete acceptance. At other points, great emphasis is placed upon the authority role of the supervisor. In one instance the student is referred to as being "under supervision" rather than "in supervision." At another point, it is indicated that inherent in a teacher's role are decisions regarding the minimum competence required of the basic student — clinical decisions involved in the student's progress, including an evaluation and grade. These inconsistencies seem to be a reflection of an attempt to use two systems at the same time.

One other point about the first half of the paper that is perplexing to me is the material that seems to indicate concern about the teacher as a model for the staff and the student. I could not tell whether this was the teacher speaking as a supervisor of a nursing student, or the teacher speaking as a psychiatric nursing integrator. It is stated that the teacher's role as a model is different from that of a staff nurse, head nurse, or clinical supervisor. I would only raise a question as to whether this is true because of a tradition, because of evolution, because of expediency, because of inertia, or because, out of careful thought and consideration, this is good and as it should be.

As we move into the second half or operational part of the paper, our authors stand upon the firm ground of their own experiences in being supervised and their experiences in individual supervision of nursing students. In this portion of the paper they write with firmness, conviction, and clarity. Tucked away in this portion are some statements which I think should have been at the beginning of the paper. "Nursing meets a need for care which is different in many ways from that met by psychiatry." "Nursing's task, then, is to provide an interpersonal experience that is different from any the patient can get otherwise. This therapeutic experience is developed through the collaboration of the psychiatrist and the nurse, and it can take place in an institutional setting or in the patient's home." I think the third sentence detracts from the second, in that I believe that part of the task is unique to the role of the nurse and not dependent upon collaboration. Collaboration with the psychiatrist should enrich the ability of nursing to fulfill the task, but, as far as the nursing student's contribution to the fulfillment of this task, the paper is not clear as to how a two-way collaboration is brought about through utilization of material from supervision of the interaction between the patient and the nurse.

Another very important statement is: "...psychiatric nursing offers a patient therapeutic learning experiences in interpersonal relationships that enable him to test out and change his concepts about himself and his relationships with others and thus further his work toward health." These quotations seem to me to represent the essence of the answer to the question I raised at the beginning of this discussion, namely: Supervision toward what therapeutic goals? But these goals are much different from the treatment goals aimed at in the supervisory process experienced by a psychiatric social work student receiving supervision of individual casework treatment, or the treatment goals of the supervisory process experienced by a young psychiatrist receiving supervision of an individual psychotherapy effort.

It seems to me that the points that I have already raised, and others that I will touch on, have to do with attempting to move individual supervision "lock, stock, and barrel" from one teaching situation to another and finding that it is not quite a tailor-made fit. Classically, individual supervision in casework and psychotherapy is aimed to prepare an individual to perform a fairly well-defined function. Efforts toward that function take place within a working relationship between two people — the case worker and client or patient, or the psychotherapist and patient. The supervisor in no way directly enters into the working relationship between the person doing the helping, and he is unknown or at least anonymous to the person being helped. In psychotherapy, the helping person in no way enters into the life situation of the person being helped except at appointed hours in a very specific place. There is a commitment on the part of the helper, and there is a commitment on the part of the person being helped. Except in the second kind of problem solving mentioned in the paper, the commitment on the part of the person being helped does not exist in the nurse-patient relationship, and the nurse-patient relationship does not have the isolated one-to-one quality of individual psychotherapy. Both of these points have important implications for individual supervision of nursing students.

In the kind of supervision just mentioned, the supervisor might well have been from halfway around the world. With the development of mental hygiene clinics and child psychiatry, some important shifts took place. Social workers and psychiatrists entered into close collaborative effort. They got so they could talk with each other clinically. This was particularly difficult for the psychiatrist with his deep roots in the importance of the one-to-one relationship and because of his great concerns about the confidentiality of what goes on in that relationship. But social workers and psychiatrists did get so they could talk with each other, and they learned how to communicate significant material without the destructiveness of having communicated or utilized inappropriate material.

During such collaborative efforts, both the social worker and the psychiatrist continue to have individual supervision, and their supervisors usually work in the same setting. They participate in case-oriented clinical interplay between the social worker and the psychiatrist mainly through supervision, although they are in other clinical contact with both supervisees and each other. If the social worker and the psychiatrist happen to be trainees, they receive grades at the end of the assigned period in the clinic, but these are grades for their total performance, and they are not graded on just the supervision aspects of their total assignment. In both instances the grading represents a broad evaluation. In casework, this evaluation is participated in actively by the trainee. In neither instance does the grade hold failure power.

During the supervisory experience, both social work student and psychiatric resident are encouraged to bring process recordings of their efforts. Some have great difficulty for a long time before they are really able to bring process material to supervision. This fact also contains implications relative to individual supervision of nursing students. I think it is important to consider because of the age and relative unsophistication of the nursing student as compared to the casework student and the psychiatric resident.

If we now transplant our psychiatric trainee and his supervisor into a good teaching psychiatric hospital of not too many years ago, we find that their job together has in some ways become more complicated and that supervision has taken on new dimensions. These changes come from the fact that the treatment process has broadened to include almost the patient's entire life situation, for the moment at least. This puts the psychiatrist into the patient's life situation, at least into a position where he must relate to the patient's life situation. It may also put him into the situation of having his supervisor for his administrative superior. But the major new ingredient in this new situation for our hypothetical psychiatric trainee is that personnel who care for the patient, and, in a very important sense, live with the patient, enter into the picture, and that the psychiatrist has some authority role with these personnel either directly or through the ward physician.

This is not a new role for our psychiatrist because of his deeper identity as a physician who traditionally gives orders regarding patients'care to the nurse and other caring personnel. But this certainly means that the supervisory process must contain much more than does the supervision of the classical or the collaborative outpatient therapist-patient efforts. In the setting we are describing, the need for staff communication about a patient was met by staff conferences in which the psychiatrist did most of the talking, and the caring personnel, particularly nursing students, were most often seen but not heard. The physician prescribed for the patient, and the nurse was so busy making certain that the physician's orders on all the patients were carried out that she had not enough time to form personal relationships with patients. The nurse had to keep the ward books and stand ready to answer to the head nurse or the supervisor. Seen in the extreme, the process would seem like supervised individual therapy with good room and board and care provided. The physician was kept informed, but the caring personnel got little or no information from the supervised therapy process.

We could transplant our psychiatrist who receives individual supervision of his therapy efforts into a contemporary psychiatric teaching hospital setting. But I would like to conclude my remarks by describing some aspects of another kind of psychiatric inpatient facility, with the hope of being provocative and of stimulating particular discussion of individual supervision of nursing students in the small groups this afternoon.

Let us transplant our social worker and our psychiatrist to a residential treatment center for severely emotionally disturbed children of grade school age. Our psychiatrist sees several children in individual psychotherapy, on a three or four times a week basis relative to matters pertaining to the parents. Both the social worker and the psychiatrist receive individual supervision. The person in charge of the total program is a psychiatrist, and he is a supervisor in the residence, in *both* senses that the word is used in this paper. There is an assistant supervisor in the residence.

For purposes of this discussion, I will call all the other residence personnel "caring personnel." For the most part, these personnel correspond in age and academic background with nursing students. These personnnel have no *model* to follow other than their philosophy of care. They provide around-the-clock care. They provide a laboratory, a proving ground, and a workshop for the insights gained in therapy. They are impinged upon by the children who impinge upon each other. These caring personnel impinge upon each other and are impinged upon by the other staff members directly and indirectly as a result of the conscious and unconscious efforts of the children to maneuver and divide and conquer. The caring personnel stand against illness by a conscious and devoted effort to be consistent, honest, fair, just, patient, incorruptible, indestructible, strong, unretaliating, and always ready to lend to a child control from without until such a time as the child's own inner controls are reconstituted. They always attempt to accept and control aggression, overt sexual behavior, regression, and so forth, along with expression of concern and appropriate affect, but without punishment and retaliation.

In addition to all of these "caring functions," these personnel also have a goal to be *therapeutic* in terms of the individual child. This further goal gives additional emphasis to the fact that individual therapy and residential care are different and separate processes with different goals, and yet are integral and interdependent parts of a coordinated treatment program. Each has a unique contribution to make to the total, yet neither can stand alone. Providing therapy for an individual child and individual supervision of the treatment process would be tantamount to attempting to stand alone, if the residential aspect of the child's existence were ignored. Paying attention to the residential aspect of the total program and the supervision of the caring personnel would be tantamount to attempting to stand alone, if the contributions of therapy to understanding of the child and to the therapeutic goals of the caring personnel were ignored. It quite naturally follows that constant, on-going, two-way communication is vital to individual therapy, to the therapeutic efforts of the caring personnel, and to supervision of both.

This vital necessity also applies to communication between the casework process and individual therapy and between the casework process and the therapeutic efforts in the residence. There are several forms of communication: face-to-face verbal communication; telephone communication; written notes from casework and therapy to the residence; written or dictated notes on interaction with a child or with several children from a caring person, for the information and utilization of the other caring personnel, as well as the several individual therapists and social workers. An additional rather special method of communication is a team meeting on each child in residence every four to eight weeks. These meetings, chaired by the supervisor and recorded for the future use of all by the assistant supervisor, are attended by the therapist, the social worker, the caring personnel, the teachers, and other personnel whose goal it is to use crafts, shop work, music, art, athletics, dancing, sewing, and club activities in a therapeutic way.

Because of the commitment of the caring portion of the total treatment program to be therapeutic in its own right and therapeutic through awareness of information from the therapy and casework processes, communication and didactic educational efforts are very important parts of the supervision of the caring personnel. This supervision is operationally oriented, in that it is on-going and directed toward the individual behavior and interaction between the children, and between the children and the caring personnel. It is directed toward the reality situation of the moment.

The supervision is given by the supervisor and the assistant supervisor by four methods: individual scheduled supervisory hours; individual unscheduled supervisory interactions; small group meetings in which one or the other or both supervisors participate; and total caring personnel meetings in which both supervisors participate. Important also is the supervisory interaction (in both senses of the word) that takes place between caring personnel.

Individual supervision is very important, and none of the above comments should be construed as critical toward individual supervision. In the clinical setting I have just described, individual supervision cannot survive as the only supervisory method of teaching the necessary mental health and psychiatric concepts.

In closing, I should like to repeat and underline two quotations from the paper. "Nursing meets a need for care which is different in many ways from that met by psychiatry." "Nursing's task, then, is to provide an interpersonal experience that is different from any the patient can get otherwise."

Nora Cline

The paper represents the experiences of nurses with imaginative and creative power to use their knowledge and experience for the purpose of cultivating nursing ability to meet nursing needs of patients. The authors discuss a method of supervision designed to help students learn nursing skills that will provide help to patients with problems resulting from emotional disturbances. The method is based on planned individual conferences between the supervisor and the student. The student brings to each conference, for discussion, a recording of her interaction with her patient. This process record provides the supervisor with information about a nurse-patient situation in which the supervisor was not an observer. The supervisor deliberately develops a relationship with the student to help the student integrate factual knowledge with appropriate emotional responses. She uses the student's experience of working with a patient, so that the learning comes from doing, with the supervision focused on the student's involvement in caring for the patient.

The supervisor has a dual responsibility: to offer the student the best opportunity for learning, and to offer the patient the best opportunity within this structure for resolving his problems.

The authors state that the purpose of supervision is to help the student learn to understand the meaning of behavior and use her own behavior as a means of helping the patient. This learning encompasses (1) knowledge of theories from psychiatry that are known to be of psychotherapeutic aid to patients, (2) use of these "talked about" theories with a patient or patients, (3) observation of the patient's reactions, and (4) understanding of feelings that block or facilitate the use of these concepts.

The individual conferences between the supervisor and the student can offer a setting and a relationship that facilitate the integration of this learning by the student. Integration of these concepts is a vital part of learning therapeutic nursing skills, and it is dependent to a great extent on the quality of supervision the student has.

What is involved in the interpersonal interaction that affects this learning is difficult to formulate. Perhaps it is impossible, amid the complexity of feelings in this working together, to convey to another exactly what occurs in the series of actions and events.

The student entering this supervisory relationship offers for scrutiny her "professional helping self." This includes what her learning has been, as well as what learning is taking place in her relationship with her supervisor in this clinical setting.

The authors convey the idea that the student moves with less anxiety in communicating and learning when the focus of the discussion is on understanding the patient's behavior rather than on the student's feelings and what she "ought to feel." The supervisor is concerned about how the student feels, and she listens to her and accepts her right to her feelings. She helps her examine her interaction with her patient, supports her in trying out her knowledge and ideas when she can, and helps her think through some possible reactions and choose another way of responding to her patient when indicated. The supervisor responds sympathetically to the student's dependency needs as she listens attentively, asks for clarification, helps her to understand the patient's behavior in relation to his disease, and helps her with her response to the patient's needs. Her acceptance gives the student permission to talk about her feelings, even angry ones.

The authors state, "...the supervisor does not respond to the therapeutic needs expressed by a student...." This discussant believes that the supervisor does respond to the therapeutic needs of the student but does not focus on the therapeutic needs of the student for the purpose of helping her work through her emotional problems or of promoting a basic behavioral change. This focus and purpose are major differences in the roles of supervisor and therapist.

As the student experiences this understanding and accepting relationship with her supervisor, she may have a beginning emotional awareness of its therapeutic value. This may be an important step in the student's feeling of trust. What the student feels about herself and other people may be expressed in the question, "How much can I feel and still be professional?" In helping this student with, shall I say, integrity of feeling — feelings that encompass love, empathy, worth — one must take into consideration the possibility of the student's need to deny the reality of feeling, a defense underlaid with anger. The student may need psychotherapeutic help beyond what the supervisor can give in her role of supervisor.

To differentiate and maintain one's role requires understanding of the difference in roles, understanding of one's self, and integrity in setting limits on the use of the supervisor-student relationship. The dynamics of dependency and its concomitant hostility provide ever-present stumbling blocks in many forms. The discussant believes, with the authors, that exploration for understanding and emotional awareness of dependency in the teaching-learning relationship is essential to the skill with which the supervisor provides guidance to the student. The authors discuss briefly one aspect of this problem, that is, patient progress through the student's imitation of the supervisor, rather than student growth through development of insight — growth that helps her maintain her professional individuality.

Some characteristics of the atmosphere that help develop the student's independence are freedom to think, to feel, and to express her ideas, and permission to act independently within certain limits, to test her ideas, to assume responsibility for working with the resulting reactions, and to use these results to deepen her understanding of the interpersonal process.

The supervisor will make errors of judgment, partly because of her "less than perfect" skill in supervision, partly because her own problems will get in her way.

Early in the paper the authors state, "It is only through the full understanding of the therapeutic use of this relationship that the nurse can give expert nursing care...." I should like the authors to consider this statement. In their discussion they convey that the teaching-learning relationship not only can survive but can move forward when the supervisor has knowledge and skill in the use of behavior that she can transmit to the student who wishes to learn, when the supervisor is sensitive and responsive to the feelings that are in the way or block this, and when she accepts her contribution to the blocks in learning. I believe this can apply also to the nurse-patient relationship.

In the statement, "The student is assumed to be a well person," do the authors wish to convey the idea that the student is functioning adequately in her student role and experiencing gratifying relationships with others? When the supervisor observes limited functioning, a degree of distortion, or other behavior indicating the need for psychotherapeutic help, she supports the student in using help that is available. It might be necessary for the student to terminate her experience in this setting. It is also possible that the student's ability to accept, understand, and relate will be enhanced as she is helped.

I should like to ask the authors about their experience with regard to the achievement by students of the goals they have discussed. The learning is complex and, according to the authors, has an emotional impact on the student. Time for assimilation is essential for the development of emotional awareness.

It is hoped that the student will learn to study behavior to understand its meaning, that she will gain emotional awareness of sources and expressions of human anxieties and tensions, and that she will develop an emotional awareness of what is meant by "to develop a relationship." Appropriate emotional response as an integral part of her therapeutic nursing skills is slow in developing, and learning the importance of unconscious emotional factors and the role they play in individual and group relationships might come much later.

Through this supervisory process the student gradually becomes more confident in testing her ideas and skills and in using her behavior to help the patient experience a kind of relationship that is useful to him in changing his attitudes and behavior. She tries out various methods and approaches and examines the patient's responses as well as her own, thereby gradually deepening the level of her nursing skill.

The termination of this teaching-learning relationship will carry with it expressions of anxiety. The separation may reactivate feelings of dependency, rejection, and so on. How much and how little was accomplished will be talked about. While accepting the feelings, the supervisor can help the student formulate some of her learnings and decide how they can be useful to her. Identifying and discussing this element of anxiety in the termination of the supervisor-student relationship help the student to work out the termination process with her patient.

In the working process between the supervisor and the student, there are innumerable reactions, reflections, and unknowns, limited only by the complexity of the problems the student brings for discussion and the understanding and skill of the supervisor.

Progress is enhanced and plagued by selective hearing, seeing, and reacting. Additional problems may be injected by other routes. The authors and this discussant believe that the process of supervision by individual conference, as it is discussed in this paper, provides an opportunity for examining the sequence of events, actions, and feelings during supervisor-student interaction and during the student's interaction with patients in a relationship and setting that give maximum opportunity for learning therapeutic nursing skills.

One criticism I have of the paper in general is that the major theme — the supervisory process — is obscured for too long by progression through statements about traditional functional supervision.

I should like to ask the authors about their statements that begin with "She needs to be aware...," "She must be able..., "She needs to understand...." Are these statements of belief, or are they intended to express that a certain level of skill will make it possible to meet a certain need? Perhaps the statements were written in a tired moment and not caught in the editing.

I should like to comment on the questions asked by the authors in the group discussion.

Summary of General Discussion

Question 1. In what ways are therapy and supervision different?

a. There is need to clarify the meanings of "giving supervision," "being therapeutic," and "engaging in therapy."

b. Is it possible for a nurse who is not a therapist to differentiate between therapy and supervision?

Discussion: Supervision and therapy have different goals. There may be therapeutic benefits in supervision, but this is not its goal.

Question 2. Is the emotional impact on the student greater in psychiatric nursing than it is in other clinical areas?

Discussion: The impact is great in the early introduction to nursing, and there is an emotional reaction to many clinical and other learning experiences in any area.

Question 3. Is the nurse-patient relationship the "essence of nursing?"

a. This statement does not define nursing. (Authors' note: It was not intended as a definition of nursing.)

b. Is it implied that the "essence of nursing" is contained only in the one-to-one relationship?

c. Is it possible, from this one kind of relationship, to deduce the essence of all nursing, since nursing has many varied relationships? Are the staff nurse and the supervisor doing nursing?

Discussion: There is a need for definitions of "nurse-patient relationship" and "interpersonal relationship."

There are verbal and nonverbal components in interpersonal relationships.

Students use observational and performance skills throughout their nursing experience.

The nurse-patient relationship is a vehicle through which we help the patient to accomplish certain things and is not an end in itself.

Scientific knowledge and technical skills are not denied in emphasizing the importance of the nurse- patient relationship.

The care of the diabetic patient exemplifies how the nurse's scientific knowledge about diabetes cannot benefit the patient if she does not take into account his feelings about his disease when she is attempting to teach him.

What the nurse communicates by touch when she ministers to the patient is also an important part of the relationship.

There are three areas of operation in nursing: (1) the individual contact with one patient, (2) the contact in a structured group situation, and (3) the contact within a fluid, changing group. The nurse has to be able to function in all three kinds of relationships with patients.

Perhaps the essence of nursing is the nurse-patient *interaction,* and the term "relationship" should refer to the abstractions which characterize that interaction.

It is this orientation to the nurse-patient relationship which lifted nursing, as we know it, out of its functional way of being performed and into a truly professional atmosphere, without leaving out what we have ordinarily thought of as the core of nursing.

Question 4. How much should the nurse be concerned with the psychodynamics of interpersonal relationships with patients?

Discussion: What would interpersonal relationships be if we did not begin to analyze psychodynamics? Even the physical care of giving a bath establishes an interpersonal relationship that should be analyzed.

Question 5. In relation to the goals of supervision, how can we provide nursing care that includes the kind of nursing relationship that gives the patient a satisfying experience?

No discussion.

Question 6. How can we counteract the many learning experiences of medical students and nursing students that make them repress and deny their humane interests in patients and that inhibit their movement toward people?

Discussion: The best way to counteract this problem is in the supervisory process.

Question 7. Was there an inconsistency in the paper in that the supervisor was both permissive and "authoritarian?"

a. Are the individual supervisor of the student's therapeutic work and the administrative supervisor the same person? (Authors' note: The supervisor has the responsibility for educational administration of the student's program as well as for individual supervision of her work with patients. She usually does not have responsibility for the nursing service administration of the clinical setting.)

Discussion: Administrative plans made by the teacher for the student's experience allow the student freedom to pursue her learning. There is no inconsistency in the fact that authority and permissiveness exist in the same situation. (Authors' note: "Authority" is not synonymous with "authoritarianism.")

The teacher gives the individual supervision and, in her ward contact with the student, handles many administrative issues with her. In the individual supervisory hour, the student and teacher discuss the work a student does with a patient; however, other issues may be brought into this conference as the student wishes.

Question 8. The individual supervisory conference, as described in the paper, seems to be a "formal" supervisor-student relationship.

No discussion.

Question 9. How often does the supervisor meet with the student in individual supervision?

Discussion: The individual supervisory conference is held weekly throughout the student's clinical experience and is an hour in length. (Authors' note: The student can see the supervisor for additional conferences when necessary, and she also has daily contacts with the supervisor in the clinical setting.)

Question 10. Does the supervisor rely entirely on what the student brings to the supervisory hour, or does she get the opinion of others about the nurse-patient episodes?

a. Does the supervisor confront her supervisee with the additional information obtained from other sources?

b. Can the supervisor accept as accurate the data reported by the student?

Discussion: The supervisor is on the ward with the student and, from her own observations, is aware of some of the things that are happening.

The supervisor may know some things from the nurses on the ward about what is taking place between the student and the patient, and, as long as there is no gross interference with the patient's progress or no potential crisis on the ward, she may not bring these up in the supervisory hour at all but wait until the student does. As the student experiences supervision as a helping process and gets comfortable within the supervisory relationship, she brings in the kind of things she was not able to look at before, and so the supervisor sees an ever-widening expanse of the kind of things she can discuss in the supervisory hour.

The student does not report only random incidents as a matter of choice. She works with one patient daily for a long period of time and reports what the patient said, what she said, what she thought the patient felt, what she felt, and what she thought was going on, and she makes inferences about the situation.

Question 11. Does the supervisor in the supervisory conference focus only on the patient's behavior, or does she focus also on the student's behavior?

a. Does the supervisor have some responsibility to pick up and deal with the student's resistance in supervision, to give suggestions out of her added knowledge, to deal with a student's problem with a patient, and to deal with the student's problems with the supervisor?

Discussion: The example of the student who has a tendency to overgeneralize is a case in point in which the supervisor would focus on the behavior of the student and not that of the patient.

Question 12. What surrounds supervision? How does it fit into other concepts? Can we define certain optimal conditions for supervision?

No discussion.

Question 13. Just how similar and dissimilar are the nurse-patient relationship and the supervisor-student relationship?

No discussion.

Question 14. The discussion of dependency in the paper was challenged on the basis that the point of regression of the patient is considerably different from that of the student.

Discussion: (Authors' note: The authors agree that the level of dependence of the patient in the nurse-patient relationship is quite different from that of the student in the supervisor-student relationship.)

Question 15. The discussion of supervision in this meeting is pointed in the direction of the professionalization of nursing.

a. How much does the argument against the more intellective approach have to do with the feeling that nurses should not move upward professionally?

b. How much does the support for the more verbal, symbolic theory have to do with the issue of professionalism?

No discussion.

Question 16. How does one become a supervisor? What are the stages of development? What practices in the organizational structure tend to develop people along directions we would like?

Question 17. The personality of supervisors has been underemphasized in the discussion. What sort of personality attributes do we think are useful for supervisors?

Discussion: It is important to try to identify early the student who might be a good candidate for supervisor-training in the narrow sense. This person is a better-than-average student who is perceptive and understanding, is willing to admit she doesn't know enough, and is willing to keep on learning in different ways. A good nursing supervisor is one who has demonstrated some skill and has had success in nursing relationships with patients; she must be willing to take a long, hard look at what she does and does not do in the supervisory process. Skill in supervision is not something one is born with, nor does it result from a formal course in supervision, but it is something one learns gradually over a period of time.

The supervisors who are healthy are able to say with the supervisee, "our patient," not in a possessive way, and not in a condemning way; to feel with the supervisee about the patient; and to feel that they are both participating in the treatment and management of the patient.

The nursing supervisor who does not continue to do some direct work with patients will not, in the long run, be as successful a supervisor as the one who does.

Question 18. Should training in individual supervision be part of the teacher-training of students in current masters-level programs that prepare teachers of psychiatric nursing? Should a masters graduate be certified as a teacher of undergraduate students unless she can carry out some of this supervisory process?

Discussion: This supervisory process has the value of helping the nurse function more effectively with patients and learn how to teach as a supervisor. The graduate student should supervise a basic student while she herself is being supervised.

Question 19. The supervisor and the clinician must be able to perform certain intellectual operations and be aware of the use of these operations.

a. Is the whole educational program focused on identifying and intensifying the intellectual competencies of the student, or does one give information, then try to get the student to think independently of that information later on?

Discussion: Students need to know when they are generalizing and when they are applying concepts and to recognize a host of other intellectual operations. This is where we should focus our efforts rather than on the personality of the nurse.

In order to apply a concept, one must know the concept, be able to make certain observations, determine which concept applies, utilize that concept to find out what further data are needed, and so on.

There is no reason to assume that there is a correlation between the ability to abstract something within a perception of the theoretical field and the ability to use clinical intellectual processes.

Question 20. At what point in the educational program should this kind of supervision begin?

Discussion: It should begin when the student first begins to care for patients.

Question 21. How can we discuss supervision without defining the theory of what we are trying to do?

No discussion.

Question 22. What kind of training must be provided for the pediatric nursing instructor and the medical-surgical nursing instructor who wish to give this kind of supervision in their clinical areas? What additional kind of didactic experience, plus supervised clinical experience, does a person need in the psychiatric area and in other clinical areas to prepare her for this supervisory role?

a. Is this method of supervision very feasible in other areas?

b. Is it as pertinent in other areas as it is in psychiatric nursing?

Discussion: In psychiatric nursing, you have exposure to concepts of behavior, psychodynamics, and psychopathology that you use in your understanding of people and apply to the supervisory process. It is not likely that graduate programs in the other clinical areas succeed in broadening a student's concepts of interpersonal relations and the concepts of human behavior through didactic instruction. We are not actually preparing teachers to engage in this individual supervisory process.

You cannot avoid having the supervisors in other clinical areas concentrate on nurse-patient interaction, since we have made the assumption that the essence of nursing is the nurse-patient relationship. One can identify certain common experiences and problems that every human being must face from birth through maturation to death. Illness of various kinds can be studied in each of these areas. Nursing educators should decide to concentrate certain learning experiences in one section of the curriculum and other learning situations in other sections. For example, one may learn most about the dying patient in a medical service and about separation anxiety in a pediatric service. Every nursing supervisor ought to be very much concerned about nurse-patient interaction regardless of her clinical field.

Question 23. Should the supervisor be a nurse?

Discussion: The supervisor of the student's clinical work should be a nurse. A psychiatrist may be used in addition to the nurse supervisor but not in place of her.

Question 24. Do nursing facilities have on-going seminars in which they can learn about new things without being placed in a student-teacher situation? Is this one way to approach the problem of educating others about supervision without making them feel competitive about a colleague?

Discussion: Examples of such seminars in two schools were given.

Question 25. What aspects characterize nursing as an art, and what factors tend to make it a science?

a. Does the practitioner contribute to the science of nursing or just practice the art of nursing?

Discussion: Nurses can make a real contribution by holding the microscope over the nurse-patient interaction in the psychotherapeutic areas and feeding what they learn about behavior into nursing itself.

Question 26. What safeguards need to be set up for students learning the supervisory process?

Discussion: Safeguards are learned in the student's experience with patients and her experience in being supervised.

Question 27. Is it possible, through the use of the group method of supervision, to achieve, more economically, the same ends that are achieved through individual supervision?

Discussion: Group supervision and individual supervision are two separate teaching methods, and one does not replace the other. (Examples of group methods of supervision now being practiced were discussed.)

Question 28. Do nurses pay enough attention to the significance of the nonverbal area of behavior?

Discussion: Nonverbal behavior is highly communicative. We know a great deal more about this area than we did five or ten years ago, but nurses have not been concerned enough about its implications for nursing. Medicine itself has ignored the nonverbal kinds of communication with patients. We need to study a great deal about what goes on in these types of communications.

Question 29. How are the concepts of mothering related to nursing? Is the nurse's role a mothering role?

Discussion: The nurse's role is a "mothering-like" one. However, she does not really mother patients. She does certain things that mothers also do to children, but she is actually not mothering patients; it is a different kind of relationship. The essence of this nursing relationship has to begin with some sort of nonverbal contact, particularly with regressed patients.

Care of the coronary patient is an example of the need for different kinds of nursing care at different stages of illness. The beginning is nonverbal and protective, the second phase is comparable to a parent's treatment of an adolescent, and finally there is the maturation phase in which the patient makes decisions for himself.

One of the chief concerns of the psychiatric nurse is the nonverbal communication area. One cannot examine the interpersonal relationship of a student with a patient without dealing with the nonverbal behavior. Work with regressed schizophrenic patients, where there would obviously be more nonverbal communication than verbal over long periods of time, illustrates this point.

Authors' Response to Discussion

The authors wish to mention again that the paper on individual supervision was written with psychiatric nursing as its clinical context, but that this in no way presupposes that the supervisory process described is limited to the area of psychiatric nursing. In addition, the clinical experiences mentioned have counterparts in other clinical fields. The fact that students have experiences that precipitate emotional responses or emotional conflict in any clinical area is a case in point.

One of the purposes of the project for which this paper was written was to discuss concepts and practices in the fields of psychiatric nursing, psychiatry, and the social sciences that might be used in teaching in all clinical areas of nursing. To achieve this purpose, both curriculum content and methods of teaching were considered. The paper on supervision was designed to deal with *one* teaching method, individual supervision, which was selected because it is one of the most effective ways of guiding a student's clinical learning. Individual supervision is one of the newest methods of teaching in nursing and one about which there is very little in nursing literature, whereas the many other teaching methods are discussed fully in nursing and educational publications.

There was much concern in the conference discussion about the following statement: "The authors believe that the essence of professional nursing is the meaningful, understanding, and scientific use of the interpersonal relationship with the patient. It is only through the full understanding of the therapeutic use of this relationship that the nurse can give expert nursing care and can assign duties to nonprofessional personnel and supervise them in carrying out the tasks." It would seem that further clarification is indicated. This statement, as such, was not intended to stand alone. The sentence which followed was considered by the authors to be an essential part of the idea we were attempting to express: "The physical and emotional components in any procedure or contact with a patient are inseparable in a therapeutic relationship." To us, an interpersonal relationship refers to all of the interaction that takes place between people. This includes what they think, feel, and do, which can be expressed by what they say (or do not say) and the ways they behave toward each other. In nursing, much of the interaction involves "doing something to" the patient that entails touch and manipulation of his body. The nurse, if she is concerned about the way a patient responds to or accepts nursing care, cannot ignore the communication that takes place on this bodily level. By the same token, she cannot deny the importance of the verbal communication with him. These two aspects of communication have to be considered as a whole. As the student learns to give nursing care, and as the supervisor guides her in this learning, all of these aspects of her interaction with patients are examined in the supervisory process.

It is equally important that the person who gives direct patient care and the person who delegates nursing care to the various kinds of nursing personnel comprehend the therapeutic potentials of all of the facets of interpersonal relationships in order to provide the best nursing care to patients. We get into many meaningless arguments when we center on only one component of the whole interaction between nurse and patient with the idea that this one is the only important one to the patient, and that we either do not have to be concerned about other factors or do not have time to consider them. These arguments, and many errors in nursing care, result from such a singular focus on either the importance of a physical procedure, a nurse's verbal ability, or her capacity for human warmth and kindness.

We stated in our paper that during the process of examining the student-patient interaction in the supervisory conference, it is the patient's behavior that is studied for its meaning. This statement precipitated considerable discussion. It was made only in relation to examining the nurse-patient data that the student brings to the conference. When one focuses on the patient's behavior in this manner, one is necessarily involved with how the nurse's behavior has influenced the patient. To this extent, the nurse's behavior is examined. We were attempting to show that the patient's behavior is examined in relation to understanding him and his pathologic condition and in relation to determining the effect of the nurse's actions.

In addition to the nurse-patient data, the student's activities in other areas of her work come to the attention of the supervisor. In these instances, as well as in some portions of the examination of nurse-patient interaction, the supervisor may be concerned with the student's learning problems and working relationships.

The paper apparently left the way open for our readers to think that we were concerned only with the verbal communication in the nurse-patient interaction, that our aim was to teach students to "be verbal" with patients and to interpret a patient's behavior to him. This was not the aim of our paper, nor is it a part of our philosophy in clinical practice. We believe that it is important for a student to think about what she does and how she behaves with a patient in order that she may plan and carry out nursing care with specific goals in mind. We are interested in helping her develop the ability to communicate clearly (both verbally and nonverbally) in her relationships with her patients and with colleagues who work with her, and at the same time continue to become more effective in the nursing tasks that are a part of her care of the patient.

A large portion of the supervision of any nurse-patient interaction is concerned with what is communicated in the behavior of the nurse in the ministrations of nursing care to patients. We believe that effective use of nonverbal communication is teachable, that even the most intuitive student can increase her skills in this area as she becomes more aware of what she does, and that even the least "naturally endowed" student can learn some of these skills. This teaching should begin early in the student's nursing program so she can gain increasing depth of understanding and skill in this area along with her development in ministering the technical procedures of nursing. The authors do not teach nursing students to make interpretations of a patient's behavior to him. We do not see this as a part of the basic student's armamentarium. The nurse deals with the patient's life as it is now being lived, in which she temporarily has a necessary part. She does not select certain aspects of his behavior or certain problems in his past experience to explore back to his generic roots as a psychiatrist might.

It becomes increasingly obvious from the discussion that if it had been within the scope of this paper to define fully what a nurse does in therapeutic situations, the discussion on supervision could have more clearly assumed its place as one teaching method of helping students learn how to give therapeutic nursing care.

Permission to reprint granted by the National League for Nursing.
Proceedings of the 1959 Conference at Boulder, Colorado of the National League for Nursing, 1960.

Toward Therapeutic Care: A Guide for Those Who Work with the Mentally Ill

Formulated by the Committee on Psychiatric Nursing, Group for the Advancement of Psychiatry, 1961

(Part One)

Theoretical Basis

I. Introduction

Therapeutic effectiveness in day-by-day nursing care depends upon nursing personnel's* understanding the patient's behavior and responding to it appropriately. The report deals with some psychiatric concepts which hopefully will lead to sounder understanding of the patient's behavior. Understanding should lead to clearer recognition of the patient's emotional needs and better corrective response to them. These concepts are discussed as current working formulations and a dynamic orientation is offered for persons, by whatever title designated, who participate in the daily 24-hour care, treatment, and rehabilitation of the mentally sick. The formulations and examples can be extended and applied to the fields of occupational therapy, physiotherapy, recreational therapy, vocational counseling, volunteer services, and other fields.

We hope that these concepts will be translated into daily action and thus will help the supervisor, teacher, or administrator to make his job assignments, conferences, and classes more purposeful. We also hope that this document will be useful to those concerned with instruction of professional nurses, practical nurses, psychiatric aides, attendants, psychiatric technicians, child care workers, orderlies, workers in the field of rehabilitation, and others who perform similar duties. All of these persons give direct patient care and are well aware of the complexity of human relationships. Too often these relationships are left anxiously unscrutinized. As a result the response and care may be anti-therapeutic.

A patient enters a psychiatric hospital because he has experienced difficulties in living which included a breakdown in relationships with other people. We assume that the behavior of the patient has meaning; that his behavior affects the behavior of those who care for him; and that the behavior of those who care for the patient affects him. The hospital must serve as a smaller world wherein new experiences in living and new personal relationships produce minimal anxiety and maximal support. Thus, the patient gradually may learn to feel that living with others is a less threatening and a less foreboding experience.

The patient's hospitalization should enable him to live more effectively with other people. Every mental illness includes the problem of the patient's particular way of relating himself to others and participating with others in activities. When a patient enters a mental hospital he has already established patterns of behavior to defend himself against anxiety-provoking relationships. Many of these defenses are pathological. In the attempt to cope with his anxiety, the patient chooses that form of expression which, in his past experience, has been most effective in maintaining distance from others for his subjective comfort.

In the hospital new personal relationships must gratify the patient's need, facilitate his communication with others, and enhance his social participation. It follows that the nursing personnel, who have the longest and most intimate contact with the patient are deeply involved in these processes. Every contact with the patient, whether in the performance of "official nursing care" or in a less directed capacity, involves patient-nurse relationships. The relationship can be therapeutic or harmful. If these relationships remain essentially therapeutic, they can become an integral part of the patient's whole therapeutic regimen. It is important for nursing personnel to understand and to be aware of the feelings, thoughts, and actions of the patients. They should have a similar understanding of their *own* thoughts and actions in any situation. Such awareness is acquired gradually. It depends upon repeated experiences with patients and the collaborative examination of these experiences with physicians, supervisors, and co-workers.

To enhance awareness of anxiety and of reactions and defenses to anxiety, we shall first discuss the theme of *regression* with symptoms of dependency which is part of every illness, mental and physical; second, we shall consider essential areas of dysfunc-

*The terms *nursing personnel* or *nurse* are used throughout the text to include all persons, whatever their titles, who are involved in the 24-hour care of the mentally sick patient.

tion; and, finally we shall re-examine the *changes in relationships* that invariably ensue when chronic and intense dependency are expressed.

These phenomena are readily available for continued observation in daily behavior. They are manifestations about which society has ideas of "normality," concepts of good and bad, and of morality and immorality. They raise problems, the mastery of which are the concern of patient as well as nurse.

Nursing personnel and physicians have different primary areas of responsibility and different techniques. It cannot be sufficiently emphasized, nevertheless, that whoever works with patients must face, and react constructively to, their behavior and the manifestations of regression and altered capacity for human relationships.

The recognition of these processes and the understanding of their dynamic significance can become a common denominator of all the different "therapies" to which the patient is exposed. Understanding of these processes offers a basis for communication among the various participants in patient care. Such communication in the hierarchy of personnel provides consistency and direction for the total therapeutic regimen. Moreover, understanding of these concepts should further facilitate the definition of different roles for personnel, and of the various levels and areas wherein each person can best make his contribution toward a plan of treatment.

It should be noted that the case studies illustrating a representative group of daily occurring clinical problems are not intended to offer definitive prescriptive models or techniques for solution of problems. Such an attempt could lead only to premature closure rather than to exploration of feelings and ideas. It is intended that the cases should serve to stimulate discussion and independent thinking. As they are analyzed they will: (1) reemphasize the already generally accepted concept of how nurses' feelings influence the quality of patient care; (2) highlight the importance of open communication among all personnel; and (3) emphasize the importance of adequate supervision. To illustrate significant and commonly occurring clinical problems we chose dramatic situations. A preponderance of these involve unsuccessful approaches.

We are describing a method for ongoing clinical practice. The nature of the patient's illness determines the treatment program. In order to get all relevant facts, treatment planning involves inadequate communication at all levels; all personnel must contribute. Conferences, discussions, and supervision will result in ongoing constructive reassessment of the treatment. As the patient changes, treatment changes, and as treatment changes, the individual contributions change. It is hoped that the selected illustrations of clinical problems will be a useful stimulant for supervisors and students in carrying out their own therapeutic programs.

II. Regression With Symptoms of Dependency

Editor's note: This section of *Toward Therapeutic Care* was published in 1955 in "Therapeutic Use of the Self: A Concept for Teaching Patient Care" almost exactly as the 1961 version. The Committee on Psychiatric Nursing of the Group for the Advancement of Psychiatry used Report No. 33 as a discussion focus in the intervening years. Please refer to pages 69 through 72 of "Therapeutic Use of the Self: A Concept for Teaching Patient Care."

III. Areas of Dysfunction

Editor's note: In the 1955 "Therapeutic Use of the Self: A Concept for Teaching Patient Care," the Areas of Dysfunction are presented almost exactly as printed in 1961. The only substantial difference was that they were reordered in their presentation. In 1961, the order was Diminished Integrative Capacity, Disturbance of the Function of Reality Testing, Change in Conventional Attitudes and Moral Standards, Inability to Control Basic Impulses, and Disturbance of Productive Activity. Please refer to pages 72 through 77 of "Therapeutic Use of the Self: A Concept for Teaching Patient Care."

IV. Decreased Capacity for Mature Relationships

Editor's note: The material in this section is not substantially different from the text as it appeared in the 1961 version. Please refer to pages 77 through 79 of "Therapeutic Use of the Self: A Concept for Teaching Patient Care."

(Part Two)

Clinical Applications

V. Function and Therapeutic Effectiveness of Nursing Personnel

In the foregoing discussion, we focused primarily on the *patient's* reaction and its meaning in the interpersonal relationship. In this discussion the focus is primarily on the *other person* in the relationship. As previously indicated the reaction of the nurse to the patient has direct effect on his progress. In this part, we attempt to analyze some of the reactions experienced by the nurse and their significance in this therapeutic relationship.

The function of the nurse is a complex one that has yet to be fully defined. Her functioning may vary from that of a controlling authority figure to a most permissive one. Traditionally, the nurse, like the physician, has been primarily concerned with facilitating more effective relationships and with utilizing interpersonal skills in the day-to-day care of the patient.

What may interfere with the therapeutic effectiveness of the nurse? The nurse must function in a situation of rapidly changing demands. She works with a variety of patients, with supervisors (nurses and physicians), with other nursing personnel, and with persons of other disciplines. She must work with individuals as well as with groups. She tries to cooperate with people of differing attitudes and responsibilities. The nurse responds to problems in ways which reflect her life experience and educational background. Each nurse has her own unique responses.

How well does she understand the way in which she responds to other people? Everything she says to the patient, everything she does for the patient, every move she makes — her very presence — exerts an influence on his immediate condition. The problem in nursing, then, is the nurse's understanding and utilization of her own natural reactions to other people rather than depending on prescribed or conventional attitudes. The nurse who examines her behavior discovers that her own attitudes, likes, dislikes, and other feelings enter into her every action, whether it be a technical nursing procedure or her very presence in the clinical setting. The nurse should be a therapeutic agent. What a nurse does, as a person, is as important as any other technical skill she may possess. Thus, when she understands her own emotions, her own motivations, and her own way of meeting and solving problems, she can function more effectively.

A patient may respond to a particular approach by a nurse in many different ways. He may react appropriately to her behavior or his response may be incomprehensible because his past life experiences and his present illness cause him to distort his perceptions of the total situation. For example, the refusal of a previously cooperative patient to comply with a nurse's request should not be responded to as an overt rejection. Rather, an assessment of the interaction should be made. In this way the feelings of the nurse about what the patient is communicating with this unexpected response can be more clearly understood. From such a realistic appraisal of the situation and her approach, the nurse should be able to gain further understanding, alter her response in light of this understanding, and thereby respond in a way most helpful to the patient.

To help the nurse in her self-appraisal is an extremely difficult task. Complete self-appraisal would require something approaching a personal analysis. Obviously, this is not possible without individual face-to-face discussion. With this limitation in mind, we evolved an approach that would effectively stimulate the nurse to reexamine the relevancies of her responses to the patient. We decided to use clinical material which helps to highlight the most common and typical situations to which the nurse must respond.

VI. Clinical Case Studies

In the material that follows, a number of clinical nursing problems are presented through illustrative case studies. In each of these cases, an attempt is made to identify the nurse's reaction to the patient's behavior and to show the relation of her response to the degree of therapeutic effectiveness. Out of an accumulation of experiences and a proper working through of such experiences, the nurse will develop the capacity for foresight — the ability to anticipate and predict. In so doing, she should be able to increase her therapeutic effectiveness.

Case 1. Withdrawal from the Demanding Patient

A handsome 21-year-old Latin American student was hospitalized with the diagnosis of paranoid schizophrenia. On the day of admission the patient was dejected and withdrawn but on the second day he became excited, appeared fearful of all personnel and several times shouted out of the window, "Help me! Murder! Murder!"

On another occasion, while personnel were preparing a cold-wet-sheet-pack, he thrust his fist through the window pane. Because of his agitation, "sleep therapy" was prescribed and, since he reacted with violence to male personnel, a female nursing student was assigned to care for him during the sleep treatment. She fed, bathed, and toileted him. Within a week the patient entered into group activities. About this same time the nursing student's assignment on this ward terminated.

The patient's only visitor was his mother, a fashionable and sophisticated woman. Mother and son were exceptionally close and walked down the corridors with their arms around each other. The nursing personnel were surprised to find that on each visit the mother left comic books and lollipops in his dresser drawer.

The patient became increasingly interested in group activities; simultaneously, he gradually became more attentive to the head nurse on his ward, although he rarely spoke to anyone else. One morning while this nurse was sitting with a group of patients, the patient after staring at her for some time said, "I have committed a sin." Following a non-directive technique that she had been taught, the nurse replied, "You have committed a sin?"

"Yes," he stated, "I have eaten my mother, and that is evil."

Glowering at the nurse, he left the room. Uncertain as to what to do next, the nurse decided to remain with the other patients.

The next day the patient began to follow her about the ward. Day after day, he waited patiently and quietly outside the nursing office until she emerged.

He would walk with her, staring intently, sometimes adoringly, and sometimes angrily. One afternoon as she gave him his medication, the patient smiled, looked deeply and intently into her eyes, touched her cheek, and said, "You are a good mother."

Again, the nurse restated his remark, "I am a good mother?"

"Yes".

The nurse reported this incident to the psychiatrist who was noncommittal in his response.

From then on, the nurse never allowed herself to be alone with this patient. Instead, she tried to interest him in group activities on and off the ward. He responded by withdrawal from any further attempts to get close to the nurse, other personnel, or patients.

In this example, when the nursing student was transferred, the patient turned his interest toward the head nurse, bidding for closeness with her and probably indicating what he may have perceived as a quite difficult relationship to his mother. This was communicated to the head nurse in disguised form by fantasies. The head nurse was too uncomfortable, could not accept the patient's movement toward her or utilize it in a way useful to the patient. The patient subsequently withdrew even further from relationships with other people on the ward.

Speculations about the nature of the problems of the head nurse which served as interferences to the progress of this patient must include the impact upon the nurse of having this handsome 21-year-old male patient following her around hour after hour. In addition, there was a disturbing effect of the patient's repeated, "You are a good mother," after having said, "I have eaten my mother." This, when associated with the patient's fluctuation between adoration and anger, aroused disturbed feelings in the nurse.

The head nurse faced a different situation than did the student. She had too many other patients to look after, while the student had only this one. The nurse had insufficient supervised experience in working with this kind of problem; also she was intimidated by the destructive nature of the expression of closeness. The student did not have to face this situation since the patient was in sleep therapy.

Under the circumstances, the nurse could not respond in an appropriate helpful manner to the patient's strong demands.

She could only respond to the patient in a stereotyped, inhibited manner as evidenced by her "non-directive" approach. This was her defense against the stress of the situation; here the "non-directive" approach impaired the therapeutic relationship.

Recognizing her difficulties she went to the physician for help. He, too, was "non-directive." As her attempts to gain support from him were unavailing, she could only withdraw.

Case 2. Meeting the Needs of the Over-Demanding Patient

Mrs. A who had been in the hospital for the past nine months had obtained a reputation for being difficult and a trouble-maker. She was transferred to Ward X, where she rapidly became the center of everyone's attention. She constantly asked the nurses to do things that in their opinion she was capable of doing herself, fetching her glasses from her room, fixing the hooks on her bra, etc. When the nurses refused to comply with her requests she became sarcastic and tried to persuade other patients to refuse medications and in other ways disobey the nurses. The nurses responded by putting her in seclusion and by making requests for her transfer to another ward.

Following a ward staff meeting, it was decided that Nurse M should give this patient special attention. Nurse M agreed to attempt to satisfy all her requests.

The other nurses were instructed to do the same when they had time. If they were busy they were to tell the patient so and refer her to Nurse M. The total situation was to be reviewed in one week. Initially, there was a rapid increase in the patient's demands. This lasted for a few days and then began to diminish. At the same time there was a marked improvement in her behavior. She ceased needling the nurses, ceased provoking the other patients to behave badly, and became relatively cooperative with all the nurses. Her dependency on Nurse M became marked. Initially, when Nurse M was off duty, Mrs. A's behavior would deteriorate. After two months of this regimen, when Nurse M was off duty, the patient became depressed instead of *acting out.* Prior to her relationship with Nurse M the patient was wont to talk loudly with other patients about her sexual relationship and exploits with her husband. Here, too, a marked change took place. The patient became reticent about her relationship with her husband, with everyone except Nurse M to whom she confided her fears about, and disgust for, the sexual act.

It is of interest to note that at no time during this period was the patient seen by any other therapist.

Case 3. Bribery Used for Acceptance

Kathy and Mary were intelligent, attractive, and thoroughly rebellious teen-agers who occasionally took it upon themselves to "test the limits" of the adolescent treatment unit. They reinforced each other in episodes of disruptive behavior and had eloped on three previous occasions. To prevent further elopement orders were written forbidding them to be allowed off the ward together. This order was especially emphasized when the treatment program for these two patients was discussed with the nursing students who received clinical experience on the ward.

The nursing student involved in the following incident was a shy, passive person who could not effectively accept or set limits. During her first two weeks on the adolescent ward she made only a few tenuous patient contacts, such as getting something for a patient or answering a direct question. This behavior contrasted with her ability to do excellent work on the geriatric ward; she had been described by her instructors in the geriatric service as alert, and conscientious, although over-compliant. After the first weeks the psychiatric patients made few requests of her and usually turned to one of the other nurses. She no longer participated in the shop talk of the other students, and had little to say at conferences about the patients.

During the fourth week, Kathy and Mary, separately and together, approached this student on numerous occasions and "permitted" her to do things for them. The student responded enthusiastically and intensified her efforts to comply with their requests until the following incident occurred.

One evening Kathy and Mary asked the student to take them off the ward and down to the lobby for a coke. She hesitated momentarily but acquiesced when Kathy said, "Oh it won't take but a minute. We can be back by the time you ask the head nurse. We knew we could count on you."

As soon as they reached the lobby and got the cokes, they threw them down and bolted for the unlocked door. Surprised and hurt, the student broke into tears and tried to catch them but was prevented by another patient who "playfully" held her until Kathy and Mary were out of sight.

The nurse returned to the ward to report what had happened. The head nurse attempted to utilize this incident to help the student achieve insight into why she had taken the patients off the ward without notifying anyone and had disobeyed the specific order prohibiting their absence from the ward. The student, however, was so overwhelmed with remorse that she could not reflect on her behavior. Paradoxically, she appeared to respond with increased guilt and anxiety to the head nurse's matter-of-fact, non-punitive attitude.

These data emphasize two related themes. First, the student's difficulty in coping with her own rebellious feelings are expressed in her identification with the two adolescents. That she had trouble coping with her rebellious impulses can be inferred from her characteristic over-compliance, her inability to function adequately when she was expected to exert control over patients who exhibited a high level of rebelliousness, and finally her direct impulsive flouting of authority. In contrast, she could function well with geriatric patients since their submission did not stimulate her rebelliousness.

Secondly, because of the adolescent nature of her conflict, she lacked sufficient inner controls and was not yet able to form mature identifications with the staff, her professional role, and its controlling effect on her own impulses. The non-punitive attitude of the staff as she interpreted it provided inadequate external reinforcement. Consequently, she tried to have only a minimum of contacts which remained superficial and tenuous. Avoidance of responsibilities would generate guilt and anxiety in such a conscientious person. Her withdrawal from the patients was followed by withdrawal from the staff and her fellow nurses.

The nurse's anxiety about her inability to relate to the patients expressed her conflict between the need to withdraw and the desire to reestablish herself professionally. Consequently, she was vulnerable when Kathy and Mary attempted to exploit her — especially since the price of their acceptance was only in terms of *doing* things for them. By catering to their requests, she effected an anxiety-alleviating compromise in which, by superficially relating to them and giving them care, she believed that they were accepting her.

The amount of anxiety and insecurity she experienced was directly reflected by her rebelliousness and the manner in which she acceded to their demands. Her anxiety was compounded by her own inability to assess the events correctly and the lack of necessary understanding and support from the supervisory personnel. This circular process of anxiety leading to withdrawal from patients and staff resulted in further anxiety and guilt, and culminated in the student's inability to respond to the head nurse's attempt to give her support or to achieve any degree of insight.

It is probable that the conscientious, highly motivated nurse is especially prone to being caught in this kind of dilemma when she is faced with a non-punitive matter-of-fact attitude by a person in authority. One often encounters this type of reaction in response to errors in judgment made early in a psychiatric experience. When supervision can intervene effectively in this process, a further step toward therapeutic use of the self occurs.

Case 4. Honesty vs. Hypocrisy

The remodelling of two wards (A and B) entailed the evacuation of all patients. Owing to uncertainty as to when the maintenance crews were going to start, numerous dates were set for their transfer. As each day for the move came round it was cancelled. The response of the patients on the wards was quite different. On Ward A, the patients remained stable even though they were annoyed by the repeated changes in dates set for their transfer. On Ward B, six patients became incontinent; there were four fights within a period of one week; a number of patients showed marked increase of psychotic manifestations, hallucinations, and delusions, etc.

On investigating the different responses of the two wards to the same situation, the following difference in nurse behavior was strikingly apparent. On Ward A, the nurses, too, were annoyed by the changing dates. Supported by their supervisor, they made no attempt to hide their annoyance and made it clear to the patients and other staff members that it was a response to administrative indecision. On Ward B, however, the nurses attempted to hide their annoyance and defended, somewhat hypocritically, the administrative vacillation, even when one of the more articulate patients was critical of the indecision. On Ward A, the nurses had maintained their fellowship with their patients through their honesty in feeling and communication. On Ward B, the patent dishonesty in feeling and communication of the nurses broke the relationship with their patients; hence, the marked increase of regressive behavior and *acting out*.

Case 5. The Professional Person as a Patient

Miss B, a 45-year-old surgical nurse, was admitted to the hospital on a voluntary basis. Her educational preparation included a Master's Degree, but she was retired from professional activity because of her emotional instability.

The head nurse was the only member of the nursing personnel able to establish a therapeutic relationship with the patient. She was not intimidated by Miss B and was able to accept the patient's truculent outbursts. Firm and persevering in enforcing ward regulations, the head nurse was able to remove a razor which the patient had obtained from other personnel contrary to ward policy. She treated Miss B as a patient despite her aggressive and patronizing behavior, but somehow she was unable to help other personnel in utilizing this approach.

The patient's behavior on the ward was characterized by a condescending and patronizing attitude toward the nursing personnel. She frequently criticized the personnel and referred to them as being stupid, lazy, and neglectful of patients. In response to these accusations the nursing personnel increasingly ignored her and permitted her to violate ward regulations.

Miss B's relationships with other patients were characterized by intimidation and condescension. She refused to participate in ward work assignments as she felt they were menial tasks and beneath her. Since she was overbearing and patronizing, the other patients on the ward did her work assignments as well as their own.

The patient was thus controlling her environment by intimidating the patients and all of the nurses except the head nurse. Furthermore, she intimidated the physicians by reporting them to the superintendent as incompetent, and adding a wide variety of other threats.

This illustration presents a common situation wherein a patient is not seen as a patient by psychiatric personnel. The patient's similar age, and professional and cultural background, may threaten the integration of the personnel. As a result, they may react to the threat by perceiving the patient as less sick than the patient really is. The person is not seen as a patient but as a hostile, bullying person.

Unable to maintain objectivity, the personnel recoil from the patient's hostility and participate with the patient in a mutual withdrawal process. The nursing personnel's position is reinforced when the physician is seen by them as being as helpless as they are in the situation.

It would seem that the head nurse's ability to work effectively with Miss B was based, at least in part, upon her ability to view her as a patient. As a result, she was able to be more objective and helpful to the patient than other members of the personnel. Although the head nurse was able to work effectively with the patient, she was unable to assist the ward staff in achieving this objective. The gratification that comes to a professional person from knowing that she is the only one who can work with a given patient may have been a deterring factor in the implementation of a successful nursing care plan. The total treatment plan was apparently not geared to meet the patient's need for a more structured ward environment. The personnel's perception of the patient's needs were distorted because of their involvement in the mutual withdrawal process.

Case 6. Placing the Blame

A young woman was admitted as a transfer from another hospital. In the previous hospital she had been closely supervised because of a severe depressive action, suicidal preoccupation, and a history of suicidal attempts. The self-destructive acts usually came in response to unanticipated separations from significant people and in response to the bickering between her parents or between her husband and her parents. Such bickering invariably distracted attention from her needs. She had little awareness of her contribution to the continuation of these behavior patterns.

In the new hospital, the more ominous depressive symptoms were not apparent, and a fairly permissive privilege program was instituted. Two weeks after admission the patient left the hospital grounds and committed suicide.

The nursing personnel reacted to the news of the suicide with two major responses. First, they made sure that there had been no negligence insofar as "orders" were concerned; no one could put the blame on them. Second, they directly and indirectly placed the blame for the tragedy upon the medical administration and the hospital in general.

The nursing complaint regarding medical administration was both general and specific. The general complaint was that the recent move towards an "open," "permissive" hospital atmosphere placed a responsibility on both patients and nurses which was not necessarily therapeutic. They felt that in a "permissive" atmosphere some self-destructive acts could not be prevented. Related to this view was their specific complaint about the administrative physician of the unit which had housed the depressed patient. Personnel stated that this psychiatrist changed his orders too hastily, was too permissive, and was not available when needed for direction. All in all, they had felt ignored and helpless in using their independent judgment. As the discussion of this problem continued, it soon became apparent that within the nursing service there was considerable conflict regarding the increasing autonomy of the nursing department entailed in the responsibilities of a more open hospital. Some nurses said, "We have to grow into the idea of being autonomous and trusting our own decisions. If we disagree with an administrator, we have to talk it out with him. We frequently fall down in setting limits because we feel we will be criticized by administrator or therapist."

With the growing awareness of inter- and intraservice conflict, the wide implications of "placing the blame" became clearer. The ward administrative physician was quite new to the hospital, and the senior administrative physician and the clinical director were not readily accessible because of vacation schedules. They were not able to supply close supervision and support for the ward administrator during this period of acclimation. Also, during this period of the patient's two weeks at the hospital, the director of nursing was on vacation and the area nursing supervisor had to extend her activities. Thus, the key personnel were not available and this played an important part in the feelings of helplessness experienced by the nurses. In addition, the more experienced administrative personnel might have diagnosed an impending crisis and taken more appropriate action.

The dissension in the staff closely duplicated the patient's lifelong experience of parental bickering and resultant inattention to her needs. That the nursing service was amply aware of the patient's need for supervision is observed in the comment of the ward charge nurse: "She (the patient) said everything was rosy, and I kept telling her things were not this way. I can't help it if she did come from a hospital where she was under lock and key; it wasn't that much rosier here." The nurse made the pertinent clinical observation that a depressed patient who suddenly, without good reason, begins stating that things are much rosier in a new situation is probably a most serious suicidal risk. During each of the two days preceding the suicide, the patient was permitted unescorted ground visits of ten hours with her mother. The mother was notorious for her belittling and demanding attitude toward her daughter. The patient's need for some protection from this was seemingly ignored.

On the day of the suicide, the charge nurse was off duty. The therapist phoned in sick that morning, and the patient was told he would not be seeing her. The nurse in charge failed to report this information to the nursing office and to the medical administration.

Once again, the patient's needs were not clearly seen even though this separation from charge nurse and therapist directly duplicated for her previous unanticipated separations to which she had reacted by self-destructive attempts. There were no limitations of privileges, no special escorts, even though both such actions can be taken by nursing personnel in emergency conditions. On this score, too, there was for the patient a duplication of adverse life experiences to which she was most sensitive.

For all persons there is increased anxiety and a lessened ability to express feelings when there is real or imagined lack of clarity in responsibility, authority, and sources of support. Such increased anxiety interferes with constructive awareness of other persons' needs. In an institutional setting, this may result in a disaster. The reaction of personnel to a disaster is often very revealing of the stresses and strains within an institution. In this case, the process of "placing the blame" was an attempt to handle an anxiety and guilt-laden situation. When the data became available, retrospective analysis made it clear that several opportunities for therapeutic intervention had been missed. In addition, the situation compounded anxieties already at play and revealed schisms in the institutional structure. Hopefully, the ultimate analysis and resolution of such a hospital-wide crisis leads to a re-evaluation of the therapeutic climate and an increased therapeutic use of self by all personnel.

Case 7. Blackmail With "Gifts"

Mrs. C is a 50-year-old housewife and mother whose present hospitalization occurred after she had presented several neighborhood children and their families with "gifts" of poisoned candy. She felt that they had not accepted her in a friendly manner. Previously, she had been hospitalized following the birth of the first of her two daughters. Her marriage had been incompatible, and her entire life history was one of considerable turbulence.

In the hospital, Mrs. C proved to be a "good patient." Although she was somewhat curious and prying, she had come to be accepted by the staff; this acceptance was, in part, through her numerous gifts of crocheting.

During the Christmas holidays, this woman was an active contender in a contest for the "most originally decorated door." Several of the judges were nursing staff personnel who had been recipients of her "little tokens." One by one, she singled them out and told them that the gifts they had accepted had been made from hospital supplies. The intent to blackmail was little disguised.

Two of the nurses thus confronted became uneasy and assured her of their support. Another angrily went to her supervisor, protesting with chagrin that she had been blackmailed; however, she did not wish to "make trouble." One judge told the patient that he would vote for the door he thought to be the most original. This particular judge was able to discuss the matter further with Mrs. C, reminding her that the staff had not been aware of the source of the gifts and, in general, was able to clarify the realistic factors in the situation. The patient was able to accept this, and her manipulations stopped. Furthermore, she acknowledged her awareness of what was going on and said that she had known the others would be frightened and would vote for her.

This incident illustrates the need for a knowledge of the motivation of the behavior patterns utilized in order to gain acceptance. Meeting such a patient's manipulative maneuvers is a somewhat simpler task in the light of her previous history and an understanding of the meaning of her many gifts. It is interesting that this was apparently not taken into consideration by many of the personnel, or utilized by them in understanding and in dealing with this particular patient. This may have been, in part, related to the rather frightening nature of the earlier deeds. However, from the theoretical standpoint, this extreme only highlights the general principle involved, namely, the need of the patient to be accepted and the subtly coercive maneuvers to gain this acceptance. The similar origin and meaning of the words *gift* and *poison* is rather nicely substantiated by the dynamics operative in this case.

Another important factor which may be noted in this case has to do with the necessity for an over-all assessment and understanding of the ward situation at the time an incident occurs. It is a well-known observation that childhood sibling rivalries and feelings of rejection by parental figures come into the foreground at the Christmas season. Of course, this is true of personnel as well as patients and may account for an increase in problems during the holiday season.

In this case, as in many instances of *manipulative behavior* in a hospital setting, one of the most appropriate and immediate means of handling the situation is clarification of the reality situation to the greatest extent practical. The judge, who was personally most secure, was in a position to comprehend, test the situation adequately, and deal with it in a manner that was therapeutic. For whatever reasons, this particular individual was not intimidated by the double-edged meaning of the gift and of the acceptance of the gift.

Case 8. The Patient as a Victim of Misunderstanding in Supervision

The following clinical observations, demonstrating nurse-patient interaction, were selected from a three-month participation-observation study carried out by a graduate student nurse. The patient was seen by the nurse one hour daily, four days a week. The nurse was supervised by the staff psychiatrist and had frequent conferences with the Director of the Graduate Nurse Program. These observations covered a period of two months, during which the patient talked of running away with increasing frequency. Approximately three weeks later the patient carried out her threat in a way that was quite disturbing to the nurse.

Over a period of one and one-half months, the patient had talked about wanting to go home each time she was seen by the graduate nurse. Most of these comments were countered with the nurse's statement, "You must have permission from our doctor before you can leave the hospital." On a few occasions, the subject was initiated by the nurse: "Do you still think a lot about going home? Why do you think you would like to go home," etc.

The day the patient ran away she was taken, at her request, beyond the hospital limits to a park. A verbatim account of the incident, taken from the participant-observation studies, follows:

> The patient said, "Let's walk on down to the river."
>
> I looked at my watch and said, "I'm sorry, but don't feel we will have any time to go further."
>
> She looked at me with a pained expression on her face and said, "But I don't want to go back. Can't we walk down to the river?"
>
> "I'm afraid that would be a little too far for us to go, and besides, we don't have time."
>
> "I'm not going back," she answered. "I'm going to walk on home now that I'm this far."
>
> "But you'll have to go back, Mrs. D, you can't go home without the doctor's permission."
>
> "No, I'm going home. You go back and I'll see you later." With this the patient got up and hurriedly started off in the opposite direction.
>
> I called as I ran behind her. "Please come back, Mrs. D, and let's go talk to the doctor about going home."
>
> She suddenly changed her course and started back towards me; I got the impression she wasn't coming back to me, but from the way she was looking around she didn't seem quite sure of the way she wanted to go. As she came past, I caught her by the arm.
>
> She was quiet for a short while as I talked to her. "Mrs. D, you don't want to go home this way. You will only have to be brought back. If you wait until you have the doctor's permission, you can stay for a while and not have to worry about someone coming after you."
>
> With this the patient broke away from me and ran. I followed her to a building where I telephoned the hospital to send some help. I then went out to the road and watched as she ran out of sight. I waited for the hospital car and we then started out to look for her. We quickly found her walking down the railroad track.

During her work with the patient, the nurse had become increasingly anxious about her relationship with the supervising staff psychiatrist. She felt he was not really interested in helping her, and this manifested itself in many ways; questioning her in great detail about her interaction with the patient (which had been recorded for him so that he could read it previous to her appointment with him); spending time during the hour explaining basic concepts of psychiatry which did not seem pertinent to her, etc. She had tried frequently to discuss with him her feelings about escorting this patient on walks because she considered her an elopement risk, and had pointed out the patient's verbalizations which seemed to reinforce this danger. The nurse felt he dismissed this too casually; he made the following statement two days prior to the patient's attempted escape: "D's just talking — she won't go anyplace. She doesn't have enough energy to walk out the door if it were unlocked. I think you're over-reacting."

Subsequent discussion with the nurse revealed that perhaps she had actually wanted the patient to run away and had encouraged this by taking her to an area considered off-limits by the hospital. She stated that the nursing service personnel on the unit had teased her about the incident and that the supervising psychiatrist had expressed amazement that it had occurred. She still felt very antagonistic toward the psychiatrist for putting her "in that position;" she could not resolve her feelings toward him and, eventually, became overtly hostile to the patient. This outburst was quite unusual for this nurse. She had immediately felt very guilty, anxious, and depressed, and said to the Director of the Graduate Nurse Program the day of the first incident, "I just can't work with this patient anymore; she's bound to suffer. All the feeling I have toward the psychiatrist is being displaced onto the patient. I know it, but I can't do anything about it."

In addition to the displaced hostility, a large part of the nurse's resentment toward the patient stemmed from the fact that the patient had in many ways rejected her attempts to form a relationship. The nurse acutely felt a sense a failure, and her rather intellectualized insights about her displaced feelings were at least partially a defense against the anger she felt toward the patient for rejecting her. The patient's *acting-out* in this particular incident appears to have resulted from the anxiety generated by being caught in the middle of the doctor-nurse struggle.

In many ways what happened is similar to the "mirror-image" mechanism described by Stanton and Schwarz. The doctor and nurse were mutually antagonistic and talked past each other. Instead of dealing with their feelings directly, they tacitly agreed to disagree about the patient. On the one hand, the doctor became less concerned about the possibility of elopement (although the patient had done so frequently); on the other hand, he became much more restrictive and withdrew many of the patient's privileges without explanation to either the patient or the nurse. The nurse followed an opposite pattern of becoming increasingly concerned with the problem of escape, but going to great lengths to cater to the patient by buying her cigarettes and stretching the rules concerning privileges. The patient, caught in this web of compounded inconsistency, perhaps attempted to run away to clarify her status. She did not know that she was a victim of disagreement between the psychiatrist and the nurse but sensed the tension. Her subsequent behavior forced the staff to take definitive restrictive measures.

Case 9. Contrasting Expectations

Mr. G was a 34-year-old man who had been hospitalized intermittently for many years. At times he was severely disorganized in his thinking, careless about his appearance, and impulsively assaultive. At other times he was in fairly good contact, friendly, and displayed a good sense of humor. Visits by his parents were often disturbing. They hovered over Mr. G, picked at him about minor details of his appearance, and criticized him for overeating. His mother was particularly guilty of this and seemed oblivious to the impact that it had on her son. He frequently became disturbed in her presence and she in all seriousness suggested that it must be because he didn't like the particular type of glasses she was wearing.

During one of his better periods, while on the way to the dining room, the patient passed his psychotherapist and ward psychiatrist in the hall. He smiled at them and then very deliberately continued to walk as though he were going to leave the building rather than go to the dining room. A student nurse who was escorting the patients to the dining room followed him to the front lobby and asked him to return. The patient gave no indication that he was making a serious attempt to leave the hospital and there was plenty of help available should it be needed. The student nurse waved her finger at him and said sharply, "Go right back and get down to the dining room." The patient raised his arm more in a gesture of irritation than as a threat to strike her. The student again shook her finger in the patient's face, saying "Mr. G, don't you dare raise your hand to me!" At this point the patient struck her in the face, knocking her to the floor. He became disturbed, confused, and mumbled incoherently. Only after several days did he gradually emerge from his disturbed state.

The student nurse in this case felt her professional competence threatened by the patient's behavior (especially because of the large audience) and she lashed out vigorously. Unwittingly she had triggered the patient's response by behaving in a way similar to his mother. Contrast her handling of this incident with that of the head nurse when she was faced by a similar situation.

Mr. G was being escorted by the head nurse to an appointment with his therapist. This made it necessary for them to walk a distance of several hundred yards on the grounds. As they started, the patient abruptly changed course as if he planned to leave the grounds. The head nurse stayed with him emphasizing that his psychiatrist was expecting him and that he did not have permission to leave the grounds at this time. Mr. G slowed up a bit but continued towards the front gate. The head nurse repeated the limits saying "Mr. G, you can't go off the grounds; you have to go to your appointment." He replied to this saying, "Well, it's going to take force." The head nurse, sensing that the patient was not too serious about wanting to leave the grounds and appealing to his sense of humor, said, "Well, I certainly can't force you; why don't we go find some aides who can?" Mr. G laughed, walked with the nurse until they found an aide, and went to his appointment without further protest. In this instance the nurse had had greater experience with the patient and was better able to predict his behavior. Perhaps even more important, she did not feel threatened and did not need to react defensively.

The student nurse expected trouble and she got it. The head nurse felt able to handle the situation and she was.

Case 10. Myth of the "Dangerous Patient" as Exploited by the Ward Personnel

Mr. E, a short, stocky Irishman, was proud of being considered the most troublesome patient in the entire hospital. He was suspicious, irritable, belligerent, and averaged at least one fight each day. If another patient so much as brushed his arm or dared to use any particular article to which Mr. E had staked claim, he would strike without warning. It was clear to all nursing personnel that Mr. E was deriving a great deal of satisfaction from the attention paid to him. He was all too willing to be "martyred" by being secluded. If he were placed in cuff restraints, he took advantage of the occasion to demonstrate that he could still beat any other patient on the ward by using his feet and forehead. Despite the fact that technically he was a poor fighter and rarely injured anyone except himself, his reputation for being "a very dangerous patient" grew until it acquired the status of fact. Rarely did the morning report fail to highlight one of his outbursts. Few hospital bull-sessions failed to cover the latest gossip about him. In fact, an outside observer would have readily seen that Mr. E consumed an almost unbelievable amount of time and energy of the staff on this three hundred bed unit.

To the new ward doctor, this patient presented the challenge of his then brief career as a psychiatrist. If he could do anything with this patient, "who everybody knew was difficult," his local reputation as a therapist would be assured.

From the beginning, the doctor let it be known that Mr. E was to receive special treatment and privileges. Even in this over-crowded state hospital ward, a private room for the patient was arranged. If the patient did not want to eat in the dining room with the rest of the patients, he was to be served in his room. When Mr. E, in one of his tantrums, kicked in the ward radio, the doctor saw to it that he got his own private radio which could be kept in his room.

The doctor then announced that the patient was to be actively encouraged to verbally express his hostility, and that any time the patient felt angry towards any of the aides, the doctor, the patient, and the aide involved would go into the office and "have it out." This arrangement resulted in an increasing series of incidents in which the patient accused the aide of having struck or kicked him while attempting to break up one of his fights with other patients. The aides viewed the "having it out" sessions as kangaroo courts where the patient took the role of prosecutor, the aide that of the defendant, with the doctor acting as judge, who always found the defendant guilty. The aides retaliated by not only failing in trying to prevent Mr. E from fighting with the other patients but by actually encouraging the more aggressive patients to "stand up for themselves." In the following months, Mr. E's episodes of assaultive behavior increased greatly, and he was injured several times by the aides while they were ostensibly breaking up a fight.

By this time, none of the personnel on the unit was impartial or un-involved, and a close look at the situation revealed that Mr. E's assaultive behavior was tacitly tolerated, if not actually abetted, by the doctor and the aides.

An observer who entered the ward at the height of the difficulty noted that the emotional reactions of the personnel when reciting their latest trials with this patient did not at all correspond to their account of how much trouble he had caused them. On the contrary, their reactions contained elements of pleasure and satisfaction.

The aides, however, were quite angry at the doctor.

The latter, on the other hand, felt that most of the aides were a calloused bunch of "bughousers" who could not, or would not, understand his treatment program. It must be said that the hospital, at this time, was undergoing extensive reorganization and that the doctor's appraisal of some of the aides was not totally incorrect. As is the case in every attempt to change a hospital from one of custodial care to an active treatment center, there was a great deal of sensitivity to anything which smacked of being "an old-time method," especially physical abuse of the patients. The doctor's conscious and unconscious motivations led him to capitalize on this intolerance of any rough handling by using the patient's assaultiveness to create incidents which would permit him to get rid of those aides who he felt were undesirable.

It is also possible that through his identification with the patient he achieved some personal satisfaction in being aggressive toward those aides who stubbornly resisted all of his new ideas about patient management.

In addition to the short-term gain which the doctor derived in achieving his ends through the assaultive behavior of this patient, there are other more general aspects of the "dangerous patient myth." It is a commonplace occurrence for the behavior of patients to be exaggerated far out of proportion and thus to be perpetuated in the verbal tradition of the psychiatric unit thereby becoming a ward myth. This is most true for the aides, although occasionally the nurses participate in this fiction. This particular myth of a dangerous patient creates an atmosphere of tension and potential violence on the ward which serves some of the inner needs of the personnel which have rarely been made explicit. Interviews with the aides on this ward revealed that job prestige ran on a continuum from infirmary or geriatric unit which was poorly regarded to "this ward" which was highly prized. Examination of these phenomena revealed some of the hidden motives for the exaggeration and the barely covert encouragement of assaultive behavior.

One of these motives was the aide's need for status. All too often the aide feels that in the eyes of others, there is nothing which he can do better than anyone else on the psychiatric team except physically restrain the assaultive patient. Further, he believes that the doctor's and nurse's technical competence in all other aspects of patient care exceeds his, and that his contribution is unique only when *muscle* is required. As a consequence, the aide believes that none but he can cope with the assaultive patient. Status and prestige are then derived from the aide seeing himself in the role of protector of the doctor and the nurse, and as indispensable to their efforts with the patient. On the other hand, aides who feel insecure and resentfully see themselves as being without status or power will often fantasy and talk about letting the assaultive patient be the instrument of their aggression — by allowing him to strike the doctor or nurse. From insights into the folklore of the hospital, attitudes can be detected which tend to foster combative behavior in the patient.

Another and more pathological of these motives which exploit the assaultive tendencies of the patient can be observed in some of the personnel who prefer to work on acute wards with combative patients. An observer can often detect elements of pleasure in the excitement following an emergency caused by an assaultive outburst. This is most clearly seen in those of the personnel who must make the greatest struggle to control their own aggressive tendencies.

Such personnel tend to externalize their inner conflicts by projectively attributing them to patients; then, by vigorously suppressing combative behavior between the patients, they are in a sense reassured of their own self-control. In addition, they strike a posture of hyper-vigilance and react to a slight scuffle as though it were a serious assault. These attitudes and behavior communicate a feeling of tension to the patients which set in motion assaultive impulses.

There is another common situation in which the staff uses one patient to give vent to its hostility toward another patient. This often occurs when the ward personnel are in disagreement with each other about the management of a troublesome patient. For example, there is the patient who is "into everything" and continuously exhibits provocative behavior such as taking things which belong to other patients, stopping up lavatories, etc. If adequate management devices are not agreed upon, the ward personnel often find themselves in an ambiguous position, and their frustration generates hostility toward the patient. In such circumstances, it is not rare for an aide to remark, "Just wait until he (the troublesome patient) messes around with Mr. So-and-So (a potentially assaultive patient); he'll take care of him." By relaxing vigilance and permitting one patient to assault another in a case such as this, the aide not only achieves some satisfaction of his aggressive feelings toward the patient but also uses the incident to demonstrate to the doctor or nurse the need for better management of the patient.

Many strains are apparent in settings in which the myth of the dangerous patient is exploited by nursing personnel to vent their anger and gain prestige. In the light of the foregoing discussion, techniques such as those employed by the new ward doctor in this case are questionable. He attempted to teach the aides a lesson only to have them retaliate in kind.

Case 11. Multiple Seduction

Mr. S, a 19-year-old veteran of two reformatories and the state penitentiary, was admitted to the hospital by a court order following the attempted rape of a 43-year-old woman on the day that he had been paroled from prison. He was of dull normal intelligence, small in stature, and unattractive. However, he was friendly, courteous, and extremely attentive to the student nurses on the ward, one of whom, Miss A, became quite involved with him. She talked at length with the resident psychiatrist about this patient. The doctor, young and inexperienced, did not report any of these discussions to the head nurse; instead, he focused on the more lurid aspects of the patient's previous sexual behavior. The doctor and this student nurse began dating regularly. These unusual circumstances provided the setting for the following disruptive entanglement.

The patient was interviewed and presented to the class of affiliate students (including Miss A) as an example of a manipulative sociopathic individual. One week later, following lunch, Mr. S eloped. Soon after, Miss A sought out the housemother to state her fear that the patient would try to see her at the nurses' residence. When questioned, she admitted having given the patient the telephone number and address of one of her relatives with whom she visited on weekends. Further questioning brought out that she felt sorry for the patient, considered him a victim of circumstances, did not feel that he was in any way mentally ill, and was convinced that the ward personnel (with the exception of the resident) mistreated him. The housemother told the student to discuss her feelings about the patient with her instructor. Miss A agreed but did not do this.

A few hours later the patient was returned to the hospital. The next morning he again eloped, and a few minutes after leaving the ward he was seen on the grounds talking to Miss A. She did not report his elopement to anyone, but some of the other students who had seen the patient talking to her told the housemother, who then reported this to the instructor. When questioned, Miss A freely, almost defiantly, admitted that she had not intended to report the patient because "he is such a sweet person and I wanted him to have a chance to go out and get a job and make something of himself." Several nights later when she and two other student nurses were together in an apartment in town, Mr. S telephoned and asked her to meet him in a downtown bar. Miss A became very frightened and notified the hospital authorities.

Later, apprehended and in jail, Mr. S made a number of accusations against Miss A, in regard to her dating the resident.

Mr. S was unusually skilled in making others feel sorry for him. In addition to obtaining sympathy, his ability to involve the nurse in conversations with sexual overtones served to reassure him that he was sexually attractive to women, and gave him stature with other patients in his age group. Always in the background was his need to flout and subvert authority.

Miss A's needs included elements of adolescent rebellion against authority; she had had minor disciplinary problems in the past.

She was not the sort of nurse who is vulnerable because of strong needs to "mother" patients. She had been influenced by her over-identification with the patient as an underdog who was misunderstood, and by the direct excitement of their discussion on sexual matters. The resident psychiatrist abetted the acting out. He had actually encouraged interest in the patient's sensational sexual escapades. In addition, his participation facilitated Miss A's flimsy rationalizations about her interest in the patient.

The needs of the resident are relevant to a more complete understanding. He was also being seductive with the student in his conversations about the patient. First, his talks with her were almost exclusively concerned with the patient's seductive behavior toward her; little was said about the management of the patient. Second, he did not report any of this to the nurse in charge of the students, which indicates some guilt on his part arising from unprofessional elements in his own behavior. Third, he began dating the nurse at this time and joined her with other students and their dates on weekend parties. The resident, as an active participant in the process, needed to prevent the student from seeing the patient as being mentally ill. He used his discussion of the patient's behavior as a part of his own seductive approach to Miss A. It was then necessary to deal with his own guilt. One way to accomplish this was by regarding the patient as not being mentally ill. Since the patient did not exhibit any of the more noticeable symptoms of neurosis or psychosis and had been diagnosed as a sociopathic personality, "depatientizing" him was facilitated.

However, if the doctor presented the patient's

behavior to the student as being that of a *psychopath*, with the moral connotations which are inevitably attached, he would seemingly put himself in the position of disapproving seductive behavior. Therefore, to avoid such sabotage of his own designs, he glossed over the sociopathic aspects of the patient's personality and presented him as deprived and misunderstood. By all of these maneuvers the resident also succeeded in denying his own problems. The student's needs made her more receptive to this view and the stage was set for multiple seduction, although it was no longer clear just who was seducing whom.

Case 12. Group Check on Reality

This case involves two female schizophrenic patients, both physically robust women, both on the same ward and, at the time of this occurrence, both nearly symptom-free. Both had grounds privileges and both attended social functions in the hospital.

At one of these functions they met a male patient, a markedly narcissistic, psychopathic, epileptic individual. This man was notorious for his flirtations with female patients. During the dance he approached the two women and intense two-person relationships rapidly developed between him and each of the females. Prior to this, the two women had been friendly on the ward. With the advent of the male patient their friendship ceased, they stopped talking, avoided each other, and there was a recurrence of persecutory ideas. The nurses became anxious and frightened, expecting a fight and other unspecified unpleasant happenings to occur.

On the initiative of a head nurse, the ward administrator arranged a meeting with the two female patients and a number of others with whom the man had had similar previous intense relationships. The senior nurse explained to all the patients at the meeting that two patients in the group were at odds over this man, and asked for their comments. The nurse's statement was immediately followed by roars of laughter from all the uninvolved patients who immediately proceeded to tell of their experiences with this man, telling how he had promised to marry them, how he would help them to obtain and pay for divorces, although he, in fact, had no money and only used females for his own gratification. In the face of this new information the two patients started to relax and began to ask questions. Initially, each insisted that the man was serious in his attentions. Gradually, under pressure of evidence given by other patients, they started doubting and cross-checking with each other. Lastly, both turned on the nurse. Why hadn't she warned them? The nurse apologized and stated that it was too late for warning by the time the situation was recognized. Why didn't the hospital protect patients from such happenings? The nurse pointed out that the man was ill and that when his privileges were refused, as they had been in the past, he became much worse.

Following this discussion, which lasted over an hour, the two patients re-established their positive relationship with each other and the over-all tension on the ward rapidly diminished.

Case 13. Vulnerability to Patient's Perceptiveness

Mr. P was a financially successful, 53-year-old real estate broker who was admitted to the hospital following a two-week period of hyperactivity, during which he had slept very little, ceased to be concerned with his personal appearance, and displayed increasingly poor judgment in his business dealings.

On admission he attempted to assume control over the situation with considerable urgency and to make it clear to the nurse that he was not to be reduced to patient status. His first remark was, "I'm very interested in seeing firsthand just what you do for these people here." He then continued at length, in a confidential and convincing way, to inform the nurse that he played a prominent part in the activities of the local mental health association, and was on intimate terms with several of the hospital officials.

Contrary to the usual admission procedure, the nurse first offered to show him around the ward. Mr. P readily agreed, and by his interested, intelligent questions and his authoritative bearing soon took command of the tour, placing the nurse in the role of guide. Within twenty minutes, he had inspected the entire ward, with special attention to the kitchen and bathrooms, had introduced himself to the majority of patients and staff, and had demonstrated how the number of chairs in the day room (with adequate reading light) could be doubled by rearranging three lamps. His speech became rapid, his body movements were accelerated, and his authoritative but polite requests became demands.

In an attempt to regain control of the situation, which she now realized was out of hand, the nurse abruptly said, "You have seen enough of the ward. Come with me, and we will complete your admission. You must take a shower. I'll take your clothes and have them marked." The patient replied in a loud voice, "Young lady, you will not take my clothes, and I do not need a shower. I've got a hell of a lot to do and, from the looks of this place, so have you. Now, I'll just move one of these tables out in the hall for a desk, and I'll need that pen and paper you have there."

The patient reached out and took the pen from the nurse's pocket and jerked the clipboard of admission forms from her hand. The nurse made no effort to prevent his taking these things and, without a word, turned and rapidly walked into the nurse's station. She immediately called three male aides, informed them that the patient was excited, and that they were to complete the admission procedure. She then added, "You may have to restrain him to give him his bath. In the meanwhile, I'll call the doctor and get a seclusion order."

The nurse immediately called the resident and told him she felt the patient was becoming "just too manicky." The resident attempted to reassure her, saying he had seen the patient forty-five minutes before, and while he might be a little hyperactive, he would rapidly adjust to the ward. He agreed, however, to see the patient.

When the resident arrived, the patient went to greet him, shook hands, and said, "Doctor, you were certainly right when you told me that we've got a long way to go on this mental health business. I've got to have more cooperation...."

The doctor interjected, "Mr. P, you *must* complete the admission routine, and then I'll talk to you in my office."

The patient turned to the resident, pointedly looking at a prominent silver capped tooth about which the doctor was unduly sensitive, and said: "All that glitters is not gold; you must be a sterling character, and I'd like to see you in *my* office."

The resident replied, "Mr. P, I'll see you only after you've done what the nurse has asked you to." He then walked into the nursing station, wrote the seclusion order, and instructed the aides to complete the admission of the patient.

The provocative behavior of the patient (his grabbing the nurse's pen and papers, etc.) does not appear to be commensurate with such an intense flight and fright reaction from the nurse, especially when this particular nurse had had considerable experience with disturbed patients. A closer look at the data, however, shows several additional sources of apprehension, some or all of which could have produced this reaction. First, the patient was successful in insidiously gaining control and completely dominating the situation. He accomplished this by capitalizing on his accurate perception of the nurse's need to accede to those in authority as well as her concern with social status. The nurse, in turn, perhaps due to these same needs, focused on the healthy, well-organized aspects of the patient's behavior, ignoring the pathological implications. Thus, the nurse relinquished her authority and thereby impaired her ability to structure the situation necessary for the patient's treatment.

The nurse, instead of protecting the patient by restricting the amount of stimulation, actually exposed him to excessive stimuli by taking him on a complete tour of the ward. By the time she perceived the patient's hyperactivity, she could no longer smoothly effect control over the patient's behavior. The patient's complete rejection of her crude and desperate attempts to set limits served to further increase her apprehension; as a result, when he jerked the pen and paper away from her she reacted as if she had been subjected to actual physical assault.

The doctor was also vulnerable to the patient's aggressive perceptiveness. The patient's cutting reference to his silver tooth and "sterling character" struck the resident, and he responded by withdrawing from the patient. By writing the seclusion order, he re-enforced the nurse's inaccurate assessment of the patient's behavior. This nurse had in the past been quite successful in caring for overactive patients. It might be helpful to view her inadequacy in the present instance.

Frequently, in nursing texts, behavioral hyperactivity is considered as an entity, and principles and procedures for patient-care do not take into consideration essential qualitative differences in hyperactivity. Excited behavior of a random, non-goal-directed type such as is often seen in schizophrenia elicits different emotional responses on the part of the nurse than the more goal-directed, more controlling behavior of the manic patient. Behavior of the latter kind, with direction and purposefulness, often arouses much more anxiety in the staff than an equal degree of disorganized hyperactivity. One explanation of this reaction lies in the fact that the diffuse non-purposeful type of over-activity is sufficiently alien to the nurse's own feelings so that there is little possibility of her identifying with this aspect of the patient. On the other hand, as in the incident above, the purposefulness and goal-directedness of the patient's over-active behavior sufficiently corresponded to feelings within the nurse so that some identification was possible, and control over her own impulses was threatened.

Case 14. Conflicting Therapeutic Goals — "Furor Therapeuticus"

Mr. J, a 38-year-old lawyer, was admitted to the hospital because of increasing signs of depression, characterized by feelings of hopelessness, self-deprecation, anorexia, and insomnia. One year prior to the current admission Mr. J had been hospitalized with approximately the same symptoms. At the time of the earlier admission, a series of disturbing external events (including severe illnesses of three members of his family and the birth of his first child) seemed to precipitate the depressive reaction. During the first admission, the patient was treated by six electroconvulsive treatments and was discharged in a somewhat improved state. Subsequently, however, his condition deteriorated and he was referred to a psychoanalyst who worked with him psychotherapeutically. Nevertheless, the depressive symptoms recurred, necessitating the second admission.

The therapist treating him in the hospital decided to institute a course of "regressive" therapy. Being aware that this form of treatment was not commonly carried out in this particular hospital, the psychiatrist recognized the necessity for communication with nursing personnel regarding his plan of treatment. On the day of admission he wrote the following note on the patient's chart:

> This patient is to be on a program of encouraging regression. He has consented to this plan, but is very frightened of his deep wishes to regress which he has to deny. Therefore, I think that the best plan to follow is to accept any tendencies and movements to regression — e.g., sleeping late, not shaving, meals in bed, etc. — but not to push him. He should proceed at his own pace and at his own time. Pay particular attention to bodily needs and wants. Milk and food-ad-lib, hot water bottles, massage, etc. should be freely given when he asks, but do not push these. It is not necessary to try to engage him in conversation or try to get him interested in things. If he initiates conversation, by all means respond, but keep to the topics he brings up. Specifically, do not talk about his work (law) or his family. If he seems to withdraw, there is no need to intervene, just note in the nurse's notes.

During the following months, problems developed in the application of the treatment plan at various phases of hospitalization. The head nurse, especially, had a great deal of difficulty in carrying out the treatment program. Mr. J's admission coincided with an energetic attempt to develop an integrated program of recreational, occupational, and group therapeutic activity on this particular nursing unit. Frequent patient group meetings were being held. Some of these were decision-making groups; others involved group psychotherapy. Morale was quite high, and an implicit attitude of "we can help these patients to get well quickly" permeated the air. However, for most of the personnel this meant that all patients ought to participate in the group activities. Consequently, the head nurse, who played an important part in coordinating the *milieu* program, found it difficult to see why Mr. J should not participate. She encouraged his attendance at the group meetings and recreational activities by simply notifying him of their occurrence. A large number of student nurses were also working on this section and frequently contacted Mr. J in a manner similar to that of the head nurse. With the backing of personnel, patients also played a role in putting pressure on Mr. J to be active.

One complicating factor which made it very difficult for the nurses to support the treatment plan was that they were supposed to watch for cues from Mr. J rather than to encourage regression. In other words, they were told to interact with him sufficiently to be able to support his wish to stay in bed, to be fed, and follow his spontaneous desires. The head nurse found herself very uncomfortable in this type of interaction, and it was impossible for her to desist from giving him verbal as well as non-verbal cues designed to facilitate his being a group member. Although the therapist was a highly respected and well-liked person, resentment developed in the head nurse and in other personnel as the treatment plan unfolded.

Despite these problems, the patient gradually deepened his regressive activity. At his own request, he was moved to a private room, remained in bed most of the day, kept his blinds down, and occasionally asked for extra food. As this type of behavior developed, the earlier problem became even more explicit, and the head nurse commented on the chart and also informally, saying, "We really aren't doing anything for this man. I don't think that this type of program can succeed." Staff meetings brought out strong differences of opinions, especially between the head nurse and a staff nurse (Nurse F) who was comfortable in carrying out the prescribed plan. The treatment finally reached a crisis phase when the dissension was at its maximum. On two occasions, meals were not brought into the patient's room, and he became panicky with fear of abandonment. At this point the therapist wrote the following:

> The patient has now come to the point of regressing to the extent of staying in bed most of the day. This regression must be supported in a practical way if he is to benefit from it. The patient fears that he will be abandoned, especially at mealtime. This must not happen. Someone must take the responsibility of seeing that Mr. J is fed. There have been two lapses in this connection to date and the patient has used this to justify his fears of abandonment. If the proper connectional experience, i.e., being looked after if he asks for it, is not given to him, there is no point to his being in the hospital and regressing. Personnel, as far as possible, should be available to him if he wants to talk, wants food, milk, warmth, blankets, etc. Do not push patient but continue to be available to look after his needs if he requires it. If the patient stays in bed all day, someone should drop in at least once an hour to see if he wants anything.

Finally, the staff resolved the crisis by asking Nurse F to pay closer attention to Mr. J since she seemed to have maintained a good relationship with him and was in agreement with the treatment plan. As might be expected, however, there was some difficulty when the head nurse (who continued to harbor latent doubts about the treatment plan) expressed concern that Nurse F was devoting too much of her time to this patient, to the detriment of the rest of the group. Eventually a compromise was worked out in which Nurse F took responsibility for the patient but was supported in this by two student nurses assigned to the patient.

After about eight months in the hospital, the patient spontaneously expressed a desire to "do more," after what the therapist called "the nadir of the regression." Shortly after this, he was able to leave the hospital and, on a three-year follow-up, has done well. It is interesting that two years later, while still in psychotherapy, he recalled his feelings at the point of emergence from the "nadir" by saying that at that point he had almost become incontinent and that was too shameful for him.

Mr. J's course in the hospital was complicated by two major problems in the nursing personnel. During the first phase of hospitalization, the problem was characterized by the staff's therapeutic ambition which was in conflict with the prescribed treatment. During the latter phase, the problem was characterized by a punitive response on the part of several nurses to the patient's wish for punishment.

Therapeutic Ambition in Conflict with Prescribed Treatment

This problem was best illustrated by the reaction of the head nurse to the prescribed *regressive* therapy, which seemed to contradict her notion that all patients should get better fast. Part of her problem was related to the therapeutic ambition of the psychiatrist administrator on that nursing unit. Together, they had developed a plan designed to reintegrate seriously ill patients rapidly. It had proven effective in treating many acutely psychotic individuals, as judged by rapid readjustment and return to the community of a significant number of patients.

Underlying problems in the head nurse, however, played a decisive role in her opposition to the prescribed treatment for Mr. J. She unconsciously envied the patient and wished that she, too, could have a "vacation" from adult responsibility. She was threatened by this envy and fearful that she could not control it. Consequently, her motives in subtly encouraging his participation in group activity largely represented a way of solving her own reaction to "regressive" therapy. Since many other members of the personnel shared in her particular problem, it was easy to get mutual support, albeit phrased in rationalizations. Nurse F did not have this conflict and she was able to function quite effectively with Mr. J.

Punitive Responses to Patient's Wish for Punishment

The patient entered the hospital with a strong need to be punished for his *childish* behavior. His masochistic orientation invited punishment, and it soon was forthcoming. To a certain extent, the encouragement for his participation in ward activities was a type of punishment, implying that he was a bad boy if he remained in bed and gratified himself. On the other hand, several actually encouraged him to regress, and this was also a form of punishment. The most clear-cut punitive response was seen at the maximal point of regression when meals were not brought to his room. It was as if the patient had provoked the nursing personnel into recreating his earliest traumatic experiences, and they almost reinforced his psychopathology instead of providing a corrective experience. Fortunately, the staff was able to overcome the problem and did provide effective care. This was largely due to the joint efforts of Nurse F along with other members of the personnel and abetted by the patience and persistence of the therapist.

Case 15. Frustration by Negative Response

During her first week of hospitalization, Mrs. O struggled against an underlying depressive reaction. She manifested symptomatology and behaved in a manner ostensibly designed to put some distance between herself and personnel. She protested that she really did not need to be in the hospital and was not "crazy like the other patients." After a short period in the hospital, however, Mrs. O's protests became less vehement, and she began to make tentative approaches to other patients and personnel.

When Nurse P spent one morning in shampooing and setting several patients' hair, she noticed that Mrs. O was observing her quite closely and was lingering near the doorway. It was apparent that the patient's hair needed to be shampooed, and the nurse assumed that the patient's behavior indicated a desire for a shampoo. When Nurse P completed her work on another patient, she walked over to the doorway and asked Mrs. O if she would like to have her hair set. Somehow frightened by this interaction, Mrs. O responded, "I am quite capable of doing my hair and I don't need you." Although taken aback by this response, Nurse P asked the patient if she had ever thought of cutting her hair shorter to bring out the natural wave. Mrs. O snapped, "Why should I look like the rest of the patients on this ward with their chopped-off hair? If I want it cut, I'll have it done." She then stormed down the hall back towards her room.

Nurse P stood in the doorway, feeling useless, helpless, and irritated by the turn of events. She was afraid to approach the patient on this subject again, deciding that it would not be of any use.

Nurse P enjoyed "doing something" for patients whom she felt were helpless. She derived a great deal of satisfaction from being looked upon as a "helpful nurse" and was easily frustrated when patients resisted her efforts. She had a strong wish to be needed and consequently placed herself in situations where she could advise patients and even other members of the personnel who needed assistance. Dependent patients who reached out for contact and pleaded for help in a direct way were a source of gratification to her. When Nurse P noticed that Mrs. O needed a shampoo, and was standing near the doorway, she correctly interpreted this behavior as a desire on the part of Mrs. O to have a shampoo and she fully expected a positive reaction to her question. When the patient responded in the manner described above, the nurse was offended and felt rejected by the patient. She interpreted the response as a personal insult and failed to understand the patient's fear about being hurt in a relationship in which she allowed her dependency feelings to emerge.

Had the nurse not experienced the interaction as a personal injury, she would have been able to explore alternatives to find an area where it was possible to provide therapeutic contact for this patient. It is also quite likely that Mrs. O perceived the nurse's offer for a shampoo as something other than an attempt to make a therapeutic relationship and could not allow herself to accept the offer under such circumstances. She was frightened that she might somehow be exploited by Nurse P.

Case 16. Nurse Slaps Patient

A young male patient, Tom, persistently followed the student, Miss M, around the ward. Each time she turned around, there was Tom. He would grab her and make sexual advances. She would blush, ask him to "stop" and then retreat to the nurses' station. When she came out, the same behavior reoccurred. She tried to talk with him, but he would constantly interrupt with verbal and physical advances. The student was too uncomfortable to report this problem. Finally, she gathered "enough courage" to discuss the problem with the head nurse, who suggested that if it happened again, "do whatever you would do on the outside." When she returned to the day room, Tom grabbed her again. This time she slapped his face. She was now angry. Tom was quite surprised and sat down in a chair. Miss M went into the office to report herself, fearful of what might happen, but was amazed when the doctor and the head nurse talked the problem through with her and did not "just reprimand her."

Tom, a young, handsome boy, delighted in embarrassing the young nurses. Originally flattered by his attention, Miss M soon became uncomfortable, guilty, and angry. She believed that she should not hurt his feelings because he was a patient. She knew she should treat him in a therapeutic manner but didn't know how. The doctor explained to Miss M that Tom was probably taking advantage of her feelings of inadequacy. He suggested that what she did should be in line with what she said and felt. This admonition was correct enough but difficult for her to carry out in view of her inexperience.

The fact that the head nurse had directed the student to respond to the patient as she would ordinarily respond in a comparable social situation increased the student's difficulty. The head nurse had not taken into account the girl's lack of experience in this kind of situation and thereby failed to give her appropriate support and direction.

The patient, Tom, had sought Miss M out because of her inexperience and vulnerability rather than selecting a more sophisticated person. In a discussion between the doctor, the student, and the head nurse the problem was clarified. Miss M was able to see the results when she demonstrated and felt anger at the same time. She learned that she could have handled the situation appropriately without slapping the patient.

Case 17. Nurse-Patient Problems Related to Class and Status Differences

Bill was a 13-year-old boy who could best be described as catatonic. He was persistently stiff, rigid, and posturing. He had difficulty coming through the doorway of his room. His expression communicated the hostility underlying the catatonic-like behavior.

He was really a "Little Lord Fauntleroy." He dressed immaculately at all times, expending much of his energy on maintaining an immaculate appearance, and becoming disturbed to the point of tears whenever a smudge appeared on his hands. In this context it is important to note that the patient came from an old New England family that had always emphasized fine manners and proper behavior.

Miss C, a nurse with five years of psychiatric experience, felt that the boy needed to engage in work and play and scuffling, and get his hands dirty as was common in her experience with other boys his age. The patient's doctor went along with Nurse C's attitude, since he knew that she was particularly effective in working with patients of this age. He felt that a lot could be left up to her own feeling and judgment in this situation. He noticed, however, that the boy often felt more comfortable when he was in the company of one of the older male attendants who treated him in a gentle fashion and acted as a friendly older companion.

The physician was very frequently consulted by the patient's mother. The mother was a very anxious, compulsive person, apparently highly disturbed about the patient's illness.

On several occasions, when the patient was beginning to relax and get more comfortable, he froze into states of immobility which lasted for days when he saw his hands were dirty and his suit rumpled after he had engaged in work or play with Miss C.

A staff conference brought out the point that the patient's whole pattern of daintiness was directly reinforced by his upbringing and cultural background. His training from his mother and father had been in this direction. He had been attending a "very proper" boys' school, at which the pupils were expected to maintain an immaculate appearance. The onset of this illness occurred in another school which was much more liberal and democratic and encouraged the boys to dress in a more informal way.

It became apparent that Miss C had little acceptance of the patient's cultural background. Her own ethnic and cultural background of a working family, half Irish and half Italian, with a somewhat tomboyish youth, gave her an acceptance of the more everyday work and play needs of younger patients but very little acquaintance with the depth of indoctrination in propriety that the patient had received.

Although the nurse could intellectually appreciate that she had pushed the boy in a direction that was painful to him, she believed that she had been therapeutic in her work with him. It was difficult for her to understand patients whose life experiences, class, and status were so utterly different from her own.

The doctor had based his acceptance of the nurse's work with the patient on the generalization that this nurse worked with younger patients, but he hadn't seen clearly the potential conflict between the norms of the nurse and the patient.

Case 18. Conflict Between Professional and Personal Moral Standards

The young, very proper student walked into the day room. Stretched out on a sofa was a young male patient, openly masturbating. The student turned, walked out of the day room, and encountered a male nurse entering the day room. He asked her what was wrong as her facial expression indicated that she was upset. She said, "That nasty Mr. X is at it again, and I wish you would do something about his acting like that in the day room." The student nurse went into the office and asked the head nurse why such activity was allowed. She further stated that Mr. X should be put in his room. The entire response was inconsistent with her previous relationship with this patient.

In this situation, the student was repulsed by Mr. X's behavior. She was rejecting him as well as his activity. She had many feelings about "such things" and could not in any way accept this as part of the patient's illness. She could see that the patient was withdrawn, that he responded to voices, that he had to be encouraged in everything that he did in regard to his appearance — this was part of his illness. This she accepted, but masturbation was something else. The student had definite ideas of "right" and "wrong," and was very much concerned about moral standards. As long as the patient did whatever she thought was morally "right" she accepted him; when he did something she considered "wrong" she rejected him completely. To disapprove of the behavior and direct the patient to other types of activity was at that time out of the question because she also disapproved of the patient. Here the student was not able to use herself therapeutically because her feelings got in her way. Her own concept of "wrong behavior" resulted in her rejecting everything about the patient and left no opportunity for her to help him.

The student's conflict was in having to deal therapeutically with the patient's needs and limitations as an expression of a whole person, while at the same time experiencing in herself considerable disapproval of the specific disturbing behavior. This nurse had previously expressed her feelings to the instructor that anything remotely concerned with sex was bad and she couldn't talk about it. In her own background, "things pertaining to sex" were not proper and they were not discussed. Therefore, she had a great deal of difficulty with problems of this type.

The nurse's reaction was not entirely inappropriate, except that she confused her feeling about sexual behavior with her judgment about the patient. The area of her problem is indicated by the fact that she was able to accept all of the psychotic activity as an indication of illness at the same time that she rejected the patient completely because of his open masturbation. This was hinted at in the initial description of this nurse as a young and *proper* student. The inconsistency in her response to difficult aspects of the patient's behavior should be the focal point of discussion in individual supervision.

Case 19. Displacement of Conflict with Senior Family Members to Geriatric Patient

Mrs. B was an 80-year-old patient, with an agitated, senile psychosis, who constantly talked about her daughter as if she were her mother. She pleaded to be taken home to her "mother," asking almost continually when somebody would come for her.

Most of the personnel found her quite easy to get along with and believed that she was a sweet and cooperative person albeit confused. She smiled very pleasantly whenever she was given special attention.

Nurse D, a psychiatric nurse with four years' experience at a large state hospital and a private mental hospital, was often the head nurse responsible for her care, and gave her quite a bit of special attention. She appeared to have a very real understanding of this older patient's needs and seemed to be meeting them.

However, Nurse D experienced a number of problems with the patient's daughter, Mrs. C, who could not relinquish Mrs. B to the care of another. She hovered over her mother and watched her every breath wondering if it would be the last. In addition, she alternated between praising the nurse for her devotion to her mother and blaming her for the slightest deviation of attention to other patients. Much of the pressure from the patient's daughter became focused upon Miss D who maintained the appearance of giving excellent nursing care in spite of this pressure.

No improvement occurred in the patient's agitated demanding behavior; in fact, her demands seemed to increase week by week. The daughter, likewise, became more critical as time passed.

In attempting to determine the reasons for lack of improvement in the patient's behavior in the face of what appeared to be excellent nursing care, it was learned that Miss D was ambivalent about this patient. If one heard her in her off-duty hours, it was apparent that what she was doing was a considerable strain and burden to her, and that the strain was mounting.

The nurse was caught up in a conflict situation similar to that of the patient's daughter; she shared much of the feeling of hostility that the daughter demonstrated, together with a sense of being forced into a compensating attentiveness. The intensity of the problem was also related to the daughter's frequent criticisms of Miss D.

Exploring the background of the nurse's attitude, it was seen that she had had a difficult time with her own grandparents and felt that she had suffered at their hands. One of the reasons that she had left the private mental hospital where she had worked previously was that there had been too many old patients. She had hoped that in this hospital she would spend more of her time with young schizophrenic patients with whom she was able to work quite competently.

Looking back over her early weeks with the patient, she was able to see that she had really overextended herself, trying to cover up her distaste for older patients, trying to be a good nurse in spite of her conflict. This had been misunderstood as real interest by the patient's doctor and the nursing director, so that she was repeatedly asked to do even more than she was demanding of herself. It became apparent later that Miss D was secretly hoping that the patient would die as she viewed this as the only solution to her dilemma.

It was determined that this nurse could not, at this time, give appropriate nursing attention to older patients without too much strain on her own resources. Until she resolved some of the problems connected with her feelings about older people, she would be unable to give good nursing care to geriatric patients.

Case 20. Conflict Between Therapeutic and Personal Ambition*

Miss Davis, a nurse, met Mrs. Johnson, a psychiatric aide, who had just left the room of Mrs. Calvin, a patient. Mrs. Johnson said that the patient didn't want to be bathed, didn't want to be combed. "I managed," she sighed, "but it isn't one of her good days." Miss Davis became distressed and disappointed by this report. She approached the patient's room with some hesitation, but on entering she behaved toward the patient as if she were unaware of what Mrs. Johnson had told her. Miss Davis said, "You look pretty today, Mrs. Calvin; your hair is so bright and shiny," (chuckle), "you look just like the weather. It's a bright, shiny, crisp day — the kind that makes a person feel full of pep and makes you want to look through a magazine at the new Fall styles." Miss Davis chattered on cheerfully, even though the patient slid down, drew the covers about her, and closed her eyes. It was as though the patient closed her eyes because she could not bear to watch this previously helpful person be so blind to what was actually going on at the moment. The patient, in effect, receded from what now amounted to an insensitive intrusion by the nurse.

Miss Davis finally noticed the effect that her behavior was having upon Mrs. Calvin. She drew herself up short and thought to herself: "Oh, oh — something is wrong. Why is she pulling away like that? Is it something I've said — something I'm doing. Why do I keep rattling on like this — what's bothering *me?*"

Miss Davis then explored this entire episode with the help of the supervisory nurse. The event was discussed from the standpoint of what was interfering with the nurse's therapeutic use of herself. It became clear that the nurse was overly ambitious for therapeutic success with this patient and searched for evidence of improvement or improved personal appearance, interest in the weather and in the current magazines. She focused upon these topics at the price of not noticing the real feelings of the patient and her own intrusion into the situation. The nurse's own need for success was threatened at first by realistic observation of the patient's problems. Her own goals became a barrier to progress. When the nurse acted on the basis of personal overambition to see immediate success, instead of meeting the patient's needs, her therapeutic usefulness to the patient was lost or, at best, greatly minimized.

Certainly, every nurse has as her goal the patient's improvement. To implement this goal, however, requires that the nurse observe and assess the patient's behavior in as accurate a way as possible, with a minimal amount of interference from her own problems and inappropriate motivations. In this case, Miss Davis' ambitiousness interfered with her perceptual and observational processes to the detriment of the patient. Fortunately, she was able to realize that something was amiss, located the problem within herself, and sought supervisory help. This type of experience was helpful in her maturation towards becoming a more effective psychiatric nurse.

Case 21. Successful Reassessment of a Nursing Plan

One month after Gretchen, age 19, was separated from her family in order to enter college she began to be troubled by rather profound feelings of inadequacy. She increasingly felt a terrifying sense of strangeness and feared that she was about to be destroyed. Following her admission to the college infirmary, it was immediately apparent that Gretchen was failing to win in her struggle to maintain her usual identity. It became necessary to arrange further treatment on a psychiatric unit of a general hospital.

Information was obtained from her family that Gretchen had been regarded as a rebellious child, difficult to manage, hard to show affection to, and painfully hesitant in any new situation. On admission to the psychiatric unit Gretchen had a perplexed facial expression. She seemed to want to reach out for

*The case is taken from the film *Psychiatric Nursing: Nurse-Patient Relationships*, ANA-NLN Film Service, New York, 1959.

something to hold on to but feared what the result might be if she did. She was careless in her grooming, and drooped her head so that her hair covered her face, almost completely hiding her features. She had an offensive body odor and her underclothes were soiled. She threatened her roommate with physical harm and destroyed her roommate's belongings. When the nurses came close to Gretchen she kicked and bit them. Patients became frightened of Gretchen and would leave an area as soon as she entered. During the ensuing weeks of hospitalization, Gretchen became more and more resistant to care and was almost completely mute and immobile except for intermittent rages. When approached she resentfully responded with, "I don't care; it makes no difference to me."

The nursing staff initially attempted to solve some of the problems Gretchen presented with a 24-hour "scheduled" nursing care plan which had been effective with other patients. This plan listed everything Gretchen would do on a time schedule. It included suggestions for possible approaches to engage Gretchen's interest in activities, her environment, and personal hygiene. She would be roused out of bed at a definite hour in the morning, bathed and dressed at a particular time, taken to meals, and given some task to complete during the morning period. Her afternoons were planned similarly and discussed with all the staff who were concerned with carrying out the plan. It was felt that during the "thawing out" period of Gretchen's stay on the unit, one could best determine her mood and communicate with her by taking cues from her changing facial expressions and other non-verbal signs. Often Gretchen looked angry, paced restlessly, and kicked furniture. Although the nurses tried to be direct and clear in their approach to Gretchen and in their expectations of her, she often found ways to end the contacts with the nurses. It had been hoped that the staff could make activities and tasks interesting enough for Gretchen so as to stimulate her to complete them, but she would shortly lose interest.

Since Gretchen was indecisive, it was often difficult to get her to commit herself even to a choice of clothing for the day. When she seemed unable to make such a decision and the staff would make it for her, Gretchen was resistant. Often her clothes would become torn in the dressing struggle.

Another problem was the way Gretchen reacted at mealtime. She would wander in the hallway and peek around the corner at other patients in the dining room. Sometimes she abruptly ran from the table, leaving the food untouched. At other times, she consumed large amounts of food after everyone had left the dining area; but in spite of these brief periods of gorging herself she lost weight.

There were many angry outbursts from Gretchen in connection with bodily cleanliness. Gretchen would sit rigidly in the tub while she was bathed, or would struggle to get out of the tub. Once she told the nurse that she was very modest and that the staff was intruding upon her need for privacy. The nurse responded by saying that she respected Gretchen's feelings about the matter but felt it necessary to help bathe Gretchen until she assumed responsibility for bathing herself. Gretchen screamed out, "Well, get out and let me finish." The nurse left but returned only to find Gretchen sitting defiant and unbathed.

During this phase of treatment, staff morale was at a low ebb because of Gretchen's success at warding everyone off. After a meeting of the entire staff, it was decided that it might be helpful to abandon the "scheduled" nursing care approach and try a less intrusive "one-to-one" way of relating. Only one nurse was assigned on each shift to work with Gretchen, to become acquainted with her needs, but not to expect her to participate in group activities. The remainder of the staff occupied themselves with other patients. In response to this individual approach, the change in Gretchen was dramatic. She started to dress without much assistance and came to meals. She talked more easily and behaved more appropriately with her peers. The next step was to suggest to Gretchen that she move to a room with another student patient. Gretchen agreed, and during a period in which her roommate had a brief but incapacitating physical illness, Gretchen assisted in her care. Shortly thereafter, for the first time, Gretchen attended a scheduled psychotherapy hour, talked in an appropriate manner with only some slight hesitation, and seemed quite proud of her efforts.

Sometimes it is extremely difficult for a nursing staff to sense, with any degree of certainty, what a patient feels as he experiences a sudden loss of his identity. Success in *feeling with* the patient is often a crucial determinant as to whether a patient elects to seek new solutions for the problem of living in the present or continues to live as if the present were identical with the distant past. No sooner had Gretchen separated from her familiar home and environment than she began to be troubled by a sense of terrifying strangeness and was able to employ only the most primitive of emotional reactions in coping with her sudden separation from her family. In the hospital she chose either to fight off what she interpreted as the staff's attempt to punish and destroy her, or to withdraw. Nevertheless, some part of her tried hesitantly to reach out. It was in the setting of her intermittent rages and withdrawals, her inability to assume responsibility, her resistive and negative feelings, that the nurses struggled to provide a sense of consistency and guidance. But in response to almost every move toward Gretchen, she complained that the nurses were intruding. She was furious when the nurses made decisions for her, but petulantly refused to make choices of her own.

Nevertheless, after a period of groping, the nurses devised a means for assisting Gretchen in coming out of her entrenched position. Instead of continuing to make unrewarding group efforts to relate to Gretchen, the staff decided to assign only a few of its members to care for her, a remedy which better fitted in with Gretchen's needs. When only one nurse at a time approached Gretchen, she was able to reach out and respond appropriately. A two-year-old, for example, is often bewildered by too great expectations from too many persons and is often much more comfortable in testing out, bit by bit, how well he can move toward just one person. Given this opportunity, Gretchen began to show signs of improvement almost immediately. She not only permitted a nurse to be near her but also trusted herself to get close to someone else, in this instance a patient, in the guise of caring for her. It was through this series of events that Gretchen was able to reestablish a sense of her own identity.

Case 22. Recognition of Staff Discouragement and Projected Blame

Maurice, a 24-year-old man, had been hospitalized several years for a schizophrenic reaction, catatonic type. Over the years the severity of the symptoms had varied, but in general he had been underactive, relatively unresponsive to questioning, and required help in feeding and dressing himself. Various shock therapies and attempts at psychotherapy had led to transitory improvement, but it had never been sustained. A few days after his transfer from a state hospital to a small private psychiatric hospital, he became mute, motionless, incontinent, and would not feed himself.

It was decided that the nursing plan should take care of the patient's obvious physical needs and at the same time should be utilized as a way of establishing contact with him. An effort was made to create an atmosphere in which Maurice would feel no pressure and would be assured that his needs would be taken care of. At first it was easy to elicit the interest of the nursing staff because his boyish appearance and helplessness evoked in most people a sympathetic desire to help. He was shaved each day and attention was given to his oral hygiene. He was bathed whenever he soiled himself and he was tube-fed twice daily. Both men and women participated in this program, but most of the nursing care involving close physical contact was assigned to student nurses because it was felt that this might be less threatening than if it were done by male attendants.

From the outset the patient's mother was hypercritical of the ward staff. She lived nearby and made frequent, often unannounced, visits. She herself had been hospitalized for a psychotic reaction and made accusations which suggested that she was actively delusional. Her complaints ranged from statements that the ward staff was not showing sufficient interest in her son and was stealing his clothing, to accusations that the staff systematically beat all patients on the ward, and so forth. Her more preposterous statements caused only amusement, but her total impact made the staff feel so uncomfortable that they asked that a limit be placed on her visits, and her complaints were generally referred to the ward administrator. Even so, she continued to be a problem, often visiting in the evening, virtually forcing her way into the ward, and berating the nursing staff.

After several weeks the nursing program for Maurice began to break down. Various details of his physical care were forgotten or neglected. Staff members were quick to criticize each other; some said that Maurice needed more sympathetic care, while others argued that he was getting more than his fair share of the staff's attention. Another patient, Paul, began to show his resentment of Maurice by teasing him. Invariably Paul seemed to have some request just at those times when several members of the staff were occupied with the tube-feeding of Maurice. On one occasion he spit in Maurice's face and on another threatened to strike him. As tensions grew, the nursing staff asked that the problem of Paul's threats towards Maurice be discussed at the weekly ward staff meeting.

At this meeting the problem was stated as, "What can we do about Paul's attacks on Maurice?" As the discussion of Paul's antagonism to Maurice progressed, a few staff members mentioned that they themselves had felt some anger towards Maurice. It developed that almost all staff members had experienced such feelings to some degree, but had never openly discussed them because the feelings of anger toward Maurice had been recognized only vaguely or had seemed too unreasonable.

Most of the staff members described a typical

sequence of events in their relationship with Maurice. Initially they had felt attracted to him and had been unusually enthusiastic in their efforts to help him. Their eagerness to help had been accompanied by the hope that he would respond favorably. When this did not occur they began to question their ability and had a tendency to withdraw from Maurice. At this point they often had been particularly troubled by the mother's complaints. Once the sequence of special effort, disappointment, withdrawal, and resentment had been recognized many things were seen in a different light. Various staff tensions and anger toward the mother were considered to be displacements of feelings toward Maurice. It was suggested that Paul's behavior might, at least in part, have been caused by the unrecognized feelings of anger that the staff had toward Maurice. By the end of the meeting the problem had been reformulated from "What can we do about Paul's attacks on Maurice?" to "What can we do about our own feelings of discouragement and resentment caused by the failure of our best efforts to help Maurice?" No answer was proposed for this question, but the general feeling of the group was that the discussion had relieved them of a great burden and things did not look so hopeless.

Later the same evening the patient's mother arrived for one of her surprise visits. As the evening attendant listened to the usual recitation of complaints she noticed that she felt more sympathetic toward the mother because it occurred to her that if the ward staff had felt terribly discouraged, the patient's mother must have felt immeasurably worse. As a consequence, she did not try to get rid of the mother but rather encouraged her to talk. At one point the attendant mentioned that she found it difficult to picture what Maurice must have been like prior to his illness. When the mother asked if it would help if she brought in some photographs and high school year books, the attendant encouraged her to do so.

The staff was astonished to see the difference in Maurice's appearance and to learn many new things about him. Knowing that he had been a popular class leader and reading about some of his interests in school seemed to change their concept of him. It occurred to one of the attendants that it might make a difference to Paul if he knew some of these things. The effect was truly remarkable. Not only did he discontinue the teasing but he offered to help in Maurice's care. He often sat with him, read him stories, and sometimes played phonograph records to him. Paul had previously resented Maurice because he felt Maurice's helplessness was just an unfair trick to get the attention of the nursing staff. Knowledge of his background gave Paul some appreciation of how intensely disturbed and frightened Maurice must be.

Neither Maurice's condition nor the problems surrounding his care were dramatically changed. His care was still quite taxing to the staff; patients and staff were still, at times, annoyed by the burden. His mother continued to have many criticisms. Nevertheless a crucial step had been made in his treatment. Having recognized and accepted many of their feelings about the patient, the staff did not have to be so defensive. Rather than dissipating their energies in conflict among themselves they could direct their attention to the patient and carry out a basically sound plan of nursing care.

Concluding Commentary

The goals of therapeutic interaction include the patient's better understanding of his needs, his greater facility in communication, his increased social participation, and his more constructive methods of attaining personal satisfactions. The therapeutic effectiveness of the nurse is directly related both to her understanding of the patient and his illness, and to her awareness of her feelings and the impact of her responses. In the face of anxiety, despair, helplessness, regression, and aggression which are ever present in a psychiatric hospital setting, a nurse needs this understanding in order to enter into effective relationships.

Twenty-two clinical case studies have been presented to illustrate, identify, and analyze some of the therapeutic problems that arise in nursing care. These problems involve personnel-patient and intra-staff interactions. There is no easy answer to such problems. The theoretical formulations and the clinical examples which comprise this guide are not intended to provide definitive answers to all problems. Rather, they provide a framework for studying and resolving problems commonly met by all involved in patient care.

Within the context of this guide, the term "nurse" is manifestly generic. The principles and theses formulated are equally relevant and applicable to attendants, psychiatric aides, occupational therapists, physical therapists, recreational therapists, corrective therapists, vocational counselors, volunteer workers, internes, residents — in short, all who participate in the daily life and activities of the sick person.

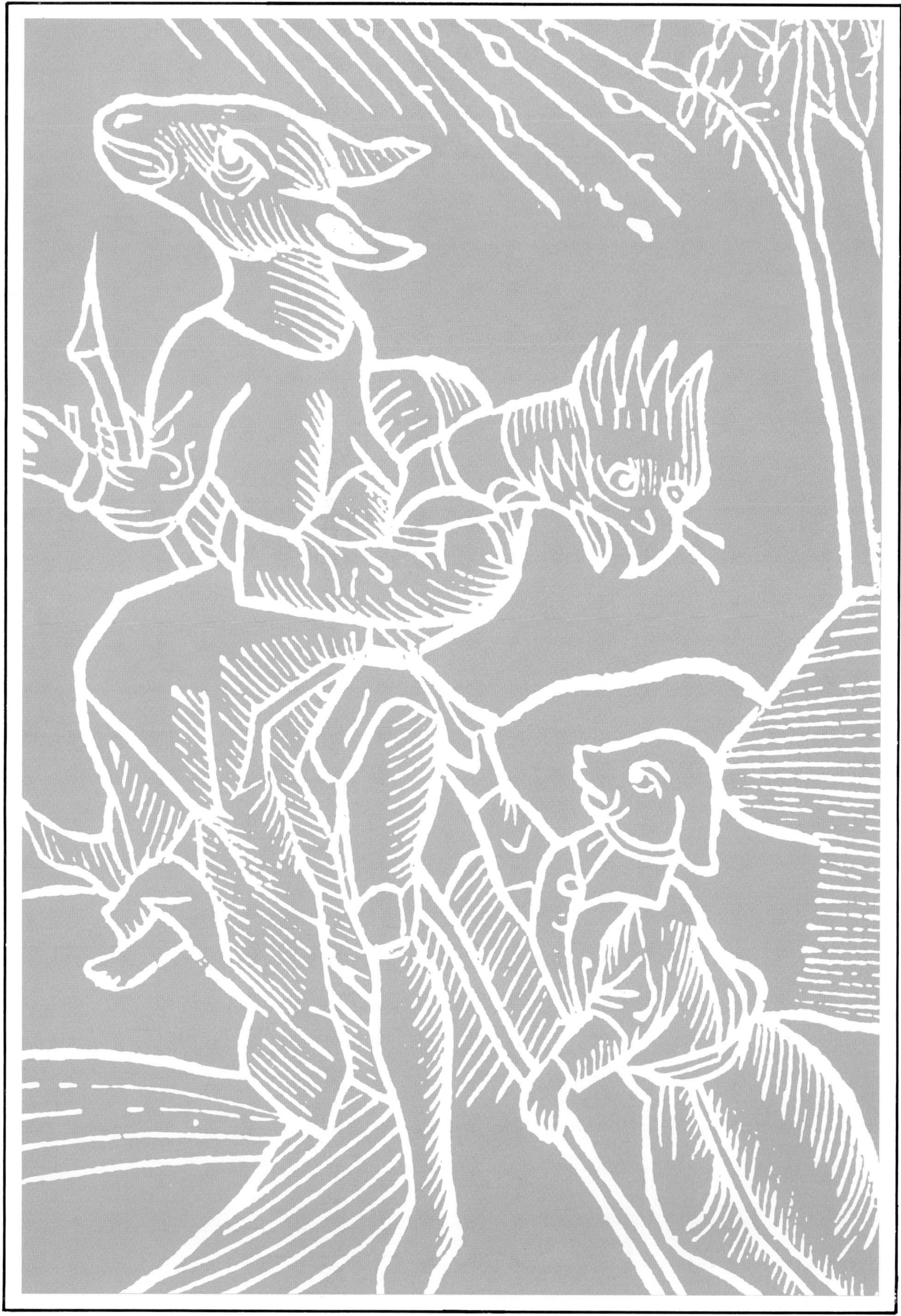

Selected Articles from Non-Psychiatric Nursing Journals Before the Establishment of Psychiatric Nursing Journals

Introduction

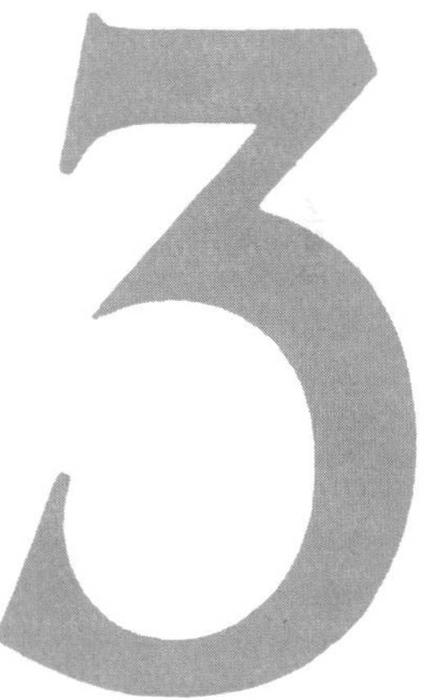

The articles included in this section span 33 years of psychiatric nursing. Indeed, the first article, "Mental Nursing, a Privilege," written in 1929 by Marie Olsen, sets the tone for the entire section. Obviously, other articles were written between then and 1950, the date of the next article presented on these pages. But none could better herald psychiatric nursing's focus: to study concepts of human behavior, to invest in clinical work, to learn from the patient, and "together. . .to reason things out." In reading the contributions from 1950-1962, it will become clear that psychiatric nursing was in the forefront of practice, although generally unacknowledged by the public and fellow mental health practitioners. Psychiatric nurses were taking leadership roles in practice — in group treatment techniques, in the analysis of sociopsychiatric problems in hospitals, in the establishment of day hospitals, and in consultation. Psychiatric nurses were engaging in early forms of clinical research, in conceptualizing clinical problems in living and dying. Through careful examination of clinical work, education, and administrative practices, psychiatric nurses were building a core of knowledge that was to build a profession.

Mental Nursing, a Privilege

Marie Olsen, R.N.

Reprinted from *The American Journal of Nursing*, Vol. 29, No. 9, 1929.

A psychiatrist at one time made an appointment for me to see one of his patients suffering from neurosis. Throughout the interview the patient asked the following questions and made the appended statements:

Are you musical?
Have you a sense of humor?
I don't want anyone who is going to tell me what comforts they have had elsewhere.
I want to spend my time with my children and husband when he is at home, and what would you do alone?
Your bedroom would be near mine, and I should dislike that.
I don't like complaints!
I want to see my friends by myself.
If I got nasty and mad and told you that I could not stand the sight of you, what would you do?

If I, at the time when I had to meet this situation, had developed no real interest in mental nursing, I would have looked at the patient, bowed my head and said, "I am sorry, but I do not think that I am the nurse you want." As it was, I had begun to realize that statements of this kind, coming direct from the patient, are very helpful to a worker in mental therapy because, before entering the home of a patient with a defense mechanism of this calibre, a nurse who is a student of the psychology of the unconscious gathers from the fragments of such a conversation exactly where other nurses have made their mistakes. She is then in a position to relieve the strain, by carefully avoiding any pressure of a similar nature until she has gained the confidence of the patient and family.

It is this attempt on the part of the nurse to sublimate her own personality, in order to gain the confidence of the patient, that the mental nurse will find a good method for approach. In a sense the patient's difficulties become the nurse's difficulties, his interests the nurse's interests. If the patient revels in poetry, the power goes to the nurse who loves poetry; if the interest is good housekeeping, the power goes to the nurse who knows a great deal about the management of a household. It is not so much the product of the effort as the sincerity that counts in the end.

We know that doctors and nurses who have never made a special study of mental therapy are inclined to punish the mentally ill by withdrawing their interest. Considering that in general hospitals one usually comes in contact only with advanced cases, who eventually are sent to institutions for the insane, and with very few incipient cases, that does not seem hard to understand. Furthermore, nurses suffer from the same lack of education in the general field of mental health as the future physicians in training. Therefore, acquiring knowledge of mental therapy for the most part still rests with the individual. The subject will have to be perused as something apart from the regular training, until mental hygiene is more effectively incorporated into the curriculum. The nurses who have worked in modern psychiatric institutions have learned something about degrees of mental illness, but they have had little opportunity to study methods of treatment. The work that apparently holds the key to modern mental therapy is done today in the psychiatrist's office. I refer to mind analysis, more commonly known as psychoanalysis; the purging of the mind of its contents, and the effort to put it together again after the missing links have been discovered.

What I know of mental therapy I have learned while doing private nursing outside of institutions. While training in a general hospital I, too, imbibed a fear of the insane, and I knew very little about the interesting, curable, first stages. During varied experiences in institutional, public health, army and private nursing, the literature dealing with mental hygiene that drifted my way did very little to change my opinion. I read psychologies for nurses, condensations of textbooks on educational psychology used in the universities. At college, a course in Psychology A covered the anatomy of the nervous system, the laws of learning, various behaviorisms, mental tests, dealing only sketchily with the mental conflicts involved in neurosis. It gave me a knowledge of educational psychology or of the psychology of the conscious as treated by E.L. Thorndike, J.B. Watson, A.I. Gates, W. James and R.S. Woodworth. There was a one-point course given in mental nursing referring to fragments of the writings of W.A. White and Bernard Harr, but even that did not awaken my interest, because *case experience is absolutely necessary* to make mental nursing piquant. And, furthermore, if we remember that educational psychology deals mainly with the conscious, it should be made clear that a worker in mental therapy must build up her interest and foundation from the study of the psychology of the unconscious.

Calling to mind the striking symbol of Stanley Hall, where he compares the mind to a floating iceberg, with one-eighth visible above the water and seven-eighths below, the one-eighth above being called the conscious and the seven-eighths below that which we call unconscious, it is evident that educational psychology is entirely inadequate as a basis for a student nurse in mental therapy. It is the unconscious, or the seven-eighths below the water, which forms the basis for a psychiatrist's investigations.

My interest in mental therapy dates from the day a New York psychiatrist called me on a case suffering from neurosis in the form of agoraphobia, or fear of public places. A neurologist had suggested me for the case. The patient was a young woman with an unusual intellect and good education, newly married to a medical scientist. She had been suffering from neurosis for some years, and at the time she was visiting the psychiatrist's office three times a week for psychoanalytic treatment. In the home of cultured patients who have been struggling with neurosis for a long time, nurses will usually find good psychological libraries. This home had an unusual collection of the latest books dealing with the psychology of the unconscious. As a rule psychoanalysts allow their patients to read only superficial, general accounts on psychoanalysis, the idea being to avoid acquainting the patient with the technic, which would be like the strategist who delivers his plan of attack into his enemies' hands. Nevertheless, my patient perused every new book; she seemed to be familiar with all the strategy, and her husband helped her by clarifying any obscure places. Undoubtedly in this case, my patient's knowledge of psychotherapy was a detriment to her because it enabled her to guard the cause for her neurosis, but her knowledge became a decided advantage to me.

Naturally I wondered where I, who knew practically nothing of the psychology of the unconscious, could be of help. From her experiences with nurses in the past, she had formed an opinion about the average nurse's knowledge of mental therapy. The nurse whom I succeeded had been with this patient for over a year. From description I got a picture of her, a kind, motherly soul, who read a great deal, but who was unable to remember what she had read. Her asset seemed to have been that she was able to keep silent whenever the patient became garrulous. It seemed the strangest and most interesting bit of nursing that I had ever done, for I was put there to give not physical care, but mental. For days I almost forgot that I was on duty. We played tennis, swam and talked whenever my patient felt like it. And then, her neurosis would crop out with renewed strength.

The patient's predicament set me thinking. I began to read the books from the library at random, psychology, mental hygiene, psychoanalysis. At first my patient seemed to resent my interest, as if the contents of those books were entirely beyond me, and, to be sure, she was nearly right. I had no knowledge of the psychology of the unconscious as portrayed in the large volumes of Drs. Sigmund Freud, Alfred Adler, Wilhelm Stekel, Carl Jung, W.H.R. Rivers, Morton Prince, A.A. Brill, James S. Van Teslaar and Beatrice Hinkle, and at the time I did not realize that every neurotic guards the secret of his neurosis as a precious possession. Nevertheless, I read the books that she chose for me openly and the others on the sly, and, at last, when she realized that I was sincere, and that I could remember something of what I had read, her attitude changed. She became my teacher, and together we tried to reason things out. There was no other way.

We tried to test the validity of the conclusions arrived at by the writers, using the total of the experiences that had entered into the making of our personalities and others. We tried to analyze the events of the past in order to understand what had made us as we were. We tried psychologically to interpret the reactions of our fellow men to certain situations, learning types of minds, such as extroverts and introverts; and inasmuch as certain actions come bobbing to the surface from one's unconscious mental life, dreams also became of vital importance as a medium that spilled over valuable material. Thus, the day came when the patient discussed with me some phases of the work done at the psychiatrist's office, and took me into her confidence. Since then I have considered nursing in preventive mental therapy a privilege, as well as a liberal education.

Psychotherapy for thousands of years has been an affair of priests and educators. And today psychiatrists acknowledge that they have much help of value to expect from keensighted educators and trained mental workers. With an oversupply of private duty nurses in the United States and half of the annually sick population suffering from some form of mental illness, which is 60 percent curable in the early stages, something ought to be done to meet the need of the most influential neurologists, psychiatrists and pediatricians who are seeking in vain for helpful, intelligent co-workers, in the form of sensitive, cultured, preferably college-trained nurses. Then, too, in this age of specialization, the nurse undoubtedly will find her economic and intellectual salvation by endeavoring to become an expert in one field. Mental nursing offers educational, financial and social recompense.

The Nurse-Leader in Group Psychotherapy

Ann G. Hargreaves, R.N. and Alice M. Robinson, R.N.

Mrs. Hargreaves (Boston City Hospital School of Nursing) is assistant principal in charge of nursing education at Boston State Hospital and is studying at Boston University where Miss Robinson (Duke University School of Nursing; B.S., Catholic University of America; M.S., Boston University) was a teaching fellow in psychiatric nursing when this article was written.

This article was reprinted from *The American Journal of Nursing, Vol. 50, No. 11, November 1950.*

Today great emphasis is being placed upon human inter-relationships in all spheres of activity. In nursing there is a special need for competence in the art of developing and maintaining good interpersonal relationships. Because the care of the mentally ill calls for outstanding ability in practicing this art, and because modern psychiatry tends more and more to utilize "group technics," it would seem that psychiatric nursing might have a unique contribution to make to group therapy. The development and application of such methods in psychiatric nursing should be exceedingly valuable in both teaching and learning situations, and in the classroom as well as in daily work.

Nurse-leaders work with 9 groups of about 15 patients each in the group psychotherapy program now being conducted at the Boston State Hospital. One of these groups is composed of patients who have had lobotomies, another of tuberculous patients, and a third is a self-governing group which meets under the guidance of a nurse. Eight groups meet twice a week and one meets three times weekly. A nurse observer records the essential data for each meeting. The nine leaders meet with psychiatrists once each week to study group dynamics. Each leader is also guided individually and advised by psychiatrists who know the patients in her group. In addition, 30 nurses serve as observers and recorders of activities in groups which are led by doctors.

Besides the groups which meet for psychotherapy, nurse-leaders preside over 12 educational groups, 8 of them consisting of nursing students. Meetings are held once a week for 7 of them and twice a week for the remaining 5. The group discussion method is used in staff teaching programs, which include all members of the psychiatric team, in staff nurses' meetings, and in classes for affiliate nursing students.

The physicians who are in charge of the various services lead nurses who work on their wards in discussion periods and give support to those who are conducting either therapeutic or educational groups. A teaching group which consists of all nursing personnel working on a ward has a goal beyond that of teaching general principles or technics. The higher goal is the clarification of patient-therapist relations and of interpersonal relations among the workers themselves.

The clinical director of the hospital and the nursing director encourage nurses to participate in group work. They believe that this use of the nurses' time and efforts is definitely worthwhile.

We do not wish to imply that the nurse should step out of her accustomed role and encroach upon the functions of the physician. On the contrary, we wish to point up the importance of the *team* as a psychotherapeutic agent, and to indicate the nurse's potentialities as an active team member.

When we consider the role of the nurse in psychotherapy, several problems are encountered immediately. Most important, a flexible pattern of teamwork must be established. Such a pattern must include not only the nurse and the physician but all others who work with the patient. Physicians can and must contribute to the establishment of such a therapeutic environment by keeping nurses informed and by helping them to use the most effective methods in caring for the patient. In this way the nurse can become a productive member of the team and can improve her already valuable contributions. The nurse's rapport with the physician is vitally important in group therapy for she must not only convey to him as much information as possible but she often needs his direction and counsel.

We know that we cannot care properly for all our thousands of patients with the psychiatric nursing personnel now available. If we claimed that we could, our yearly statistics would belie us. It is logical to assume that more individual attention will some day push down the incidence of mental illness. Until that time, however, we must be encouraged by the advent of the group therapies. Through this media, one person can help many patients and many patients can help each other.

Participation of nurses in group activities with patients has been a more or less unrecognized potential for many years. Now many nurses are actually taking part in group therapy *per se* as leaders, observers, recorders, and visitors. The nurse who serves as a *leader* in group therapy is presented with a new and specific challenge. In working with the mentally ill, we sometimes feel as if we were working in the dark. This is a good feeling to have, however, for one is always more careful in the dark. There is always some danger when we are dealing with the complex psyche of another human being. This constantly reminds us, too, that we do not *cure* patients; we do well if we can help them to help themselves.

What sort of preparation will physicians require of the nurse-leader? What will the psychiatric nursing field itself require?

Twenty years' experience in nursing the mentally ill, or a degree from a recognized university, will not necessarily qualify the nurse to participate in group therapy. But certain basic qualifications need to be considered. The total personality of the nurse is the first of these. She must evaluate herself honestly. How has she been able to adjust to her own problems? How stable is she under stress? How much aggression does she manifest when it is necessary to proceed slowly? Does she accept direction and guidance? Does she repeatedly attempt to intellectualize? How much of her personality does she project onto others? To what extent does she use other people to meet her own needs? What is her philosophy concerning mental illness?

After her own evaluation of such reactions, she should ask for and be able to accept an equally honest evaluation from the physician. Then she must review her experience. How much does she know about mentally ill patients? Has she worked with patients having many different types of psychiatric illness? What have been her reactions to patients and their behavior as she went about her daily work? What are her relationships with other personnel?

Helena W. Render has said, "The patient regardless of his behavior is a human being who thinks and loves and hates and who has quick and acute sensibilities."[1] The "quick and acute sensibilities" make it necessary for us to do more than just "get along" with the patient. Everyone who comes in contact with him has some effect on him. The aide, the physician, the nursing student, the supervisor, all those who are a part of the patient's environment, even temporarily, directly or indirectly affect his actions and his feelings. We must take stock of our own reactions and we must fit them into a mature pattern of behavior which will enable us to understand the patient and, in consequence, help to meet his individual needs. The nurse as a person affects the patient as a person, either psychotherapeutically or psychonoxiously (non-therapeutically).

In working with groups of patients, the nurse must be keenly aware of what is significant in their behavior and reactions. Many times, especially with very ill patients, there is much role-playing and symbolic language but little verbalization that can be readily understood. It is frequently necessary to interpret these non-verbal behavior patterns while the group is in session. This requires acute perception and intelligent insight.

We have found that some nurses tend to govern rather than to guide the group discussion. For instance, it seems only natural to them that a long silence must be broken. With each session, however, they learn that the group functions more cohesively when it is not prodded. This skill in knowing when to speak develops through experience.

Often groups are not ready to accept material which the leader feels they "should" have. When, for example, one nurse (who later voluntarily gave up her group) read selections from Kahlil Gibran's *The Prophet* to the group, they were unable to accept this projection of the nurse's own esthetic taste and her more or less intellectual approach.

We believe that the group should be selected by the nurse-leader, with the assistance and approval of the ward physician. She should select patients with whom she is familiar, from an environment with which she is not working every day. She should make sure that the patients are likely to remain in her group, as constant changing of group members quickly disorganizes a security-giving environment. Other treatments which are in progress or are proposed for patients while they are participating in group therapy should always be discussed with the nurse-leader.

The question of whether a group should be homogeneous or mixed is an open one. Ordinarily, life situations are not set up to provide homogeneous groupings. In our society many personalities are thrust together and must function together. To assemble a group of people who have very similar problems and reactions to problems creates strained and unnatural relationships.

Why does a group leader choose one patient instead of another? This is a fruitful question for investigation and the choice is certainly a highly individual matter. Very ill patients are chosen by some because they are particularly interested in long-term group therapy. Others choose convalescent patients because they feel more secure in the "near-normal" atmosphere. We do not review patients' histories because we do not wish to have preconceived ideas concerning their past life. Rather, we want the patients themselves to tell as much as they can within the group.

As to differences in sex and age, we have had one mixed group (in a tuberculosis unit) which has been very successful. Good standards of social behavior have been encouraged, and many problems involving emotional difficulties between the sexes have been worked out.

We have found that including patients of different ages promotes identification transference. In one group, a young girl needed someone to take the place of her mother whose sudden death had precipitated the patient's illness. She received support in working out her problems from an older woman who seemed to have particularly good insight into the situation. This identification was gradually lessened as the group became more cohesive.

Manifestations of transference relationship can be observed within the group when a patient indicates that she feels toward the nurse-leader or another patient as she has felt toward her mother, her father, or someone else closely connected with her life. The patient needs to be helped, of course, to work through these transference relationships.

Getting the Group Together

Some will maintain that this is the only real contribution the nurse can make to group therapy. Although such a statement is quite false, the nurse does have an important responsibility for encouraging patients to attend. They are invited by the ward nurse to come to group therapy sessions. The question of whether or not to "force" a patient to attend must be met and decided upon by the nurse-leader. Generally, "social pressure" is much more valuable. Sometimes the patient needs to remain away from the group temporarily for the sake of his own comfort. Often this will give the leader a clue to the emotional problem which is distressing the patient.

If a patient is missing, the group can be helped to feel responsible for his return at the next session. The nurse-leader should ask about the patient and a group member from his ward should be urged to talk to him and encourage him to return. If a patient has felt threatened or rejected at a previous session, the nurse-leader may go to his ward and extend to him a special invitation to return to the group.

Environment and Group Methods

We believe that group sessions should be held in the building where the patients live. Any room can be used but it is best to select one with which the patients have pleasant associations. This is not always feasible, however. One of our groups, for instance, meets in the room where electric shock treatments are given, an arrangement which is necessary but not desirable.

Chairs are arranged informally in a circle for the first meeting. The nurse-leader arrives after the group has been assembled. She introduces herself to the group and carefully explains that the purpose of the get-together is to talk over common problems and, through united effort, attempt to understand and solve them. Patients should understand that the goal is *better adaptation to everyday life.*

The development of security within the group is exceedingly important. Relationships must be established in which the group does not defensively resist the leader but rather finds in her a source of confidence and support in times of stress. When patients begin to feel secure they will discuss problems as realistically as they would in individual therapy.

The nurse-leader must encourage the patient to tell more about his hurts, insecurities, and conflicts. In time, with her help, and with the help of the group, he will reach a solution — an outcome which will be especially satisfying to him since he has achieved it through his own efforts.

She must be willing to listen and able to show real interest in what the patient is saying. Even the most disorganized conversation and behavior may be considered later and found to have a great deal of meaning but, at first, the content is not as important as the establishment of a comfortable relationship.

The group often serves as a support for an individual member but, as is sometimes seen in the cruelty of children, they are quick "to call the score" in reverting to reality. The nurse-leader should not let one patient suffer at the hands of others; nor can she let the patient fail. It is possible to turn the discussion in another direction, or at least to offer the group a substitute topic.

A patient will frequently be anxious about an immediate situation and will use denial and projection to console himself. At these times he is quite likely to accept the opinions of fellow members, who have had similar painful experiences, rather than those of the nurse.

The nurse-leader should not give up because she does not understand what is going on within the group. The group frequently will repeat actions as well as questions and discussion.

During the first few sessions, patients usually ask the nurse-leader many personal questions. This is common in establishing good rapport and should not cause anxiety. The importance of such questioning lies in the reasons for the patient's interest. Frequently the questions can be referred back to the group or to the individual patient. The leader retains a kindly attitude toward such questioning but an attempt must be made to maintain an attitude of friendly objectivity.

The group leader has been described as a catalyst who constantly promotes interaction within the group.[2] This is especially important at the stages when regression takes place. The leader may enter into the regression but must keep a balance between reality and fantasy.

Dr. Strecker touches on this problem when he asks, "How should the nurse go about convincing the patient that, all in all, reality is more attractive than unreality, sanity better than insanity?" His answer contains excellent advice. He says, "It cannot be done abruptly and aggressively. It is a painstaking, gradual, tactful, and often devious work, and there are many 'detours.'"[3]

The nurse-leader should always be sincere in her behavior and conversation. Patients, especially schizophrenics, are quick to sense any superficiality just as they are quick to sense lack of interest.

There is likely to be considerable tension within the group for many sessions. It is better to let such a feeling ride and to let the group decide what can be done about it. They can be encouraged to understand and work through such feelings. It is often impossible to maintain a stable atmosphere where emotionally-laden problems are being discussed. When tension is released by one member, it frequently serves as a very convenient outlet for others in the group. In one case, the group had been extremely tense for two sessions, and feeling had mounted to a high pitch. One very homicidal patient picked up a heavy wooden chair, intending to throw it at another patient toward whom she was momentarily hostile. A few quiet words from a third patient dispelled the highly charged situation and the entire group obviously felt immediate relief. It is at times like this that the nurse-leader needs to remain calm and composed. From her experience in working with patients she will be able to judge just when and where she should step in.

Undoubtedly, the nurse-leader's most important responsibility is to allow the group *freedom of expression*. She must not be troubled by aggression, nor should she retaliate when it is directed against her. Rather, she needs to feel so secure within herself that she can accept the aggression and recognize its real meaning.

Some group therapists advocate complete neutrality but others believe that this tends to produce an abnormal situation. One day a patient began twisting the sleeve of the nurse-leader's sweater and continued until she was actually damaging it. The nurse remained neutral until she felt that the situation had become unnatural; then she asked the patient to stop, and pointed out the damage she was doing.

Another patient made homosexual advances toward the nurse-leader. This is a common occurrence when the leader and the patients are of the same sex, especially with patients who are very ill. The nurse should not moralize in such a situation but neither should she condone such behavior. She must let the patient know as tactfully and kindly as possible that such actions are not acceptable, either to society or to her. She must realize that the patient needs a sounding board on which to test her feelings. These examples clearly indicate that limit setting is one of the skills a nurse-leader must acquire.

Some General Considerations

We have found that a group of from 10 to 15 patients is ideal for good group functioning. With a group this small, the nurse-leader is better able to observe the emotional relationships and reactions of all members. If the group is too small, however, the nurse is hampered by a limited interplay of reactions and a tendency toward individual psychotherapy.

The presence of visitors always has some effect on the group. This effect can be minimized if the nurse discusses the coming visit with the group beforehand. If the visitor is present over a long period of time, the group eventually will tend to accept him as a non-participating member.

If the services of a recorder are used, this procedure should be initiated from the very first session. Then, as with the visitor, the group will accept the recorder as time goes on. We have concluded that the recorder's notes should be written outside the group session. This is based on our observations that many patients feel they cannot discuss confidential material which may be "used against me," or that they feel they are being "used as guinea pigs."

The nurse-leader will often need and seek the psychiatrist's advice for her group of patients. She will also want to meet with other group leaders from time to time to discuss problems, pool experiences, and glean information. In this way leaders gain support from one another.

Besides helping patients to help themselves and

each other, the nurse-leader can make another very important contribution as a member of the psychotherapeutic team. She may frequently be able to stimulate the patients' interest to the extent that they will ask for the assistance of a psychiatrist and for the more interpretive, intensive psychotherapy that he is able to give.

References

1. Render, Helena W. *Nurse-Patient Relationships in Psychiatry.* New York, McGraw-Hill, 1947, p. 3.

2. Fidler, J., Jr. and Standish, C. Observations noted during the course of group treatment of psychoses. *Dis. Nerv. System* 9:24-28, Jan. 1948.

3. Strecker, Edward A. *Fundamentals of Psychiatry.* 4th ed. Philadelphia, Lippincott, 1947, p. 299.

A Sociopsychiatric Nursing Approach to Intervention in a Problem of Mutual Withdrawal on a Mental Hospital Ward

Gwen E. Tudor, R.N.

Ms. Tudor is Director of Nurses and Assistant Professor of Psychiatric Nursing, State University of Iowa, and holds a B.S. from the University of Iowa and an M.A. from Teachers College, Columbia University.

This study was done under the supervision of, and in collaboration with, Dr. Morris S. Schwartz, Research Sociologist at Chestnut Lodge Sanitarium and the Washington School of Psychiatry. It was reprinted from *Psychiatry — The Journal of Interpersonal Processes*, 1952.

Psychiatric nurses in a mental hospital are increasingly expected to manifest their competence in nursing by an awareness of and an ability to handle their interpersonal relations with patients in a therapeutically useful manner. Such expertness with the patient in his daily living is oriented primarily in three directions: The nurse functions to *facilitate the patient's communication.* Since mental illness is, in part, a defect in communication, any understanding of the patient's nonverbal gestures or symbolizations and in turn the conveying of meaning to the patient should be of therapeutic value. Secondly, the psychiatric nurse functions *to facilitate the patient's social participation.* Since the predominant characteristic of the mentally ill person is his withdrawal, both physical and social, the nurse who is able to "make a contact," to convey to the patient through mutual participation that social relationships need not be frightening and anxiety-provoking, but can be both satisfying and security-giving, has enabled the patient to take the first step toward mental health. Finally, the psychiatric nurse functions *to fulfill the patient's needs.* The form of expression these needs take, the manner in which they are fulfilled, and the appropriateness of the fulfillment in terms of the manifest need are all matters which the nurse must consider in relating herself to the patient.

There is a growing awareness on the part of some psychiatric nurses that the traditional skills of the psychiatric nurse, although they are important, are not sufficient for fulfilling these three functions most effectively. It is the contention of this paper that the psychiatric nurse must use, to some extent, the tools of the social scientist and combine these with the skills of the nurse. It is hoped that from this liaison will emerge a new skill which will enable the nurse to function more effectively. The social context as it determines and affects the nurse-patient relationship has been insufficiently explored and taken into account in psychiatric nursing. Although a particular nurse may establish effective and satisfactory relations with a patient, this can be easily undone by what others do with the patient, by the formal and informal social structure on the ward which tends to maintain the patient in his mental illness, by the interpersonal relationships among the staff members, and by the general institutional context which orders and forbids certain activities. The social context within which the patient lives is that pattern of interpersonal relations which is the network of reciprocal activities of all those on the ward. It is this social context which both determines in large part the nurse's attitudes and modes of behavior and also facilitates or deters the patient's mental health. The first step is for the nurse to realize that she is part of the social context. She is affected by it and, in part, determines and maintains it. Thus the envelope of characteristic attitudes and activities which constitute the nurse's formal and informal participation is an integral part of the patient's living and will move him toward health or away from it. In turn, the patient also contributes to this context, resulting in a reciprocal influence between patients and personnel; both are affected by and maintain the social context, which, in our study, is the ward, which is itself imbedded in a wider social context called the hospital.

Within this general theoretical framework, our first general assumption is that *"the patient's mental illness is a mode of participation in the social process."*[1] What has ordinarily been considered a symptom — the patient's assaultiveness, incontinence, hallucinations and delusions, demandingness, withdrawal (physical and verbal), and destructiveness — we view as his characteristic pattern of relating to other people. The interpersonal situations he characteristically integrates constitute his mental illness. The second assumption follows from the first: *This mode of participation — the patient's mental illness — can be altered and influenced by the activities others direct toward him.* And the third assumption is that *an alteration in the patient's participation can come about if the nurse is aware of, and acts upon the awareness of, two sets of phenomena:* (1) the nature of the specific interpersonal situations she integrates with the patient; and (2) the nature of the general social context within which these interpersonal situations take place.

Thus not only does the psychiatric nurse need to include the perspective of the social scientist in her operations, but she also needs to become as skillful an observer as she is a participant in psychiatric nursing. Her observations must include an awareness and evaluation of as many as possible of the relevant factors in order to best work in the direction of a therapeutic social context. Without this observational ability, the nurse cannot adequately meet the needs of the patient and facilitate his communication and social participation. Thus, the nurse must become a participant observer, free to see the actualities and potentialities in patient-staff situations and, at the same time, able to deal with the current requirements of the situation. From our point of view, psychiatric nursing can be conceived of as a continuous interpersonal process consisting of these overlapping and definable components: *observation, evaluation of the observations, determination of the various alternatives possible within the situation, intervention, evaluation of the intervention with reference to the reasons for success or failure, and further intervention on the basis of the new data obtained.*

Problem

The problem undertaken for study was twofold: first, to determine the social context and specific social situations with which the patient in a psychiatric unit was integrated and in which he maintained a recurrent pattern of participation, and to identify the various modes of such participation; and second, to determine the ways in which, and means whereby, appropriate intervention might be instituted so as to alter these modes of social participation in the direction of increased security, satisfaction, and higher self-esteem for the patient.

Setting

The data were collected in a 14-bed ward for disturbed women, which was part of an 80-bed private psychoanalytic hospital.[2] The patients in this ward all have the clinical diagnosis of schizophrenia, with the exception of one diagnosed manic-depressive psychosis. Data pertaining to the rest of the hospital were considered only when they seemed to be related to the patients or personnel in the selected unit. Because these patients were severely disabled by their illnesses in terms of caring for themselves or following ordinary social conventions, the personnel-patient ratio was high. The physical facilities provided for patients' living were minimal, consisting only of the bare essentials.

At the beginning of the study, the ward organization was such that the investigator characterized it as authoritarian as compared to the general attitude in the hospital. It was highly organized around the ideas and wishes of the charge nurse. A rigid routine had been established, to which few exceptions were made. Rules and regulations regarding the patients' living were numerous, and maintenance of these rules was stressed repeatedly with the personnel. This allowed little spontaneity or initiative on the part of the personnel, because they were kept so rigidly in line by the charge nurse's orientation; nor did it permit the undertaking of alternative attitudes and activities on the part of the personnel with patients. Patient-personnel contacts were largely limited to essential care or occasions when requests were made by the patients. These contacts appeared to be quite stereotyped in that most activities were governed by regulation, or, if not, a decision for such an activity was made by the charge nurse in accordance with a preestablished set of ideas and characteristic prevailing attitudes. One characteristic attitude which prevailed was that a "good" nurse or aide was one who "did not have any trouble with patients."

During the second month of the study, a change in charge nurses was made. The new charge nurse was a very permissive person and the ward changed rapidly from a rigid, authoritarian constellation to one in which much disorganization and confusion existed, both among patients and personnel. However, this regime did allow for greater flexibility in dealing with patients and did permit various alternatives to be used in their care. At the end of the study, the ward organization had not crystallized into a highly organized form, but there was evidence that this might occur in the future.

From the point of view of the study, however, it should be noted that the initial period of observation occurred in the authoritarian context, whereas the final period of observation, evaluation, and intervention occurred in the more permissive context.

Method

A method for study was evolved through the joint planning of the sociologist[3] and the investigator, both of whom felt that merging of sociological concepts and psychiatric nursing skills might lead to a new approach — a product of both disciplines —

which might be termed sociopsychiatric nursing. In addition, a new method or technique for social psychological investigation might be evolved.

The techniques used in this study were: (1) the systematic collection of data on the interpersonal situations surrounding the patients and the noting of factors indirectly related to the situations; (2) participant observation by the investigator; (3) analysis and evaluation of the data with the sociologist, who was outside the situation; (4) formulation of plans for intervention, in accordance with the analysis and evaluation of data.

The total length of the study was 6 months. For the first month the investigator made general observations of the ward as a whole. These were then discussed and evaluated with the sociologist. Out of this larger body of data, a particular focus of interest developed. For the rest of the time, the investigator concentrated on the problems surrounding two patients who presented similar modes of participation on the ward.

Roles of the Investigator

The investigator changed roles from time to time during the study, according to plan.

Collaborator. — Six hours each week were spent in conference with the sociologist, during which time the data were reported, discussed, and analyzed.

Observer. — During the first month the investigator attempted to maintain the role of observer without actively participating, and made as complete observations of the total social situation as possible in the 34 hours which were usually spent on the ward each week.

Participating member of the staff. — For the next 2 months, the investigator made herself available to patients and staff for 34 hours each week, although she was not held responsible for nursing service. In this role the nature and amount of the data obtained were altered. By being available to patients, the investigator was able not only to observe, but also to experience their modes of participation, and to evaluate more closely her own reciprocal response. Out of this role there seemed to develop another role which might be referred to as "float nurse." Because the investigator was not in a position to make administrative decisions regarding patients' living, she sought out, or was sought out by, patients whose needs apparently were not being understood and/or fulfilled.

Instructor. — During the last 3 months of the study definite plans for intervention were formulated, introduced, and followed through. To facilitate intervention, the investigator assumed the role of the instructor to the personnel on the ward, conferring with groups and individuals in order to clarify attitudes toward patients in terms of the patients' present mode of social participation, and to stimulate the formulation of alternative attitudes and ways of dealing with patients. The investigator observed the results of the intervention and discussed this in turn with the personnel; and a continuous process of reformulation of personnel activities occurred in accordance with the changing situation.

Data

The data presented in ths study are taken from the larger body of data collected. The patients who were selected for focus presented problems which revolved primarily around the fact that there was a constant tendency on the part of the personnel to *avoid* them. The patients' dominant pattern of participation was that of *withdrawal.* It was because of this recurrent avoidance on the part of the staff of these patients with the concomitant isolation and neglect of them and indifference toward them that these patients were chosen for study. We believe that this pattern of avoidance-withdrawal is a dominant reason for the maintenance of these patients' illnesses. It should be noted that the patients were integrated at different levels of participation in the social process. The second patient participated only on a nonverbal level, and was withdrawn physically, while the first patient communicated verbally in a highly autistic manner, although in variable amounts, and was not as withdrawn physically.

The investigator's notes on each patient will be presented separately and in chronological order.

Mrs. Smith

Mrs. Smith was a 43-year-old woman who was admitted to the hospital following the death of her husband in an airplane crash. She was an attractive, feminine person. Her clinical diagnosis was paranoid schizophrenia.

At the end of the first part of the study, at which time the observations on each patient were being systematically collated, the investigator discovered that no data were recorded for Mrs. Smith. In discussing this with the sociologist, the things recalled by the investigator regarding Mrs. Smith were vague and irrelevant and no specific experiences with her could be remembered. The investigator felt, during this initial discussion with the sociologist, that the patient must not be a nursing problem and that she must take care of her own dressing, eating, and so on, although later it became apparent that this was not true. Because of the systematic approach that had been taken in making observations on *all* patients, the fact that no observations were made on Mrs. Smith suggested that the problem surrounding this patient indicated the need for further investigation and study.

The investigator quickly discovered that other personnel responded similarly to this patient; that is, they avoided her, but their withdrawal from her was in such a quiet, insidious way that they, too, were not aware of their response. Preliminary inquiry indicated that the problem surrounding this patient could be a challenging one, since she was so effectively excluded from the vision of the personnel.

The following questions were formulated as guideposts: (1) Is the recurrent avoidance response a pattern with everybody, or is it peculiar to certain people? (2) Are the personnel aware that they avoid the patient? (3) What are the reasons behind the avoidance? (4) What can be done to alter the situation? (5) Can new ways of participation with the patient be conveyed to the personnel? (6) What changes in the social structure will be necessary in order to prevent this avoidance pattern?

In order to give a clear picture of the process type of approach to psychiatric nursing problems, a chronological view of the procedure followed is given below.

A plan was formulated by the investigator and the sociologist in which (1) systematic observations would be made on Mrs. Smith, in an attempt to evaluate her present mode of participation; (2) the investigator would spend considerable time with her in order that interpersonal contacts might be experienced and evaluated; (3) personnel would be observed and their responses to this patient noted by the investigator; and (4) casual conversations with personnel regarding their experiences with Mrs. Smith would be initiated, in order that existing attitudes might become clear.

At the next meeting with the sociologist, two days after the plan was formulated, the investigator presented data on various patients for evaluation. The sociologist asked about Mrs. Smith, and the investigator realized that she had made no observations on this patient, nor had she contacted the patient, even after having a conscious plan to do so. This was again discussed at length.

The next day, upon the investigator's return to the ward, the following observations were recorded:

> Mrs. Smith was observed sitting on the porch. I approached and asked if I might join her. Mrs. Smith was agreeable. A conversation about the weather's being "so hot and humid" resulted. A long silence ensued, and I became more and more uncomfortable. The patient made no further attempts at conversation, but stared fixedly at me. I finally excused myself. Later I observed the patient sitting in a far corner of the porch. Mrs. Smith coughed and spit on the floor; this was repeated at frequent intervals. There was some explosive laughter. She called loudly, "Bring me a cigarette." Aide approached with cigarette, lit it, said nothing. Another aide and student came on the porch; they sat near Mrs. Smith, not paying any attention to her. Mrs. Smith was incontinent of urine through clothing and onto floor and uttered, "Oh, gee," in loud, shrill voice. Student approached another patient on porch and started to converse. Aide looked at large pool of urine on floor and got up and walked into ward. [This type of activity is unusual. When a patient urinates, the floor is usually cleaned immediately and the patient is changed.]

After four or five minutes, Mrs. Smith got up and went to her room. She returned shortly, having changed her clothing. "Nurse, bring me a cigarette and some milk." Student brought milk and cigarette but said nothing to Mrs. Smith, who giggled loudly, and rocked in the chair, repeating, "Jesus."

Later, I went to Mrs. Smith's room. She was on her bed, with legs apart, moving her hips. I offered her a cigarette and smoked one with her. Mrs. Smith covered up, remained still, giggling and staring at me. I had no success at conversation. I remained with her thirty minutes, at the end of which time she voided in bed. I said nothing, got dry clothing for her, changed her bed, and left.

Later, Mrs. Smith came out of her room for cigarette, and sat in hall, smoking. A nurse and an aide were present. Again she voided onto floor. Aide: "Is anything wrong, Mrs. Smith?" Mrs. Smith giggled loudly, "Oh, my." Aide walked away. Mrs. Smith sat for ten minutes, got up, went to room, crawled into bed with wet clothing on. Later I heard her shout, "Unlock my drawers." I entered room and unlocked dresser drawers. After Mrs. Smith had selected dry clothing, she stripped, put it on, and walked onto hall.

[The following day (Sunday), I planned to go to ward for a brief period only, to observe Mrs.

Smith. This plan was completely forgotten.]

During the three subsequent days, although on the ward, the investigator made no observations and had no contacts with the patient. This, again, was not in keeping with the plan that had been formulated. The investigator, in discussing this with the sociologist, could give no reason for avoiding the patient: "Was very busy with other patients." "Spent time with personnel." (Mrs. Smith was not discussed with them, however.) "Seemed to forget about her."

The above makes it quite apparent that, in spite of much interest and enthusiasm of the investigator regarding this problem, and in spite of a definite plan of approach, the avoidance persisted.

During the evaluation of data with emphasis on the persistent avoidance of this patient, the sociologist speculated that the patient's behavior might have a sexual significance, of which the investigator was apparently unaware. Although the investigator experienced anxiety and discomfort with the patient, their source was not clear to the investigator, and the patient continued to be avoided. The investigator had been greatly puzzled by this and by her persisting anxiety in the presence of the patient and her inability to maintain this patient in focus, despite her curiosity about the problem.

Following several discussions with the sociologist, some understanding was reached regarding the possible meaning of this patient's symbolic mode of participation. With the discovery that the anxiety concerned itself primarily with what was felt to be a sexual appeal being made by the patient, the investigator's anxiety with this patient disappeared, and subsequent contacts with her were markedly different. Thus when the problem came into focus, the anxiety disappeared, and the investigator was able to see this patient's total behavior as an attempt to form a human relationship. The patient, in turn, seemed to become correspondingly less anxious and to notice and seek out the investigator's company.

It cannot be emphasized enough here that this sort of finding is nearly impossible to discover in day-to-day nursing care of a patient. It is only when this "process approach" (observation, evaluation, intervention, observation, and so on) is attempted, that one becomes aware of this type of recurrent response in relation to a patient's mode of participation. It also points up the importance of having this type of supervision, in which inquiry is made into minute details by a person who is far enough removed from the situation to be able to evaluate the data in a more comprehensive perspective.

Although the investigator had discovered a disturbing and separating aspect of the interpersonal situation and thus was able to alter her mode of participation with this patient, none of the other personnel had examined their participation in a similar way, so that they persisted in their usual pattern.

The following excerpts indicate the nature of the interpersonal contacts and the type of participation undertaken by the investigator and Mrs. Smith.

Mrs. Smith was on the porch, sitting in a chair. I sat down beside her. She did not respond to my greeting, but continued to stare, giggle, and spit at regular intervals. I made several attempts to converse with her, but she gave no evidence that she heard. She occasionally looked directly at me, and went into hysterical laughing. She continued to cough and spit about once per minute. I sat quietly for about thirty minutes.

Investigator: "You seem quite bothered by the cough."

Mrs. Smith: "Oh, it's nothing much, but very uncomfortable."

Investigator: "It is uncomfortable?"

Mrs. Smith: "Yes. You know what it is, don't you?"

Investigator: "No, I don't think I do."

Mrs. Smith: "I have this thing in my throat, and it makes my throat hurt and burn. The spit is not from my nose or stomach, but from the pus of this infection. The same thing is the cause of this vomiting." (Gets up and goes to her room. Returns and sits beside me. Does not speak. Giggling and spitting continue. I remain for about twenty minutes.)

Mrs. Smith was in the living room with a nurse, Mary (another patient), and me. Mary was telling about her trip and dinner at the Flamingo. Mrs. Smith asked an occasional question, laughing explosively on four or five occasions. Mary continued her story. Mrs. Smith voided on the floor. There was silence for several minutes.

Mary: "You're having quite a discharge, Mrs. Smith." (Leaves the room.)

Nurse: "Do you want to change your things, Mrs. Smith?" (Mrs. Smith rushes from the room, strips her clothing off, and puts on a robe. I go to her bed, and attempt to chat with her for a minute. Mrs. Smith asks for a cigarette, which I give to her.)

Investigator: "I was wondering how you were feeling when you urinated in the living room a little while ago."

Mrs. Smith: "Oh, I didn't urinate! That is life water, and not the same at all. You think it is urine, but it is not. It is life water."

Investigator: "You think it is life water?"

Mrs. Smith: "Certainly. Would you light my cigarette again? It has gone out."

Investigator: "Surely." (Lights cigarette.) "Do you mind talking about this life water?"

Mrs. Smith: "No, I don't mind, but I'd rather discuss it later, if it is the same to you. I'd like to have a bath before I go for a visit. You know I'm having a visitor this morning."

Investigator: "Yes, I know you are. I'll get your bath ready. What do you want to wear?"

Mrs. Smith was in her room on the bed. She was very thoughtful, and did not notice me as I came in.

Investigator: "May I come in, Mrs. Smith?"

Mrs. Smith: "Yes, of course, Did you bring my cigarettes?"

Investigator: "Yes, I did." (I light a cigarette for her. She looks in the other direction, staring at the wall, smoking in silence.) "Did you have a pleasant visit yesterday?"

Mrs. Smith: "Yes, very pleasant."

Investigator: "How long is she planning to stay here?"

Mrs. Smith: "As long as she wishes."

Investigator: "I see." (There is silence for about fifteen minutes, interrupted only by explosive giggling.)

Mrs. Smith: "May I have another cigarette?"

Investigator: "Yes. You seem very thoughtful this afternoon."

Mrs. Smith: "Yes, I have been for a while now. I was thinking of that Greek who killed her children. Do you remember that?"

Investigator: "Yes, I remember — is it Greek mythology?"

Mrs. Smith: "I'm wondering now if this idea to kill the children was really Medea's, or whether it was really her husband's. You know, because of the trouble they were having."

Investigator: "Why would it be her husband's?"

Mrs. Smith: "Oh, I don't really know. Maybe..." (Her talk is rapid and undistinguishable for several minutes.)

Investigator: "I can't understand you. I can't hear what you are saying."

Mrs. Smith: "I was just inferring that the basic conflict is between man and woman, whether it be interpersonal, interdependent, or interaction." (She goes into a long, involved discussion about men and women, the equality of their rights, and so on. I am not able to understand most of this, or even to identify the main theme.) "Could I have another cigarette, please?"

Investigator: "Yes. Mrs. Smith, I'd like to talk to you about some things."

Mrs. Smith: "Yes, what is it?"

Investigator: "I want you to feel free to tell me if you don't want to discuss it."

Mrs. Smith: "Yes, I will tell you."

Investigator: "I was wondering if there is anything that we could do to understand more about your urinating — you know, like yesterday morning in the living room."

Mrs. Smith: "Oh, that. Well, I don't think people should make a fuss and ask you for reasons. Were you there yesterday?"

Investigator: "Yes."

Mrs. Smith: "And who else?"

Investigator: "Miss Brown and Mary."

Mrs. Smith: "Well, I didn't urinate. That is life water, and it's a lot different."

Investigator: "It is different?"

Mrs. Smith: "Yes, it is a clear, heavenly fluid. It's good. It is not urine. I want you to understand that."

Investigator: "What was going on at the time this life water came, or just before? Do you recall?"

Mrs. Smith: "Yes, I can remember Mary was talking about the Flamingo and having dinner there. Miss Brown was looking at her tangerine nail polish that matched her lipstick. You were encouraging Mary. I could see that."

Investigator: "How did that make you feel?"

Mrs. Smith: "You kept getting Mary to talk. I was wondering why, and about Mary."

Investigator: "What about Mary?"

Mrs. Smith: "Well, first I thought she was just talking and hadn't really been to the Flamingo. Then I realized she had been. She kept getting the bar, cloak room, and the ladies' room mixed up. I was trying to put together what Mary was saying — What do you think of Mary's breasts? There is a word for them. I can't think of it."

Investigator: "A word for Mary's breasts?"

Mrs. Smith: "Yes, it is like a bower, or something. I was wondering what you thought."

Investigator: "You were wondering what I thought about what?"

Mrs. Smith: "About life and the pursuit of happiness. You kept telling Mary to talk and this kept coming up in my mind. Life — life and happiness. Then I thought about the book I had told you about the other day. You kept looking at Mary."

Investigator: "How did you feel?"

Mrs. Smith: "Oh, fine, I guess."

Investigator: "You weren't upset?"
Mrs. Smith: "Oh, no, I felt wonderful — sort of floating."
Investigator: "This was when you urinated?"
Mrs. Smith: "Yes, but I told you it was not urine. It is a purer fluid."
Investigator: "Where does it come from?"
Mrs. Smith: "I'm not just sure. But not from the bladder. From the womb, I suppose."
Investigator: "Is this different than when you go to the bathroom?"
Mrs. Smith: "My, yes. Very different."
Investigator: "How is it different?"
Mrs. Smith: "It floods, is very warm and very pleasant. When I urinate, it isn't like this. It is a sharp thing, and you feel indifferent to it. Oh, it is not the same at all."
Investigator: "Is it like anything else, this feeling you have with the life water?"
Mrs. Smith: "Well, not exactly, but nearly like it. I don't know how it is different. There is much more fluid, I guess. Do you think it comes from my womb?"
Investigator: "I can't see how it could."
Mrs. Smith: "You can't?"
Investigator: "No."
Mrs. Smith: "Well, isn't the bladder connected to the womb?"
Investigator: "No, it isn't."
Mrs. Smith: "Do you know how it is — I mean, the kidneys, bladder, and womb, and all that?"
Investigator: "Yes, I guess I do."
Mrs. Smith: "Can you tell me something about it?"
Investigator: "Yes."
Mrs. Smith: "Draw it for me. Then it will be clearer."
Investigator: "All right." (I explain, with drawings, a little about anatomy, and so on. Mrs. Smith asks many questions, requesting all the technical names.)
Mrs. Smith: "Now tell me about the ovaries, tubes, and the womb." (I tell her briefly in a very simple fashion. She asks about menses.) "Well, now if that is the way it is, I'm not so sure where this life water does come from, are you?"
Investigator: "I think that it comes from the bladder. It must be urine."
Mrs. Smith: "Yes, maybe. But it doesn't seem that way." (A nurse comes in to tell Mrs. Smith that her visitor is waiting downstairs to visit again.)

I am seated in the living room. Mrs. Smith comes in, and pulls a chair up beside mine, and offers me a cigarette.
Mrs. Smith: "How are you today?"
Investigator: "Fine. And you?"
Mrs. Smith: "I'm feeling much better." (She stands up and pulls her dress up. Then she sits down again, making sure that none of her dress is underneath her.) "I was hoping you would be here, so we could have a short talk."
Investigator: "Fine." (Mrs. Smith talks rapidly in a rather disorganized fashion about various places, plays, and college days. I say very little, making listening sounds for the most part. This continues for about 45 minutes. Suddenly she leans back in her chair, laughs in an explosive fashion, stares straight ahead, and voids.)
Investigator: "Mrs. Smith — "
Mrs. Smith: "Yes, what were we talking about? Oh, yes. You say you have been in Alaska." (An aide comes in and tells Mrs. Smith that it is time for her hour. She excuses herself, goes to her room, changes her pants, and goes down to her hour.)

Mrs. Smith continues to sit for long periods, laughing, spitting, and voiding. She voids three or four times each day, usually when seated in a group or with one person. Today she voided while off the ward with a student nurse. They were seated on a bench in the yard. Later, on the ward, Mrs. Smith comes and sits by me.
Mrs. Smith: "Just what are you doing on the ward? You are a nurse, aren't you?"
Investigator: "Yes, I'm doing a study here." (Explains.)
Mrs. Smith: "That's interesting. I wondered why you always carried the notebook. You talked to all the patients. I thought maybe you were a student doing something. What did you find out about me? At first you never talked to me. I wondered why."
Investigator: "That is true. I guess I avoided you at first. I had been meaning to ask if you had noticed, and wondered why."
Mrs. Smith: "I surely did. That's the way it goes. Were you too busy — or what happened?"
Investigator: "Not entirely. I was busy, but I don't think that was the reason."
Mrs. Smith: "Well, you'll probably find out." (Conversation shifts.)

The investigator continued to spend time with the patient each day. Careful analysis of the contacts revealed that the type and level of communication changed during this period in the following ways: Periods of silence became infrequent (other than natural lags expected in any discussion). The amount of autistic thinking decreased markedly (the patient was well informed and had abundant topics for conversation). The patient began to take initiative in making contact with investigator, would call to her upon hearing her come on the ward, or say, "Let's have a cup of tea and talk a while." Most personnel on floor were referred to as "Nurse," "Hey," "You," but the patient always called investigator by name, sometimes Miss Tudor, and sometimes by her first name. The investigator always informed patient when she would return, and on several occasions when the time of return was altered, Mrs. Smith would ask, "What happened? I thought you were coming this morning." It became possible to include another person or personnel in our contacts, by inviting the patient to have tea with us, or by going with Mrs. Smith into a group of other patients and personnel.

The type of interpersonal contacts with Mrs. Smith ranged from participating in daily care (bathing, fixing hair, helping her with meals, taking her to her therapeutic hours) to more social activities, such as visiting, singing, reading together, and so on. An average of two and a half hours each day was spent with the patient. Because the investigator had gained this new perspective, which enabled the relationship with the patient to improve, the patient's behavior changed so markedly that the therapist was led to comment about it to the investigator, pointing out the therapeutic usefulness of this relationship to the patient.

It soon became apparent that, despite the increased patient-investigator participation, the constant personnel response was still that of avoidance. A summary of the data collected on this patient revealed that no approaches were made to this patient other than for eating, bathing, dressing, and going to her hour. Despite the fact that the patient would respond and participated freely with the investigator, she often refused to get up, eat, bathe, and so on when approached by others. The result was that much of Mrs. Smith's daily care had indirectly become the responsibility of the investigator.

In a discussion with the sociologist, the following question was raised: If the investigator were to withdraw and the personnel continued their pattern of avoiding the patient, would the withdrawal of the patient be reinforced? If the patient resumed her isolation, we would have additional evidence that the specific interpersonal relationships between patient and investigator had contributed to the change in the patient's level of participation. It would also suggest the importance of the general social context (the staff's avoidance of the patient integrates with the patient's withdrawal) in maintaining the patient's illness.

At this point in the investigation the investigator withdrew from the ward to go on vacaction. The following data indicates the course of the patient's behavior:

> [Prior to going on vacation, the investigator informed Mrs. Smith of her plans; the patient became interested in where the vacation would be, what the investigator would be doing, and so on. On return from vacation, the investigator asked the charge nurse for a detailed verbal report of all patients.]
>
> Charge nurse: "Mrs. Smith has been staying in bed almost constantly, she has been incontinent four to six times per 24 hours in bed, or in her clothing, if up. She has been tearing her clothing and hospital sheets and blankets. The vomiting and spitting have increased. For the most part, she is mute, and unresponsive, 'out of contact.' Has not eaten or bathed regularly. Does come onto hall for cigarette [patients are not permitted to smoke in their rooms unless specialed] but for the most part remains in bed with her head covered. Her analyst has been coming to the ward for her hours."
>
> [I approached patient, who was in bed with head covered, and called her name several times. There was no response. I remained seated on bed for fifteen minutes, occasionally calling her name or touching her. I then got a cup of tea and returned.]
>
> Investigator: "Mrs. Smith, I want to talk to you. Let's have some tea and a cigarette." (She sits up in bed abruptly.)
>
> Mrs. Smith: "Hi, how are you? How was Iowa? How was your sister's wedding? What did you wear? Tell me about everything!"
>
> Investigator: "We have plenty of time to talk, Mrs. Smith. I'm interested in how you are, too." (The visit continues for thirty minutes. Mrs. Smith remains alert and interested, asking many questions.)
>
> Investigator: "Mrs. Smith, are you tired?"
>
> Mrs. Smith: "Yes, very. Mind if I go back to sleep? I've not been sleeping at all nights — just think, think, think, all night. I'll tell you about it later."
>
> Investigator: "All right. You take a nap and I'll be back later. Maybe you'd feel like a hot bath."
>
> Mrs. Smith: "Yes, I'd really like that." (Turns face to wall, covering head.)

After this initial response, the patient lapsed into withdrawn, autistic behavior. It was not possible to elicit responses from her as previously, and giving her care required much special ministration. The personnel response continued as before — avoidance. The following notes indicate the second phase of the interpersonal relationship between the patient and the investigator.

> I have been unable to gain Mrs. Smith's attention for past three days, even with repeated attempts. Have remained with her, mostly in silence, occasionally making a comment or calling her name. Have changed her bed and clothing as often as necessary (voiding). Have told her when I was leaving and when I would be back.
>
> Today I began taking Mrs. Smith something every hour — juice, milk, pieces of apple, a cigarette, hot tea. She responds by accepting what I bring. No conversation. She stares into space, never looking at me, and continues to spit and vomit. She is frequently incontinent in bed. When I asked her about a bath and took her hand, she went with me. It was necessary to bathe her. She made no verbal responses, but followed simple suggestions.
>
> Mrs. Smith continues mute and unresponsive. She has been tearing clothing and blankets, and spitting and voiding much. I continue to spend time with her and take her things periodically.
>
> Patient began to talk a bit again today. She also giggled and said, "Oh, God," "Oh, dear," "Oh, my," and so on. Attention is difficult to maintain. It is often necessary to take her hand or arm to make her aware of my presence. Also, if I shift position, and get in line of her vision, she will then speak and remain in contact for a short period.
>
> Data of the next several weeks show that I spent an average of one and one-half hours daily with the patient. Her communication progressed from silence to fluent conversation and became less and less autistic. Other aspects of her mode of social participation also changed. She stopped spitting and vomiting. Voiding continued, but was less frequent. Giggling persisted and was louder. She screamed, "Oh, my, oh, my," louder and more frequently throughout the day.

Thus the types of interpersonal experiences were changing. At first there was just sitting, with little conversation; then participation in her daily care; then reading together; finally singing together and with the group. Mrs. Smith learned to play the Autoharp and enjoyed playing and singing with the investigator and the group.

At this point, the patient's mode of social participation had again changed. She was spending much time out of bed, she was conversing with other patients, joining some group activity (singing and dancing), her incontinence had decreased — she was going to the bathroom sometimes on her own initiative, and sometimes at the suggestion of the investigator, frequently being continent for an entire 24-hour period. It was assumed that the interpersonal experience the patient was having with the investigator was an important contributing factor in this change. In order to validate this, and again to evaluate the effect of the ward's avoidance on this patient, a plan was formulated whereby the investigator (with much personal misgivings) would avoid the patient for a period of one week, and observe her response. The following are excerpts from the data collected during this time.

> *First day.* Mrs. Smith remained in bed much of day. She did not respond to aide who asked about bath. She came onto hall, loudly demanding. "*Nurse,* get me some tea and a cigarette." (I withdrew from hall.) In p.m. she was gotten out of bed by another patient, giggled loudly, and repeated, "Jesus." She voided twice in bed during day, and then once shouted, "Hey, change this bed." She was reported to have voided two times in bed during the night.
>
> *Second day.* Mrs. Smith had her head covered in bed at 8 a.m. and refused breakfast. She was approached for bath at 10 and did not respond. She came onto hall on several occasions. She shouted, "Nurse, nurse, get me a cigarette." Later, "I want tea — hot tea, not lukewarm." She voided two times while sitting in hall, sat for long period in wet clothing, exposed self while on hall, and did not seem in contact except when shouting requests. She did much loud giggling and shouting, "Oh, dear!" (I remained away from patient.) She was observed to be spitting on floor.
>
> *Third day.* I was not on ward. Report on patient was much the same as the previous day.
>
> *Fourth day.* I was in hall outside Mrs. Smith's door, talking with another patient who was demanding to get out. Mrs. Smith got out of bed, came to hall, and said, "Gwen, let's have a cigarette. What the hell is wrong with you? So damn snooty — get us both some tea and come in here." (Very irritated.) I complied and visited with her for thirty minutes, then helped her with her bath. Later, when I was playing records on hall

with group of patients, Mrs. Smith brought a chair up to mine and listened to music. She patted my hand on several occasions. In p.m. she was in bed for a while. She came to nursing station and said, "Gwen, get the harp. Let's get some singing going. You play and I'll sing. Maybe some of the rest will, too." We played harp and sang. I told her that it was time to leave. "Will you be back tomorrow?" "Yes." "What time?" "In the morning at 8:00." "All right, we will have coffee in the morning."

Fifth day. I could not avoid patient, since she made requests almost continuously as she did yesterday, until I started taking things to her before she asked. She then became less demanding.

The significance of this is that the ongoing social process may disrupt the best laid plans of investigators; that once having established a relationship with the patient, it was not easy to avoid her, even for purpose of research. From the first few days, however, it was evident that the avoidance of the patient by the investigator contributed to her withdrawal and more disturbed behavior.

In the situation of mutual withdrawal between the patient and personnel, the patient played her part by spending long hours in bed, occasionally making demands on the personnel, spitting and vomiting, which repelled them, yet at the same time forced some contact in the clean-up process. Personnel would not, however, talk to her during the cleaning. Mrs. Smith would giggle and shout, "Oh, Jesus," or some similar expression, making the personnel quite anxious, and reinforcing their need to withdraw from her. The following extract indicates a fairly typical response to it:

Investigator: "Why do you think Mrs. Smith says things like 'Oh, dear,' 'Oh, God,' 'Oh, my,' and so on? What does it mean to you?"

Aide: "I don't know. I wish she would stop."

Investigator: "How does it make you feel?"

Aide: "I really don't know. Like something is very wrong. Maybe she is laughing at me, making fun of me, I don't know, except that I get very uncomfortable. I just want to run."

The staff's avoidance was so excluded from their awareness that they were reluctant to talk about her, although this was in direct contrast with their collaborative attitude with the investigator about other patients. When the avoidance was pointed out, they refused to accept its validity. The following excerpts indicate the staff's attitude.

Investigator: "About Mrs. Smith, I was wondering what your ideas were. What has your experience with her been?"

Nurse: "What do you mean? She seems to get along all right. What is the problem?"

Investigator: "People seem to avoid her. I was wondering why."

Nurse: "I don't agree that she is avoided. She often refuses to do things, but people do make an effort to contact her."

This was discussed repeatedly with this nurse, who continually questioned the point that patient was avoided.

Investigator: "What about Mrs. Smith's incontinence? What could we do about it?"

Nurse: "It may be just a phase."

Investigator: "I wonder if she would discuss it."

Nurse: "I don't think so. It is representative of something."

I talked to the entire ward personnel about some of the things I had been doing on the ward and asked for their cooperation in relating the experiences they had been having with three specific patients, of which Mrs. Smith was one. The other two patients were discussed fully. Mrs. Smith was not mentioned.

In a small ward conference (five personnel), I again talked with personnel, asking for experiences with the *three* patients. The entire conference time was spent on two. Mrs. Smith was again omitted.

Investigator: "I was wondering what you thought about Mrs. Smith. What kind of experiences do you have with her?"

Aide: "I don't have any trouble with her. I like her quite a bit."

Investigator: "Have you had any chats with her?"

Aide: "Oh, yes, she is interesting to talk with. I do spend time with her."

Investigator: "What do you talk about?"

Aide: "Oh, the usual things. Let's see — Well, I can't remember any specific thing right now."

Investigator: "Do you usually initiate the experiences or does she?"

Aide: "Oh, it's fifty-fifty, I guess."

Investigator: "When was the last time you had a five- or ten-minute contact with her?"

Aide: "Well, let me think. (Pause.) I can't remember when I really talked with her that long. I take her tea and cigarettes."

Investigator: "Does she usually ask, or do you take them on your own?"

Aide: "Oh, she asks. Let's see — When did I talk to her? I guess I haven't lately. I can't really say for sure."

The above mentioned aide was always fairly accurate in reporting her experiences with other patients. She was quite free with the investigator in expressing how she felt about patients — such as whether she liked them or not, sought them out or not. The investigator had not observed this particular aide making a single contact with Mrs. Smith other than when a demand was made of the patient, or by the patient. This is an example of the aide's not really being aware of how she functioned with this patient. She distorted at first, and when questioned more closely, could not remember. This is the sort of inquiry that may lead the personnel to really question how they do respond to patients.

With some personnel, it was found that evasion was used when this patient was mentioned:

Investigator: "I was wondering what we might do with Mrs. Smith. Tell me a little about your experiences with her."

Aide: "We get along just fine. She makes a lot of requests, but that is what I'm here for. I like all the patients, and I enjoy doing things for them — even Miss Brown." (Goes into lengthy discussion regarding this other patient. Her observations are accurate and she is free to express her feelings.)

Investigator: "To get back to Mrs. Smith. Have you visited with her lately?"

Aide: "I've noticed that she is becoming very friendly with Miss Brown. They seem to be great pals."

Investigator: "Yes, I've noticed that."

Aide: "I think it is good for Miss Brown. I'm always glad to see the patients getting on so well." [Several more unsuccessful attempts were made to bring the discussion around to Mrs. Smith.]

Investigator: "I wanted to ask you what you thought about Mrs. Smith's giggling and the way she says 'Oh, my,' 'Jesus,' and so on. What does it mean to you?"

Aide: "I think it is disturbing to the others. They get tired of it. I've heard them tell her to shut up."

Investigator: "Do you think she is amused, or what?"

Aide: "I really couldn't say. It is hard to tell."

Investigator: "How does it affect you?"

Aide: "Well, I know she can't help it." (Laughs and walks away.)

Mrs Smith was discussed with a student nurse who had been on the ward for ten weeks. At first the student felt she had a good relationship with this patient. After further discussion, she became aware that she had not made a single contact with the patient during her entire ten weeks, other than to take her food, cigarettes, and so on. This student was an exceptionally sensitive, imaginative person, who had unusually constructive interpersonal experiences with the majority of patients on this unit.

The reaction of the patient to this avoidance and her awareness of it is indicated below.

Mrs. Smith was approached by a nurse in regard to an appointment for an eye refraction. She did not respond, and nurse repeated her request. Mrs. Smith became very angry, "Go to the doctor; go to your appointment. I'm not going, and you can get the hell out of here. I'm sick in bed, and not getting up." Nurse left.

I later went in to talk to patient regarding this.

Investigator: "Mrs. Smith, what about your appointment for an eye refraction? You can't read with those old glasses. We should take care of it real soon."

Mrs. Smith: "Yes, I know. I want to get it done. I've got to real soon."

Investigator: "I was wondering why you got so upset when Miss Nelson asked you about it."

Mrs. Smith: "I get sick of their paying absolutely no attention for months, then, 'Get up, get up; go to the doctor.' They don't care if I'm living or dead until they want me to do something. I've got the flu, and they don't even know it." [Patient had a cold and was probably chilly and achy.]

Investigator: "I see. Well, I don't want you to let your glasses go too long."

Mrs. Smith: "I intend to go to the eye doctor. Tell them to make the appointment. It's just that I get mad when — well, you understand."

Investigator: "Yes. Want some aspirin and a water bottle?"

The incident of the appointment for an eye refraction was discussed with the nurse involved. She had been rather surprised at Mrs. Smith's reaction and stated that perhaps this "patient is being avoided." This was contrary to her previous feeling regarding this pattern.

Our interpretation of this situation was that continued avoidance of this patient by the personnel was a result of both the lack of awareness of the staff of their pattern of avoidance, and the sexual connotation of the patient's behavior — her use of the terms "Oh, my," "Oh, God," "Jesus," and so on, and her incontinence, all of which seemed to contain orgasmic qualities.

Throughout the study, the investigator had frequent contacts with the therapists whose patients were living on this ward. Mrs. Smith's therapist was contacted at the point in the study where the investigator wished to begin fairly lengthy and consistent contacts with this patient.

The pattern of mutual withdrawal was discussed, emphasizing the subtle nature of this problem, including the investigator's failure to recognize this pattern initially, and the fact that this was currently true of the rest of the personnel. The therapist felt that because a strong, positive (good mother) relationship had finally been formed between the patient and the investigator, her negative feeling was beginning to come out and be worked out with the therapist. This was something that had not been accomplished previously in the therapy. Because avoidance was no longer necessary on the part of the investigator, she was free to form a relationship which focused on the healthy part of the patient. Because the patient could begin to be aware of some of her health, she could then begin to deal with her sick part with more comfort.

The therapist also felt that the investigator had been able to give an unconditional type of care to this patient, making almost no demands of her, anticipating her needs, and setting limits only as determined by the situation. This had communicated the investigator's acceptance of the patient on a level she could understand (taking her things, sitting with her for long, silent periods, bathing her, feeding her, and so on). This type of acceptance was a prominent need in this patient, and could not be conveyed on a verbal level. It was felt that the fulfillment of this need was appropriate to the patient's present level of participation.

Summary

In reviewing the course of the participation with this patient, it became clear that without the *joint analysis* of the data with an outside person possessing a perspective of the social structure and who was not involved in the interaction, the subtle nature of the avoidance pattern might never have been uncovered. The following steps constituted the joint process undertaken by the sociologist and the investigator:

(1) Recognition and observation of the interpersonal situation surrounding this patient — the avoidance-withdrawal pattern.

(2) Evaluation of these observations, including the reasons for the avoidance, resulting in a reduction of the anxiety of the investigator, which then permitted the problem to come into sharp focus.

(3) Recognition of the problem as one in which the staff's mode of participation maintained the patient at a withdrawn, autistic level.

(4) Intervention in the process of avoidance by the investigator's providing those interpersonal experiences that both fulfilled the patient's needs and were appropriate to her present level of participation.

(5) Observation and evaluation of these interventions: it was seen that the interpersonal situation with the investigator permitted the patient to participate at a higher level.

Miss Jones

Miss Jones is a 28-year-old woman, who has been hospitalized for the past 10 years. The onset of her illness was acute, and the diagnosis at time of admission was schizophrenia.

Miss Jones is a tall, very thin, attractive girl, with long blond hair, worn either in pigtails, or piled high on top of her head. She appears much younger than her stated years. Miss Jones' mode of social participation at the beginning of the investigation was one of almost complete physical and verbal withdrawal. The investigator's first introduction to Miss Jones and her difficulties was during the investigator's initial orientation to the unit. The following are verbatim comments made by the head nurse:

> "Marian Jones has been here for 10 years. She is about 30 years old. She is mute and inactive, and, for the most part, remains in bed. She will not talk to you. She has ceased being assaultive, but will blow up and attack you if you get too close to her. She cannot tolerate *closeness*. She will accept routine nursing care, like bathing and having her hair combed. She eats poorly and has to be reminded about this — or forced to eat. She sometimes refuses to go to her hours, and we do not force her to go."

Daily observations were made on Miss Jones by the investigator. The following gives a picture of Miss

Jones' usual day, abstracted from observations made early in the study.

Breakfast finds Marian in bed, not asleep, but with her eyes tightly closed, as if dreading the prospect of another day. The covers are pulled tightly about her, her body in a rather shrinking position, denoting in itself withdrawal from the surroundings. "Here is your tray, Marian." There is no sign of interest, the only response being that the covers are pulled more tightly about her. Her facial expression seems to combine apathy and distaste. "Now, you must eat your breakfast," continues the voice in a very automatic fashion. The tray is placed beside her. Her eyes close even more tightly, and she relaxes slightly after she hears the footsteps leaving the room. After 4 or 5 minutes, she opens her eyes and glances at the tray, reaches for her nearly cold coffee, has a few swallows and sinks back into the bed. Then, as if compelled, she eats a few bites of breakfast, swallowing hard with each bite. Turning over in bed, she assumes her former position. It is almost as though she eats just enough to keep alive, not really to satisfy her, but just to exist.

Around 9:00 or 9:30, Marian is again approached for her bath and dressing. She physically clings to the bed, but after much urging, starts toward the bathroom, being more pushed than going on her own. A hot bath with perfumed bubbles is ready. There is no pleasure in this, despite the fact that, other than eating and perhaps a silent walk, this is to constitute her day. Her clothing has been selected. Marian dresses automatically, with help, and allows her long, thick blond hair to be combed and piled attractively on top of her head. She then is led to the porch to a chair. She sits here, legs and feet outstretched on the floor. Sliding down in the chair, she rests her head and face on her right hand, carefully covering her mouth. Her gaze is directed at the floor; she does look around occasionally, but if you catch her eye, she quickly looks at the floor, as if frightened at the prospect of exchanging a smile or glance.

Little is said to Marian, other than at meal time, or if it is time for her hour or a walk. Then, "Marian, it is time for your hour." No response. "Marian, come on, let's go to your hour." Then she is taken by the hand and led to the door. Often, she shakes her head, "No," as she goes out the door. At times she holds onto the chair and does not go. Her eyes remain on the floor. She knows that she will not be forced to go. Occasionally, persons will sit beside her for a short while and leaf through a magazine or say a few words, but they soon leave. Marian may glance quickly up as they go. In the evening, she sits in front of the television. At times she watches, but the major portion of the time her eyes are on the floor. Soon it is bedtime. Marian goes willingly, hurrying into her pajamas and toward her bed.

Periodically Miss Jones becomes upset. Over a period of time it was observed that (1) the upsets always occurred after a contact with the personnel; (2) the upsets occurred when some sort of demand had been made of the patient; and (3) the content of the verbalizations was always very similar. The following is a fairly typical upset taken from the data collected by the investigator on this patient:

> Marian has remained in bed all day today, refusing her meals and her bath. At 2:00 p.m. she is approached for her hour. She refuses to get out of bed. The aide urges her, as usual, and then leaves the room. Marian begins to scream, and this continues for about twenty minutes. I can get only part of the content of this upset, since she is screaming and shouting at a very rapid rate.
>
> Marian: "Why I put up with this, I don't know. Nothing to drink but water since I was a baby. I'm not taking it any more. I'll marry Winston Churchill or anyone else that they say. That dirty rotten whore. I never had trouble with people in my life before I came here. They try to teach us how to live and they don't know how to live themselves. Filthy whores, filthy bitches, horrible old prostitutes dressed in white satin and shoes. I was brought up by a lady, never treated like this. They will apologize or know the reason why. No one understands anything around here. I can't stand this. Eat this, do this, do that. Come on, now, Marian, you know you must do this. She yells and screams when I don't feel well. How in hell can I put up with this? Throws a fit at me. There is no reason in the world why she has to act like this. This place is a dirty, filthy whore house. It's the dirtiest filthy whore place in the country. They don't have any respect for living. They don't have manners, or live on Fifth Avenue, or pay their bills. I tell the truth, but no one will listen. They try to train me to do something I can't learn. I can't be this way. How can you walk in high heels when you haven't learned to walk yet? Most people sit up to eat. Most people do this and that. Throw her out; knock her down. I don't want her. She is filthy. She doesn't pay her bills or live on Fifth Avenue.
>
> I can't do anything about it. I can't wear high

heels. I'm sick of all of this. I won't stand it any longer. Get rid of it. I can't do it any longer. They tell you how to walk. Then they say, 'Poor girl, she never got well. She can't walk. I don't want Miss Jones. I can't stand her.' I can't understand why I do things wrong. Miss Jones, Miss Jones, do this, do that, do this, do that. I can't stand this. They tear up my clothes, my hair, my body. They slobber on me. Slobber all over me. I can't do it any longer. I don't want her. Her father throws her in a mental hospital and lets her rot. He can't understand. She is crazy. I can't have it. I'm sick of it. Miss Jones. She has been trying to learn how to walk in a mental hospital for years. If Miss Jones can't learn how to behave, then why doesn't she leave? I can't stand her. Her background is horrible. Wears ridiculous clothing. She hasn't a bit of taste in food. Not a nurse in the world could take care of her. She has the worst family. Her mother screams all the time. I've had enough of Miss Jones. Old, broken-down person. No one wants to help her. No one wants to know her."

Data were also collected regarding the recurrent responses of the nursing staff in their relations with Marian. The most frequent experience personnel had with Marian was that of *failure*. Because of this repetitive experience of failure, the staff became indifferent and apathetic and developed much guilt. By labeling the patient "hopeless," this guilt could, to some extent, be alleviated. Her upsets were dismissed as being caused by "too much closeness with people." In casual conversation, the personnel would point out that they did try, they did make a few approaches, but they felt that there was no hope. There was also some evidence of hostility and contempt toward Marian, probably derived in part from the repetitive failure. The following extracts from the data illustrate these attitudes on the part of the staff.

Three days out of four, Marian remains in bed the greater part of the day, and the personnel report that she refuses to get up. Her eating habits are very poor and any attempts to urge her to eat are unheeded or precipitate an upset. Verbal responses are completely absent. [The first notation in the data of any verbal response is "uh-huh," which was made 8 weeks after the study began; this was the first verbal response any of the personnel at the time had experienced other than during an upset.] Consequently, the personnel make few approaches to Marian other than those absolutely necessary for her care — that is, for baths, meals, analytic hours, and bathroom. She is frequently incontinent of urine and feces, although she usually responds to toileting when approached.

Aide: "Marian refused her breakfast tray. What should I do?"

Nurse: "Well, let it go. I don't know what we can do about it."

Aide shrugs shoulders and walks away.

Aide: "Marian, would you like a bath?" (No response.) "Come on, honey. You have to take a bath." (No response.) "Marian, do you hear?" (Aide pulls at bed covers. Marian makes no verbal response, but turns toward wall and holds tightly onto covers.) *"Marian."* (Aide leaves room. Marian remains in bed the entire day.)

Marian is incontinent of feces in bed. This is reported to the nurse. "Well, invite her to go to the bathroom. We can't be cleaning that stuff up all the time."

Investigator: "I noticed that Marian Jones is up and dressed today. I wonder what happened. What was done differently?"

Nurse: "Oh, periodically she will. Nothing particular happens. This has been going on for ten or so years. She takes spurts and will do things, but she will be back in bed tomorrow. It's the same old pattern."

Aide: "She has been sick so long. She seems to be happiest when left alone. I hate to upset her, and you know it will happen if you get too close."

Nurse: "Marian is a good example of a hopeless patient. One would never realize that she was well educated, and had traveled abroad, to see her now."

A new aide on the floor made several approaches to Marian. The aide then asked Marian to take a walk with her. Marian became upset, shouting and screaming, "This dead body of mine! Marian Jones, that crazy person. You're insane. You're crazy. Such behavior is expected of you. You'll never get well. You'll never learn how to walk. You can't be a lady. You can't act right. Do this. Do that...[and so on]." She pulled the aide's hair and beat her. The aide discussed this incident with a nurse, following the upset.

Nurse: "Marian attacked you because you got too close. This is a repetitive pattern. Marian always turns on those who are good to her."

Marian was rarely consulted as to what clothing she might like to wear or what kind of juice and sandwiches she would like for lunch. Even though she probably would not respond, most

> patients on the ward were given a choice in these matters.
>
> Personnel were observed combing and brushing Marian's hair, without making any verbal approach to her.
>
> Marian was incontinent of urine and feces in bed. The nurse cleaned her up and changed her bed. In doing this, there was no explanation made to the patient.

The above illustrations certainly would raise the question as to whether or not Miss Jones existed as a person to the personnel. In her very disturbed periods, Miss Jones did refer to "my dead body," which may have revealed how she felt about her existence as a person, and in a reciprocal fashion, personnel, too, treated her as if she were nonexistent.

New personnel soon fell into the same types of response to Marian that were predominant on the ward.

> *Monday.* New aide oriented today. In afternoon she was observed sitting with Marian on porch. She attempted to converse. Marian frowned and turned head. Aide withdrew.
>
> *Tuesday.* Marian in bed. Aide approached Marian with a magazine. "Let's look at this Marian." Marian frowned and turned toward wall. "Don't you want to read the magazine?" Marian made no response. Aide walked away.
>
> *Wednesday.* Aide made friendly approach to Marian, who turned away. Aide asked nurse about patient. Nurse, "She can't stand you to come too close. She will turn on you and attack you, if you get too close."
>
> *Thursday.* Aide's interest seemed to be lessening. Today she did not give Marian her warm greeting. Made only the necessary approaches.
>
> *Friday.* Aide observed to pass patient several times. Gave no evidence of seeing her.

In evaluating the data, from which the above was abstracted, the interpersonal situation surrounding this patient could be readily visualized. Her mode of participation was withdrawal, both physical and verbal, interspersed with very disturbed upsets. Her communications, other than during upsets, were entirely on a nonverbal level. Her responses to contacts were minimal and gave evidence of much anxiety. The response of the personnel in this situation was reciprocal to the patient's mode: staff withdrawal, minimal communication of personnel when making demands on the patient, no respect for her as a person, and evidence of anxiety when contacting this patient.

The predominant attitude on the part of the personnel (and it can be assumed that this was conveyed to the patient) was *hopelessness,* which grew out of repeated failure, indifference, guilt, and hostility.

Thus, the interpersonal context, as observed, consisted of failure with regard to the patient, indifference and apathy toward her, guilt about avoiding her, labeling her as hopeless to avoid this guilt, and, finally, rationalizing the avoidance by saying that the patient could not tolerate closeness. This patterned attitude-response prevailed with such intensity that new personnel were almost immediately indoctrinated into it. If a new aide started with a different approach, he was easily persuaded, both directly and indirectly, into adopting the prevailing attitudes of both the staff and the patient.

Four main problems became apparent in attempting to formulate a method of intervention into the above described mode of social participation. (1) How does the nurse become aware of her feelings regarding this patient? The attitude that the patient was *hopeless* had blocked the personnel in their ability to engage in any interpersonal contacts other than those which maintained the present mode, or the illness of the patient. (2) What needs does the patient communicate through this type of social participation? If these needs are anticipated and fulfilled, will they foster a higher level of participation? (3) What kinds of interpersonal activities can be engaged in with this patient? (a) Does one begin with nonverbal communication? (b) What is the way of moving on from nonverbal communications? What specific forms of communication can be used? (c) What types of interpersonal situations can be structured? (4) What type of social structure will best facilitate an alteration in the staff's mode of participation regarding: (a) the staff's taking Miss Jones into their purview and moving in her direction, in contrast with their present moving away and ignoring her; (b) the staff's looking upon her mode of participation as a problem which is constantly to be grappled with; and (c) mobilization and maintenance of enthusiasm and interest on part of staff that will promote this?

The first step in this plan was to have the investigator herself experience the patient, consider the various alternative ways of responding to her, try a number of these alternatives, determine the one or ones which were most successful, continue this process, and observe the effect on or changes in the patient's behavior. As envisioned, the plan would comprise a series of steps in which the patient was responded to and with, at the level she was capable of at the time. Once having achieved an integration at this level, higher levels of integration would be attempted with the patient.

The second step was to communicate the procedure to another staff member who would then attempt to participate with the patient in the mode similar to that of the investigator. In this way, the following questions could be answered: Is the method of participation developed by the investigator intrinsic to her type of personality, unique experience, and skills, or can another staff member be trained to participate with the patient in this mode? Can a staff member maintain an attitude toward the patient counter to the general staff attitude? If this is possible, what are the consequences of maintaining the counter attitude?

This process, as it was carried out, is stated in the following abstracts from the investigator's notes:

> *First week.* I sat with the patient for two hours — one in a.m. and one in p.m. I made very minute observations, but during this period was silent. Marian remained turned toward wall, with covers pulled tightly about her, her body tense and in curled position, her eyes tightly closed, and her fists tightly clenching the covers. Respirations were fast. If I moved, Marian frowned, closed eyes more tightly, and held onto covers. At the end of 30 minutes, Marian began to relax, straightened legs, changed position in bed, and no longer clenched the covers. After 45 minutes had passed, Marian glanced at me several times, but looked quickly away when I met her glance. At end of hour, I touched her hand and left.
>
> In the afternoon, this was repeated. Patient began to seem comfortable at end of 15 minutes.

These interpersonal contacts were repeated on three subsequent days. The patient's response was increased, in that many glances were exchanged; she allowed the investigator to take her hand for long periods, although she did not return the grasp; she followed with her eyes when the investigator entered or left the room.

The response on the part of the investigator is also significant. The patient began to become quite real; there was much more awareness of the patient's expression, and a real feeling that the patient was being experienced as a person.

> *Second week.* I went to the patient, sat on her bed, and began to talk with her about the weather and other general topics. Marian frowned, her body became tense, her eyes closed tightly. I talked on, becoming more and more uncomfortable, for 30 minutes, at which time Marian turned her face to the wall and pulled the covers about her. She did not become disturbed to the point of an upset. I made no overt demands on her during the monologue.
>
> For the past two days I have been sitting with Marian, saying nothing. Her response similar to those reported during first week. At end of 40 minutes, I said, "Marian, I'm going to be going in 5 minutes." Marian looked at me and nodded, "Yes." "I will come back later. All right?" Marian nodded, "Yes."
>
> I left and returned later that day.
>
> I asked, "Marian, do you want me to stay with you?" Marian shakes head, "No." "O.K., I'll go now, but I will be back." Marian nodded, "Yes."
>
> [The investigator assumes here that a demand was made on patient — to make a decision about the investigator's sitting with her. If she had said yes, she would have been assuming some responsibility for the contact, and therefore might have had to participate with the investigator.]
>
> I returned and said, "I'd like to be with you, Marian." Marian said, "Uh-huh." (Verbal.)

As a result of the initial contacts, it was easily determined that the first steps were merely sitting with the patient, or being with her in silence. Verbalization at this point only made her uncomfortable and succeeded to disrupting the relationship. However, after a long period of nonverbal participation had occurred, a word or two could be interjected and would be responded to by the patient. After two weeks of contact, verbalization was more readily accepted, as is indicated below.

> *Third week.* Subsequent contacts were initiated by statements such as: "I want to stay with you," "I'd like to show you this magazine," "I'd like to brush your hair," "I'll help with your bath."

Miss Jones' response continued to be a verbal "uh-huh," nothing more, but she watched the investigator, smiled readily, and returned the investigator's grasp. The type of interpersonal activity changed from sitting with patient (with no verbal communication) to physical contacts, holding hand, brushing hair, looking at book, reading, singing with patient. This was the next step in the process. Physical contact with the investigator brought appropriate responses from the patient. Such activities at the beginning were not responded to at all.

> Investigator: "Marian, I brought the Autoharp.

I'd like to sing with you." Marian smiles and says, "Uh-huh." Other patients gather around and begin to sing with me. Marian smiles, is very alert, rocks in chair in time to music. [Patient does not sing, but her rocking indicates a further step in participation.]

Fourth week. Marian is spending more time out of her bed. Personnel are observed to say "Hi" or sit beside her for a moment in the hall, or take her a magazine. Marian responds by smiling or saying, "Uh-huh."

As a result of the investigator's interest in the patient, and as a result of direct propaganda, personnel developed a greater interest and approached the patient more frequently. In addition, as a result of the investigator's interest, the patient became more active. As she became more active, personnel dealt with her more easily. Thus, the reciprocal process of staff-patient interaction started to move slowly away from the avoidance-hopelessness state. The patient, however, moved slowly, taking only minute steps — the distance yet to go was great.

Fifth week. A new student nurse approached Marian for her bath. Marian responded well. This student was observed to spend one hour sitting with patient today. She made some inquiries of the investigator regarding the patient, and often observed the investigator when she was with the patient.

At this point, it was decided that the investigator would attempt to work through this student.[4] A plan was formulated in which the investigator would supervise the student in the same way that the investigator was being supervised by the sociologist. Being a new student, she had not become indoctrinated with persisting attitudes of the ward, nor was she "caught in the hopelessness" surrounding the patient. Could she be prevented from falling into the reciprocal responses to this patient's mode? If so, what type of interpersonal experience would it be necessary to structure, and what sort of direction would be necessary? What type of changes in the social organization would be necessary? If this student should experience successful interpersonal contacts with this patient, how would this be viewed by other personnel on the ward?

It was felt that much could be gained in understanding not only how to interrupt a certain mode of participation on the part of the patient, but how this skill could be transmitted to another person.

With the cooperation of the nursing service and education departments, and agreement by the student, arrangements were made for this student to spend ten consecutive weeks on the ward, to be partially free of responsibility to the rest of the ward, and to have time for conferences with the investigator which would enable her to discuss fully her experiences with Miss Jones, and her feelings about Miss Jones' reaction to her.

The remaining data on Miss Jones consist of the investigator's and the student's observations of the experiences with this patient, the joint evaluation, and the subsequent action on the part of the student.

Sixth week. For the past three days, Miss C [the student] has spent varying lengths of time with Marian, just sitting, making an occasional comment. In conference with Miss C we have discussed these interpersonal experiences, stressing what happened, Marian's response, Miss C's feelings, and alternatives that might be considered in future contacts. The role of the therapist was discussed with Miss C and how the varying roles became integrated in the interpersonal situation.

Miss C goes to Marian, who is seated in hall.

Miss C: "I've brought some juice."

Marian: "Uh-huh."

Miss C: "Which do you want, pineapple or tomato?" (No response.) "Tell me, Marian, which do you want? Hear, Marian? — you choose."

Marian becomes upset, starts to scream: "Tomato or pineapple, grapefruit. It doesn't matter. Give the sick girl tomato or pineapple or grapefruit." (Hits and kicks Miss C.) "Men try to rape her. She keeps bleeding. It is all mixed up. Menstruation, babies, egg salad sandwiches. She will never get well. That poor insane Marian Jones. Stay away from me. Get out, get out. She'll never get well." (This continues for about 20 minutes. Miss C stays near.)

In conference between investigator and student, the upset was discussed, with emphasis on the following points: how Miss C felt, the possibility of a choice (pineapple or tomato) at this point being perceived by Marian as a demand, the positive effect of just staying near rather than leaving, and how this relates to future experiences.

The twofold significance of this incident was pointed out to the student: (1) that at this point, a choice for Miss Jones is too much of a demand upon her; and (2) that the most important thing about the upset is not that it occurred, but how it was handled.

The latter point served to allay the student's guilt about the upset, and indicated a method for handling it.

Seventh week. Miss C was in another room. Heard Marian beginning one of her upsets (precipitated by another personnel, regarding eating her dinner). Miss C went to Marian, took hold of her arms.

Miss C: "Marian, I'll stay with you."

Marian: "Go away. Meat and potatoes, eat this. She doesn't know how to live. She can't even walk. Get out. Stay away."

Miss C: "Marian, do you know who this is?" (Marian continues to scream.) "Marian, I'm staying with you. It is Miss C. Hear, Marian?" (Marian becomes quiet.) "It is Miss C and I'm staying with you."

Marian: "Uh-huh." (Relaxes and sinks back on bed. Miss C remains with her, holding onto her hand.)

Miss C: "Marian, I'm going now. I'll see you tomorrow. I'll be back tomorrow. Goodnight."

Marian: "Goodnight." (Whisper.)

[Here the student put into practice the result of previous discussions — that is, staying with Miss Jones during an upset.]

Marian attended tea dance with Miss C today. They held hands and skipped over to another building on the hospital grounds. Marian was not verbal, but smiled much and was very alert. She danced two numbers with Miss C, but refused invitations of others to dance. [The student was still participating with the patient on a nonverbal level, but getting much responsiveness from the patient.]

In conference with Miss C, the attitude of a nurse on the floor was discussed. The nurse had been interrupting Miss C's interpersonal contacts with Marian by asking her to do other assignments on the ward, and had made inquiries of Miss C as to why she talked to investigator so much, and criticized her for interrupting Marian's hour with the therapist (hour being held on hall, Miss C speaks to Marian as she passes).

In discussing this situation with the head nurse, it was determined that the difficulty could be attributed to the fact that the plan had not been communicated to the nurse involved. Following a discussion between the head nurse and the nurse in question during which she was taken in on the plan, this difficulty immediately cleared up. Miss C began (on her own initiative) to share some of her experiences with this nurse. This nurse became very interested in the situation and was observed to do a number of extra things to further the interpersonal experience of Miss C and Marian.

The above is an example of what happens when the communication between the personnel breaks down. It is also an illustration of what happens when certain members are "left out." It should be emphasized that the entire plan can be disrupted and thus the possibility of failure increased if both of these points are not considered. It poses the important question as to what type of organization must be maintained within the social structure to avoid this kind of breakdown in communication, and as to the need to bring personnel in on any special plans being carried on so that they will not disrupt them, directly or indirectly.

Eighth week. Miss C reported several more upsets during her interpersonal contacts with Marian. These were discussed and evaluated. The upsets are changing in nature: (1) they are shorter now, lasting approximately 5 minutes, in contrast to 20 or 30 minutes; (2) there is little physical striking out or kicking; (3) there is some difference in content (that is, more reference to "I" — "I don't understand," "I'm so ugly," "I can't get well" — rather than to "that insane girl," "that Marian Jones. She can't even walk"); and (4) Miss C has little anxiety during upsets, is able to stay with Marian in relative comfort.

Here, again, it was concluded by the investigator and student that the important fact was that *an upset was successfully handled* rather than that *an upset was avoided.* In future interpersonal experiences with Miss Jones, we would not attempt to avoid all upsets, but would concern ourselves with noting the factors precipitating them, the nature of the upsets (length and content), and what we did during and immediately following the upset.

Miss C reported that she now talks fluently with Marian during her bath, combing her hair, and sitting with her. Marian looks directly at her, nods and smiles in response to her remarks. They have read together, sat looking out at the rain, watched the moon together in the evening, and Marian participates by keeping time to the music when Miss C sings. The investigator suggested that the student let her imagination "run wild" in thinking of activities in which Marian might participate more actively. In sharp contrast to a few weeks previously when participation was minimal (when any verbalization would result in evidence of much anxiety and withdrawal), the patient's present response to verbalization is acceptance and nonverbal responsiveness. How can this type of participation be further altered?

Miss C's enthusiasm and interest was very apparent. She appeared to anticipate her contacts with Miss Jones and reported them to the investigator in detail and with much satisfaction. This enthusiasm was accompanied by a change in her role. From this point on, she began to be much more imaginative and resourceful in her relationships with the patient.

Ninth week. Miss C reports: "Today we sang for a while. Marian kept time with her hands to my singing. Her eyes were shining and she smiled. Looked me straight in the eye most of the time. Then I got the idea of the old patty-cake game — you remember — slapping your knees, then clapping your hands, and then meeting the other person's hands." (Demonstrates.) "I began. Marian giggled, watching me; then she began. She would hit her legs, then clap and hold her hands up. At first, I'd always have to meet her hands — she wouldn't come to meet mine. Finally, she did. It was really exciting. Later when I went to go, I stopped to say goodbye and tell her when I'd be back. I took her hand and actually felt her squeeze mine back. Do you suppose she will ever talk to me? I'd really be thrilled." [Here the patient has moved to another level. She now participates more actively, but is still on a nonverbal level.]

This type of contact continued. Miss C reported: "Today we listened to records. I said 'Come on, Marian, let's be orchestra leaders.' She did, right away, keeping real good time, and laughing."

Miss C: "We were just sitting. Marian was very sober. She had her hands clasped together. I started to play with my hands. 'This is the church and this is the steeple. Open the door, and see all the people.' Marian laughed and would go through the motions with her hands as I said the words."

Miss C reported: "Marian gets up nearly every day now. She went to the patients' floor meeting. She kept looking at me and smiling."

Miss C reported: "Birthday party for Marian on the ward. She smiled and laughed when we sang happy birthday. The personnel were all so interested. The other patients, too. She wouldn't blow out the candles, but she seemed to like the cake." [Not only was the patient showing greater responsiveness to the student, but to the others on the ward.]

Tenth week. Miss C reported: "Today in the bath I said, 'Wash yourself, Marian.' She took cloth and began. I washed her back. Helped her get out of tub. 'Want to brush your teeth?' She said, real plain, 'Yes.' I was so surprised I said, 'What?' Then I said, 'It feels good to brush your teeth, doesn't it?' Marian said, 'No, it doesn't feel good to brush my teeth.' 'It doesn't?' 'No, it doesn't.' She really spoke. Very calm. Her voice is different than when she is upset. I was real thrilled. When we finished, I asked if she wanted to go to the hall. 'Yes.' 'Want to sit here for a while?' 'Yes.'"

Miss C reported: "We were playing records. Marian danced with me. She seemed to enjoy it." We discussed at length the entire experience, including how Miss C felt. "I was so excited when she began to say 'Yes,' and then the time she said the whole sentence. She seems so much more like a person than she did seven weeks ago, when I first met her. I am much more aware of her every response. Another thing — I'm not apprehensive about her upsets. I was afraid at first, and dreaded them. More dread than fear, I guess. I felt I was doing something wrong, and I couldn't relax with her. Now, it's different. She knows me and I think she knows I'm really interested."

Investigator: "How do you think you maintain this feeling with her?"

Miss C: "By being with her. I always tell her I'm here when I first come to the floor, and say goodbye when I leave, and when I'll be back. I never go past her without speaking. She follows me with her eyes."

There has now been an evolving mutual relationship in which the student's continuing enthusiasm and interest in the patient is maintained by her satisfaction in direct participation with the patient, by approval by the discussion with the investigator, and by feeling that she is doing a worth-while piece of work. In turn, the patient has now reached the point where she can be asked to make a choice, and instead of "blowing up," she can respond with words. This is at the end of five weeks of contact between the two. In addition, the student is shaping time for the patient, making it more definite, announcing her arrivals and departures, and is maintaining her awareness and interest in the patient, even when not with her.

Eleventh week. During the eleventh week, Miss

C was not on duty because of illness. Other student reported to her that Marian was remaining in bed. This caused great discouragement on the part of Miss C, who felt, "When I leave, everything will go back the way it was before." This was discussed, and the importance of sharing these experiences with others was emphasized. It was felt that the nature of the interpersonal relationship existing between Miss C and Marian was such that interpersonal situations which would bring Marian and Miss C into the group should be structured. Also, both the investigator's and Miss C's activities would focus on the other personnel in an attempt to stimulate interest and enthusiasm regarding Marian's mode of living on the ward. Miss C would also continue in her contacts with the patient.

Thus as soon as the student withdraws, the patient returns to her old pattern of behavior. This may elicit and reinforce the old feeling of failure and hopelessness. Thus we see the importance of organizing the social context to provide for the simultaneous participation of several staff members, so that the absence of one person does not disrupt the increasing participation of the patient in the social process.

Twelfth week. Miss C's report: I was going to class. I said goodbye to Marian. Asked her to tell me goodbye. "No." "Come on, Marian, tell me 'bye.'" "No." "Will you tomorrow?" "Yes." Next day, when I left for class, I said, "Bye, Marian." She smiled and looked away and then said, "Bye, bye." The following conversation then took place.

Miss C: "Anything you want before I go?"

Marian: "No." (Hesitates.) "Yes."

Miss C: "What, Marian?" (No response.) "Want some juice?"

Marian: "Yes."

Miss C: "What kind?"

Marian: "Pineapple juice." (Student brings juice.)

Miss C: "Anything else, Marian?"

Marian: "Yes. Do you have a little piece of cake or something?" (Student brings some crackers and jelly.)

Miss C: "I'm going now. I'll be back after class." (Marian starts to be upset, throws some juice across hall.)

Marian: "I don't understand. I don't understand. . ." (Miss C sits beside her, begins rocking chair.)

Marian: "Go away from me. Get out."

Miss C: "I'm going to stay with you. I'm not leaving you." (Marian relaxes and stops screaming.)

Miss C: "You all right now, Marian?"

Marian: "Yes."

Miss C: "Tired?"

Marian: "Yes."

Miss C: "Want to take a nap?"

Marian: "Yes."

Miss C: "All right. I'm going to class. I'll be back in an hour and then I'll stay with you a while."

Marian: "Yes."

In this incident, the patient was apparently objecting to the student's departure. No provision had been made for the patient to participate in this decision. When the student stayed with her for a short while, the patient was then able to accept the second attempt at departure of the student.

Miss C has been talking the past few days about cutting Marian's hair. This was discussed with all the personnel. Marian smiles when this is mentioned, but does not answer. Today during bath:

Miss C: "Want me to cut your hair, Marian?"

Marian: "Yes."

Miss C: "Want it parted in the middle, or on the side?" (No response.)

Miss C: "In the middle?"

Marian: "No."

Miss C: "On the side?"

Marian: "Yes."

Miss C: "O.K. As soon as we finish your bath, we will cut your hair." (Marian gets out of tub. Miss C starts to whistle.) "Can you whistle, Marian?" (No response.) "Want me to teach you?" (Marian frowns and looks real disgusted.) "Oh, you can whistle?"

Marian: "Yes." (Begins to whistle, smiles. Someone begins to play music on ward. Miss C begins to do Charleston to music.)

Miss C: "Come on, Marian, Charleston with me." (Holds out hands. Marian takes them. Charlestons with Miss C. Much laughing and smiling. Finishes dressing, goes to room.)

This afternoon Miss C cut and fixed Marian's hair.

Miss C: "You should have seen how everyone on the ward reacted. She looked so well. Like a different person. She is so pretty. When she looked at herself in the mirror, she was really pleased. Kept touching her hair and smiling. All the patients remarked; so did the personnel. They really seemed to be interested in her. I notice everyone pays a lot of attention to her. I've noticed them sitting with her. We talk a lot about her."

Although no one has actually taken over from this student, personnel are paying more attention to the patient. The patient now talks more than she has in years; her greater response is reciprocated by a livelier interest on the part of the staff; the patient is now even making some beginning gestures to talk in the presence of other people.

Group was singing Christmas carols on the ward. Miss C and Marian joined group. Marian moved lips, but did not sing out loud. Watched everyone. Personnel remark to each other about her moving lips in singing.

Thirteenth week. Since this was to be Miss C's last week on the ward, plans for termination were formulated. Miss C would be assigned to O.T. for the last two weeks of her time at the hospital, so would be coming to the ward for short contacts. In addition to explaining this to Marian, Miss C would continue her contacts with the patient. The following are excerpts from the data collected during this week, and they give positive evidence of a constructive change in Marian's mode of social participation as well as a corresponding change in the personnel's reciprocal response:

Marian starts to bathroom with Miss C. Both bathrooms are busy, so they sit in the hall.
Miss C: "Want me to stay, or get your things ready?"
Marian: "You can come back."
Later, in bathroom, tub is nearly full of water.
Miss C: "Like this, Marian?"
Marian: "Yes, I like lots of hot water."
Miss C: "Want to wash yourself?"
Marian: "Yes." (Washes self.)
Miss C: "I'll do your back?"
Marian: "Yes."
Marian dresses herself without help. Combs own hair, and puts on make-up. Goes onto hall with Miss C.
Miss C: "Would you like some coffee now?"
Marian: "Yes."
Miss C: "How do you want it?"
Marian: "With cream and sugar."

Marian is dancing on hall with Miss C.

Miss C: "What do you want to wear, a dress or skirt and blouse?" (Standing at Marian's closet.)
Marian: "A dress."
Miss C: "Which one?"
Marian: "A dress. Any one will do."
Miss C: "A red one?"
Marian: "Yes."
Miss C: "Which?" (Has two.)
Marian: "This one. This red dress."
Miss C and Marian attend the dance. At first Marian refuses to dance with anyone else. Later, several of the men (both patients and personnel) cut in. Marian dances every dance. At one point, ends up across room from Miss C. Looks all about, finds her, nods and smiles. Goes on dancing with one of the men. Later in dance, Miss C asks if she wants to jitterbug. "Yes." They jitterbug to "Slow Boat to China." Miss C begins to sing it softly. Marian smiles and moves lips with the words. They go to table for refreshments. Marian says, "Tea with cream and sugar."

Marian continues to say "Bye" when Miss C leaves the ward.

The patient's participation is now spreading to others. She can now sustain a separation from the student and still participate with another person.

During Marian's bath, Miss C begins to hum "Slow Boat to China." Marian smiles.
Miss C: "Remember this at the dance?"
Marian: "Yes." (Smiles.)
Miss C: "Let's sing it."
Marian: "Yes." (Sings out loud with Miss C. Marian knows all the words.)

O.T. worker came onto ward to make programs for Christmas party. Miss C and Marian join the group. Marian participates in making programs by cutting the paper.

Miss C is playing piano. Marian comes to piano and joins group who are singing. Moves lips in words of Christmas carols, occasionally singing out loud.

Group dancing on the ward. Marian joins group with Miss C. Patients are dancing alone and with group. Marian begins to tap dance after seeing Miss C tapping. Later does the hula with the group.

Marian joins group in living room. Nancy (another student) is reading aloud from a new book. She passes the book to Betty (another patient) who reads a bit, and then passes it on to Miss C. Book is the passed to Marian who takes it, reads paragraph silently, and passes it back to Nancy.

As seen in the above notes, Miss Jones is moving toward the group, whereas her participation previously has been limited to one person. The reciprocal response of the group, both personnel and patients, is to begin to include her in their activity. Because of Miss Jones' constructive experiences with Miss C, Miss Jones is able to move with Miss C into a more complex interpersonal situation and begin to participate with a group.

The "whirlpool-like" interpersonal activities as seen in the events with this patient can be synoptically described as follows: The sociologist offers advice and suggestions to the investigator in evaluating the interpersonal situation surrounding this patient; the investigator offers guidance, counsel and suggestions to the student; the student participates in a spontaneous fashion with the patient; the patient's greater responsiveness toward the student enables her to engage in more activities with other persons on the ward. The staff personnel respond both with qualitative and quantitative differences to the patient.

Miss Jones' therapist was approached as to the types of interventions the investigator felt might be successful in altering Miss Jones' present mode of social participation. At the termination of the study, an attempt was made to evaluate with the therapist the relationship between Miss Jones' interpersonal experiences on the ward, and the progress made in the analytical hours. The therapist felt there had been three major changes in the analytical hours that could be directly related to Miss Jones' experience on the ward.

1. There was an increase in the capacity to follow an idea or thought from one meeting to another. Prior to the intervention on the ward, the therapist felt that between hours "Marian seemed to drop out of existence." He no longer felt this way; probably because of the more consistent environmental support she seemed no longer a person lost on the ward, but had more positive experiences in her living between therapeutic hours. There would seem to be a direct relationship between this change and the fact that Miss Jones was having experiences on the ward that enabled her to carry a thought from one day to the next — or one hour to the next. "I'll sit with you a while." "I'll be leaving in five minutes, but I'll be back tomorrow morning." "Maybe you will say 'Bye' tomorrow," and so on. This aided in shaping time for Miss Jones, and in helping her to identify people and experiences in her living.

2. It was much easier for the therapist to deal with deep, regressed feelings and needs in the analytic hours as the patient became more comfortable in her relationships on the ward and as her participation on the ward became more socially acceptable. Miss Jones' experiences on the ward were planned to facilitate communication and participation at whatever level was possible, always watching for cues that indicated her ability for a higher level of participation. This was accomplished because of the constant observation-evaluation process.

3. The therapist's dealings with the ward personnel had changed completely. Before, he had much hostility and resentment toward the personnel. Now he felt much backing and support. The interest and enthusiasm in the patient was very apparent to the therapist. The therapist also felt more comfortable on the ward and had little anxiety in leaving Miss Jones after an hour, even if she had been quite anxious during the hour.

While exploration of this is not within the scope of this study, it raises some assumptions or speculations: Hopelessness on the part of the nursing personnel must be conveyed to the therapist. Either he takes on this attitude himself, or he has resentment toward the nursing staff. This could have two ramifications: (1) this hopelessness is conveyed to the patient, and reinforces her withdrawal; (2) the staff perceives this resentment and may interpret it as "the therapist feels we are no good." Thus, there is additional confirmation of their failure. The whole process of hopelessness regarding the patient is reinforced.

Thus, the significance of the *total social context,* in affecting a variety of interpersonal relationships in regard to the patient, is evident.

Summary

In summarizing the data on this second patient, a progression of steps becomes clear: observation of the interpersonal situation of the patient and the relationship of this to the total social structure; evaluation and analysis of this situation; formulation of alternative interpersonal experiences; intervention; further observation and analysis of the results of the intervention; and further formulation of alternatives, in accordance with the results of the intervention. From this process, the following steps evolved in attempting to solve the problem of mutual withdrawal surrounding this patient: recognition of the pattern of avoidance withdrawal existing between patient and personnel with the resultant attitude-response of hopelessness on part of both; participation with patient on nonverbal level (just sitting with patient in silence); physical participation of patient in form of gestures (frowning or smiling), body tensions (rigid or relaxed), body position (turning back to wall); verbal communication to patient as she begins to respond with appropriate nonverbal gestures (shaking and nodding of head, pressure of hand); physical participation of patient in response to verbal requests (get up, take bath, and so on); hand games — patient begins to participate and to move actively; one- or two-word remarks initiated by patient; response by patient to making a choice; hesitant response by patient to participation with others in group; greater response by patient to participation with others in a group; reciprocal response of entire staff, whose approaches to patient are more frequent and of a different kind.

Conclusions

The problem of mutual withdrawal was selected for investigation because of its critical significance in the maintenance of the patient's mental illness within the ward setting. Not only does this process reinforce and stabilize the patient's mental illness, but it also enters into other problems of patient-staff interaction on the ward. Thus, the labeling of patients as "hopeless," "assaultive," "unresponsive," and "unable to tolerate closeness" serves as a convenient rationalization for avoiding the patient, and thereby perpetuating the process of mutual withdrawal. We have demonstrated that this deeply ingrained and subtle process, often running its course outside the awareness of the participants, *can be systematically observed, evaluated, and interrupted.* In order to do this, we have attempted to develop a *sociopsychiatric nursing* approach, combining the knowledge and conceptual tools of both the sociologist and the psychiatric nurse. A perspective has emerged in which the specific interpersonal relations that the nurse engages in with both patient and personnel, and the ward context with its social structure, are viewed as a total interacting process, and in which this interaction is kept under constant scrutiny in order to determine and evaluate the interventions instituted. As a guidepost for this type of approach, we have asked the following general questions in the course of the study:

1. What is the nature of the social structure as it exists on the ward, and what are the dominant attitudes and patterns of activity which characterize this social structure?
2. What is the relationship of this structure to the therapeutic progress of patients? What criteria can be used in evaluating this relationship?
3. What is the role of the psychiatric nurse? What contradictions are there in this role? What alterations can be made?
4. What is the nature of the interpersonal relations engaged in by the personnel? How do they relate to other aspects of the social structure and to the patient's progress?
5. How can these interpersonal relations and the social structure be altered, and in what direction, to facilitate the patient's recovery?

Evidence for the value of this type of approach resides in the fact that the investigator was able not only to employ this approach herself, but also to communicate it to another nurse and to enable this nurse to utilize the approach. Through this procedure, the process of mutual withdrawal was interrupted, and significant alterations in the patient's mode of participation occurred. While the problem of maintaining and carrying forward favorable change among these mentally ill patients has not been dealt with in this study, its significance is manifest. In order to capitalize on the favorable change, it must be carried through to the eventual "cure" of the patient. Psychotherapy — the intensive investigation of the patient's difficulties in living — must be integrated and coordinated with sociopsychiatric nursing care in order to consolidate and continue the improvement.

Chestnut Lodge
Rockville, MD.

Teaching Psychiatric Nursing in the Psychiatric Unit of a General Hospital

Marion E. Kalkman

Ms. Kalkman (Army School of Nursing; B.A., Brown University, Providence, R.I.) is director of the advanced program in psychiatric nursing at the University of California Medical Center School of Nursing.

Reprinted from *Nursing Outlook*, Vol. 1, September 1953.

The psychiatric unit of a general hospital offers some excellent opportunities for teaching psychiatric nursing. When such a unit is part of the total hospital service and one of the essential departments of the hospital, it no longer has the disadvantages of seeming remote and different — qualities that are commonly ascribed to institutions which care for psychiatric patients exclusively. When the psychiatric unit is regarded as an integral part of the total treatment facilities of a modern hospital, it becomes extremely helpful in the preparation of medical personnel who are getting their first introduction to psychiatry and psychiatric patients. It gives the students a kind of emotional security to receive this instruction in a setting similar to the other medical specialties.

Patients in the psychiatric unit of a general hospital are usually acutely ill. Frequently it is their first hospitalization, and some have been admitted primarily for diagnostic study and evaluation. Patients who are admitted for treatment are usually those who are likely to respond to treatment rapidly or who require only a short period of hospitalization. No such unit, with its limited bed-space, can afford to carry patients requiring long-term therapy. In other words, although psychiatric treatment in general is notoriously long and time consuming, the patients admitted to psychiatric units of general hospitals offer the student the best opportunity to see change and improvement in the short space of time she, or he, is assigned to the service. This selection of patients also helps to overcome the false impression, which is common among the uninitiated, that psychiatric disorders carry a poor prognosis. The best way to overcome this misapprehension is to give the student the opportunity to see patients get well and go home.

Patients on the psychiatric unit of a general hospital often have a combination of mental and physical symptoms, or they may have been admitted originally to some other service of the hospital for a physical complaint and later transferred to the psychiatric service. This gives the student the opportunity to move from the known to the unknown, for by the time she has reached the psychiatric service she is already familiar with many medical and surgical conditions, and feels fairly competent to deal with these aspects of the patient's difficulties. Now she will learn to acquire the new skills of psychiatric nursing, which makes for an easy and natural introduction to this subject.

Several types of psychiatric nursing programs are well-suited to the psychiatric unit of a general hospital. They may be grouped for convenience under three headings: (1) a basic program for student nurses, (2) an inservice staff program, and (3) an outservice program for personnel in other departments of the hospital.

The Student Nurse Program

Students from the school of nursing associated with the general hospital may be assigned to the psychiatric unit as an integral part of their clinical nursing experience; also, affiliate students from other schools of nursing may be accepted for psychiatric nursing experience. Many psychiatric nursing educators feel that three months or twelve weeks is a desirable length of time for a basic or introductory psychiatric nursing program. Not only must a considerable content of psychiatric information be given to the uninitiated student if she is to have any understanding of psychiatric patients and their conditions, but also a certain length of time is needed for the student to assimilate this information, to acquire the rudiments of a psychiatric point of view and, even more important, to make the necessary emotional adjustments in her own personality. Experience has shown that this takes about twelve weeks for most student nurses, though this may be insufficient for some. It is important to remember that this is only an introductory course to the subject. In some university schools of nursing, courses in clinical psychiatry, abnormal psychology, and other related subjects are offered before the student is assigned to the psychiatric service; the psychological aspects of treatment have also been integrated in other clinical areas such as pediatrics, obstetrics, and psychosomatic medicine. In these schools the period of student experience on the psychiatric service may be shortened to two months.

For the nursing school with a 3-year program, however, in which the student does not have a psychiatrically oriented program, three months' experience on the psychiatric service is recommended. Some psychiatric nursing educators feel that even three months does not prepare the student sufficiently for beginning positions in psychiatric hospitals. Much depends on how the course is taught, and what experiences are planned for the student in this period.

The introduction of a program for student nurses in a psychiatric unit carries with it certain responsibilities for the personnel of that unit. Students must have opportunities for learning experiences and must be taught and supervised by qualified personnel. Opportunities for learning experience should include access to charts, case histories, and library facilities. Students should be able to attend some of the staff conferences, ward rounds, clinics, and lectures. Their assignments should include experiences with different types of patients. Although they may contribute a great deal to the nursing care given to the patient, they should not be depended upon to carry the load of patient care, nor should they be required to perform routine activities which no longer have value as learning experiences. That is, students should not be used to relieve the regular personnel of monotonous ward duties. It is usually undesirable to have student nurses work after the evening activities have been completed and the patients have gone to bed. Learning opportunities are minimal then, and the responsibilities are too great for student nurses to carry.

Even more important than the provision for learning opportunities is the presence of adequately prepared personnel. Students learn psychiatric nursing more quickly and effectively by observing its practice by competent psychiatric nurses, aides, and attendants. A qualified staff that works well together as a team is a necessity before students can be introduced to the unit.

The psychiatric nurse who is responsible for the student program should be chosen carefully. If the unit is small, consisting of one 12- to 16-bed ward, and if there will be only a few students (not more than 8) assigned to it, the psychiatric nurse supervisor may also function as the instructor. This, however, takes an experienced supervisor who is able to see that neither the patients nor the students suffer from lack of attention. Even an experienced supervisor faces the ever present possibility that a ward class or a student interview may be interrupted, or even cancelled, if some unforeseen situation arises on the ward. Generally a more satisfactory plan is to take a few more students and give the responsibility for the student program to a qualified psychiatric nursing instructor. One instructor can give adequate instruction to 15 or 20 students. With more than 20 students, additional instructors should be employed.

Even when an instructor is responsible for the student program, the ward supervisor and head nurse play an important role in the student education program. The instructor is responsible for the student records, attendance, contacts with the nursing school office, and the student health service. The instructor must also outline the curriculum, arrange for lectures, teach the classes in psychiatric nursing, and assign students to wards, classes, and other educational activities. In addition to this, she checks experience records and evaluation reports, and holds individual conferences with students. The nurse who observes the students most closely in her contacts with patients is the head nurse on the ward. It is very important for her to be interested in students, and also to be willing and able to teach. Although her teaching is often very informal, and is imparted in small discussion groups or on-the-spot supervision, it is extremely valuable to the student and cannot be delegated to the instructor. No one can know the details of the patients' care as the head nurse does. A hostile head nurse or one unable to communicate her skills to a student nurse can seriously hamper an educational program.

Good staff nurses are also important to an educational program. They demonstrate to the student nurse how good psychiatric nursing care is given and they also help students in their first contacts with patients. Though students may learn much from observing skilled aides, they should always be supervised by a graduate nurse, and never should be assigned to work under the direction of a psychiatric aide or attendant. In some psychiatric units, students are assigned to work along with designated staff nurses for their first few days on the ward before working with patients independently.

It is difficult to estimate the number of students that can be accommodated on a psychiatric service. This depends on the size of the service, the variety of conditions demonstrated by the the patients, the variety of treatments available, and the number of special departments within the service — occupational therapy, physical therapy, outpatient service, somatic therapy, neurosurgery, and similar adjunctive therapies. A 30-bed unit, comprising only one ward with the same type of patients and therapy, could absorb far fewer students than another 30-bed unit comprising three 10-bed wards, with patients of varied psychiatric conditions receiving different kinds of therapy. It is important also that there are sufficient permanent members of the staff to maintain the therapeutic ward milieu and to give the patients a sense of security and continuity of nursing care.

The advantages of introducing a student nurse program into a psychiatric unit more than compensate for the expenditure of money for the instructor's salary and the time spent by the staff in teaching students. One of the most important advantages is the program's effect on the patients and the permanent staff. Every member of the staff, from the chief of service to the kitchen maid, responds to the interest, lively curiosity, and youthful enthusiasm which most students bring to this new and fascinating experience. A teaching program makes for an atmosphere of greater mental flexibility in the staff and a willingness to examine and try out new ideas. Work which one may have been doing in a competent, but routine, fashion for years suddenly becomes fresh and interesting as one attempts to present it to young students. Their questions make one constantly re-evaluate material which otherwise would remain undisturbed in the back files of one's mind. New ideas, new ways of doing things are tried. The staff reads current articles more frequently in a search for the students' reading material.

Students are important to the patients, too. They often find students easier to talk to, and they prefer engaging in social activities with students rather than with the more psychiatrically sophisticated staff, with whom they are always more or less on guard. Students change fairly frequently; this means new faces and new personalities. The patients can often get extra time and attention from student nurses — both of which the busy ward personnel are not always able to give. Patients often feel freer to make requests of the student than of the staff, and also they may become very much interested in the student program, asking the instructor when students will leave or be assigned to their ward. Often they tell an instructor about a particular student who, they feel, is doing a good job or whom they particularly like.

In planning the educational program for the undergraduate students one should neither attempt to include too much in the curriculum nor to stress the most infrequent or most pathological aspects of psychiatry. The majority of students will be going into fields of nursing other than psychiatry, but they need very much to learn to recognize the more common forms of mental disorders, which they may see in the psychiatric unit. They need to gain skills in psychological nursing which they can apply to any patient, whatever his diagnosis. To be sure, if one has planned a good basic program, the student should have acquired enough skills in psychiatric nursing to be employed as a staff nurse in a psychiatric facility. She should understand, however, that to continue psychiatric work in a professional capacity she will need added inservice training, an advanced psychiatric nursing course, or both.

One should not leave a discussion of the student nurse program without mentioning a few other important factors. One is the necessity for adequate housing facilities and a good housemother for the students, especially if the school has affiliate student nurses. Such a housemother should be aware both of the problems the student has as a growing adolescent girl, with her possible attendant homesickness and loneliness, and also of the problems related to her psychiatric experience. The student is often shaken emotionally by some of the problems which she encounters in her contacts with patients. The subject matter of her lectures and classes in psychiatric theory and her growing awareness of her own emotions and personal conflicts often create considerable anxiety in the student. An understanding housemother, as well as others associated with the student's program, can do much to help her with these difficulties.

The instructor, the head nurse, and the staff nurses should be able to recognize when a student needs professional help from a psychiatrist. The housemother is in a position to see the student during off-duty hours, and she should know what to expect from students during this educational and "growing-up" period. Students often prefer to confide in the housemother, rather than an instructor or supervisor, and the housemother can often do much to ease the student and guide her to seek help. One psychiatrist who is interested in students and their problems should be available to any students who may need his help. Though only one or two students in each group might require psychiatric help, these are just the ones who can benefit greatly from an interview or two with a psychiatrist.

Inservice Educational Program

Only the very rare institution can staff its wards with experienced psychiatric personnel. It is necessary for most units to employ nurses and aides with varying degrees of psychiatric knowledge and skill, including some individuals without previous psychiatric experience. It is imperative, therefore, to have some type of inservice educational program.

This can be done in many ways, depending upon the administrative organization of a given unit and the particular problems of the staff. Sometimes it is a matter of giving the staff a good background in psychiatric theory, or filling in gaps in previous experiences, or getting the staff to accept newer and more modern techniques; and sometimes it is none of these things but rather teaching the staff some principles of supervision and administration, and helping them to learn to work together more effectively.

In the psychiatric unit of a general hospital, the problem of the nurse or aide who has had no previous experience in psychiatry is common. Often these individuals have been employed in some other service of the hospital and have been transferred to the psychiatric unit. Such persons need a very careful and comprehensive orientation to both the ward and the patients. This is best done by the head nurse, or her assistant if she has one. Then comes the problem of giving them a working knowledge of psychiatry and psychiatric nursing. If a student program is already established, it may be possible to have the new staff nurse or aide attend some of the student classes, such as the lectures in psychiatry, or the demonstrations in hydrotherapy. Attendance at staff conferences and ward rounds may also help. Sometimes it is possible for the new staff nurse to be in the psychiatric nursing classes which the instructor gives the students, but usually it is a better plan to arrange for separate instruction in psychiatric nursing for staff nurses and for aides. Their ward duties and problems with patients differ somewhat from those of students, and instruction given by the ward supervisor, rather than by the instructor, is often more useful to the staff nurse or aide.

Another important aspect of inservice training for the inexperienced staff member is rotation through all the services and departments related to the psychiatric unit before giving a permanent duty assignment. In order to function most effectively, the new member needs to get an over-all picture of the treatment facilities. Evaluation of his work on each of the wards or departments, and periodic discussions — with the supervisor — of his potentialities, progress, and short-comings during the critical learning period often make the difference between a competent employee and a failure.

The second group of nursing personnel needing an inservice educational program are those staff members with varying degrees of psychiatric experience. Student nurses are on the service primarily for education; the new employees must have instructions to function safely and effectively; but for nursing personnel who have worked for some time either in their present staff position or on the staff of some other institution, an educational program often has not been regarded as necessary.

This group, which is most often neglected in the total educational program, constitutes the backbone of the nursing service. They have close and prolonged contacts with patients. They remain while student nurses, residents, and interns come and go. It is they who create the psychological environment, the milieu in which the patients live. They carry out the psychiatrists' instructions and maintain the administrative policies; yet, generally, little or no attention is given to what they know of psychiatric concepts or what their attitudes are until the rigid ideas or the superstitious beliefs of one or another of them suceeds in frustrating the psychiatrist's efforts in treating a patient. Unless an educational program is provided in which such problems can be discussed with staff nurses and aides, it will be impossible to develop an effective therapeutic program for patients.

The purpose of an educational program for experienced personnel is not so much to impart psychiatric information — though keeping abreast of modern psychiatric developments should not be neglected — as it is to modify untherapeutic attitudes, to acquaint the staff with the rationale of psychiatric treatment used at the particular psychiatric unit, and to pool the experience gained in other institutions, agreeing on what could be used profitably in this one.

Methods used in teaching staff personnel cannot afford to be didactic or formal. Such methods are often misinterpreted as attempts of the instructor to make the personnel appear stupid or inferior. Informal discussion groups, often over a cup of coffee with the ward psychiatrist or the ward supervisor, are much more satisfactory. Problems of dealing with individual patients, ward problems, and questions about existing orders or suggestions regarding new or needed orders may be discussed profitably. Such a discussion allows an exchange of information about patients and helps to develop new ideas about how to deal with a nursing problem. It also serves as an outlet for pent-up feelings of irritation and frustration which the staff members have accumulated, and gives them a feeling of being supported by the psychiatrist and the supervisor.

Ward conferences which all the ward personnel attend are a valuable educational activity for the permanent personnel. At these conferences, patients and their problems and problems of interpersonal relationships among staff members may be explored thoroughly, especially if each member of the group has an equal opportunity to express his thoughts and feelings. The conferences should take place weekly at an hour when the majority of the ward staff can attend. It is most important that the educational program for the staff nurse or aide be as carefully planned as that of any other group working on the psychiatric unit. Staff members should also be encouraged to attend staff conferences and special lectures whenever possible.

Others of the permanent nursing staff who need some type of inservice educational program are the head nurses and supervisors. It is difficult to make specific suggestions regarding this group because much depends on the number of nurses on the supervisory staff and their psychiatric background. If, for example, the unit has only one head nurse and one instructor, further educational growth may come from meetings with supervisory staff in other departments. A group composed of the supervisors in psychiatric nursing, social service, occupational therapy, psychology, and adjunctive therapies may participate in the psychiatric unit's special group activities and work projects such as a journal club at which new trends in the various disciplines are reported on from the literature. They should be encouraged to attend nursing school faculty meetings, head nurse meetings of the general hospital, meetings of professional nursing organizations, and psychiatric institutes and meetings in particular.

If the staff consists of several head nurses and supervisors, head nurse seminars should be organized. Members of the group should plan their own programs, which may include single sessions of speakers on special subjects or a planned course of study of some aspects of psychiatric nursing. Reviewing current psychiatric articles and books is a program well suited to this group of nurses. Discussions of the problems of supervision on a psychiatric unit — which are somewhat different from those in general nursing supervision — and discussions of the teaching aspects of psychiatric nursing are always helpful.

Outservice Educational Program

No discussion of educational programs on the psychiatric unit of a general hospital is complete without emphasizing the responsibility of the unit to the nursing services of other departments of the hospital. The psychiatric unit sets the standards of psychological nursing care in the hospital, but it also should be a source of information and assistance when psychological problems in nursing care arise on other services. Furthermore, it can do an important educational job in helping to overcome the fear and misunderstanding that most nurses unfamiliar with psychiatric nursing have about psychiatric disorders.

When a psychiatric unit is first opened in a general hospital, the most common reaction is to give it a wide berth, as though it harbored patients with some peculiarly virulent contagious disease. A little later, the psychiatric unit becomes a wonderful place where one can send patients who suddenly become psychotic during hospitalization. Soon the nursing staff may discover that "difficult" neurotic patients, or troublesome patients with personality disorders, often can be transferred to the psychiatric unit where "the nurses are better equipped to handle such cases." At this stage of tolerance of psychiatry, referring all psychiatric nursing problems — flattering as this may be to the psychiatric unit — is neither practical, because of the limited number of beds available on the psychiatric service, nor healthy for the rest of the hospital nursing service. Therefore some type of educational program for the general hospital nurse needs to be evolved.

The student nurse is often an excellent "psychiatric missionary" to the older, more experienced graduate nurse. The student nurse who has completed her psychiatric service writes better observation notes on the patients' clinical charts when she returns to other clinical services. She is likely to note signs of depression, suicidal trends, evidences of hallucinations, delusions, and other psychopathological symptoms, as well as to comment on the patient's reactions to medications and treatments. Thus the graduate nursing and medical staff have psychological observations brought to their attention. Many head nurses, pleased with the improved clinical notes of students, and the increased sensitivity of the student to the patient's emotional needs, encourage this; however, some head nurses who are unaware of the significance of such psychological observations, or who are conscious of their own lack of knowledge in psychiatry, may ridicule the student, so that she is discouraged from putting into practice what she learned in her psychiatric experience.

It is important, therefore, that nurses in the general hospital have some understanding of psychiatric nursing, or at least have some sympathy with the psychiatric point of view, if the student is to integrate her psychiatric experience in her general nursing care. The best way to accomplish this is to make some psychiatric information available to the general staff nurse. How this is to be done will vary according to the resources available at the particular hospital. Elizabeth Bixler has recommended that a psychiatric nurse be employed on the nursing faculty of every school of nursing, not to teach the psychiatric nursing program, but to assist the other clinical services with the psychological problems that arise on their services or to point out psychological aspects of nursing care that are being overlooked. The psychiatric nurse, in such instances, would function as a consultant.

Another method, then, is to have the instructor or the supervisor of the psychiatric unit discuss emotional problems and mental illness with the general staff nurses periodically at their meetings. Generally those aspects of psychiatric nursing which the general staff nurse is most likely to encounter in her patients prove more interesting and helpful than discussions on purely psychiatric conditions. There is an awakening interest among nurses in the so-called psychosomatic illnesses. The psychiatric nurse could be of great assistance to her colleagues in nursing regarding the care of these patients. Films such as *Emotional Health,* produced by McGraw-Hill Films, *The Feeling of Rejection, The Feeling of Hostility,* and *Overdependency,* produced by the National Film Board of Canada, can often be used to good advantage, particularly if an opportunity is given for discussion afterward. With the increased interest in psychiatric problems in general, many excellent films are being produced, which are good material for general staff meetings.

In some psychiatric units it might be possible to work out opportunities for direct observation experience for those graduate nurses who are without previous psychiatric experience. Perhaps an orientation period of a week, or an 8-12 week period of instruction and experience similar to that given the undergraduate student nurse, might be developed. This latter course should carry academic credit if possible. The psychiatric unit often can utilize special events — such as opening a new ward, a tea honoring a new instructor, or a special lecture or conference with a well-known guest speaker — to break down the barriers between the psychiatrically oriented and the nonpsychiatrically oriented nurse.

Conclusion

Several nursing education programs have been discussed which could be instituted without too much difficulty in any well-organized psychiatric unit of a general hospital. These programs, however, do not by any means exhaust the educational opportunities such a unit offers. Many problems in psychiatric nursing urgently need investigation. Nurses must be found who are willing to advance the skills of psychiatric nursing further, as well as being eager to do research in psychiatric nursing problems. It does not take a large number of patients to make a good teaching and research laboratory. But it does take a nurse with imagination and creative ability to see the potentialities for education in such a unit and to develop them.

Bibliography

Babcock, Charlotte G. Emotional needs of nursing students. *Am J. Nursing* 49:166-169, Mar. 1949.

Barrett, Mary V. An in-service educational program for nurses. *Am J. Nursing* 51:388-391, June 1951.

Barton, Walter E. The nurse as an active member of the psychiatric team. *Am J. Nursing* 50:714-715, Nov. 1950.

Beck, Sister M. Berenice. Is more education necessary? *Am J. Nursing* 51:207-208, Mar. 1951.

Bixler, Elizabeth S. Psychiatric nursing in the basic curriculum. *Ment Hyg.* 32:89-101, Jan., 1948.

Cameron, D. Ewen. *General Psychotherapy.* New York, Grune & Stratton, 1950.

Ellis, Albert, and Fuller, Earl W. The personal problems of senior nursing students. *Am J. Psychiat.* 106:212-215, Sept. 1949.

Haigh, Gerald A. Staff conferences make a difference to psychiatric aides and patients. *Mod. Hosp.* 69:74-75, Oct. 1947.

Kalkman, Marion E. Psychiatric principles applied to general nursing care. Contained in the 54th Annual Report of the National League of Nursing Education, 1948. pp. 146-152.

———. The psychiatric affiliation. *Am. J. Nursing* 47:399, June 1947.

———. What the psychiatric nurse should be educated to do. *Psych. Quart. Supp.* 26:93-102, 1952.

Mereness, Dorothy. Meeting the students' emotional needs. *Am J. Nursing* 52:336-338, March 1952.

Preparation of the nurse for the psychiatric team. *Am J. Nursing* 51:320-322, May 1951.

Naes, Estelle B. Clinical courses for graduate nurses. *Am J. Nursing* 2:338-339, Mar. 1952.

Reiter, Mary. Educating adolescents to become nurses. *Am J. Nursing* 47:117-120, Feb. 1947.

Stevens, Leonard F. and Bombard, Pauline L. A training program for psychiatric aides. *Am. J. Nursing* 52:472-476, Apr. 1952.

U.S. Public Health Service. *Training and Research Opportunities under the National Mental Health Act.* Washington, D.C., U.S. Government Printing Office, (Public Health Service Publication No. 22).

Wallace, Grace S. Joint planning for psychiatric affiliation. *Am. J. Nursing* 51:409-410, June 1951.

The Psychiatric Nurse's Role

Dorothy E. Gregg

Miss Gregg (B.S., University of Colorado School of Nursing; M.A., Teachers College, Columbia) is assistant professor and coordinator of psychiatric nursing and mental hygiene at the University of Colorado School of Nursing.

Reprinted from *The American Journal of Nursing*, Vol. 54, July 1954.

The work of the psychiatric nurse is to help create an environment in which the patient will have an opportunity to develop new behavior patterns that will enable him to make a more mature adjustment to life. This change in behavior is a growth process in which the patient learns through his experiences with others to examine his beliefs with a new perspective and to work with his problems with new capacities.

If we assume that recovery from mental illness is essentially a growth process, then the kinds of experience through which growth may take place must be provided in the ward life of the hospitalized patient. Skilled persons within the patient's environment must be able to detect the kinds of experiences he needs and to create them in ways that he can use them with his capacity to function at the moment. We assume that the accomplishment of each task opens the possibility that a more advanced task can be met (1). Through this process, the patient gradually accomplishes the tasks that allow him to mature.

These learning experiences take place within the patient's relationships with people, and therefore our focus is on the interpersonal relationships in his environment. We are interested in the interaction between people and how interpersonal relationships can be used to extend the therapeutic process to the patient's life in the ward. The goal is to help him work through his problems by providing learning experiences that give him new tools and a new perspective with which to meet them.

This orientation is different from another kind of ward environment in which the emphasis is on helping the patient conform to accepted social behavior by keeping him occupied with activities and routines that are planned to keep him in touch with the familiar patterns of daily living. The goal in this orientation is to try to make reality more desirable than illness with the hope that he will choose the former. This type of environment has value, but it is somewhat limited.

There is a third kind of ward environment in which the patient is merely confined for a course of psychiatric treatment or for custodial care. The goal here seems to be to provide a protected living area for the patient.

Therapeutic Environment

Our concern is with the first kind of ward in which the environment is a part of the therapeutic program. In the therapeutic ward, first, the patient is allowed to express conflict; second, the staff tries to understand him and his problems; and third, there is an opportunity for interpersonal relationships in which the patient may test his beliefs and possibly change some of them through experiential learning.

If the hospital ward is to be a place in which the patient can express conflict, it must be free from unnecessary limitations, inhibiting routines, and attitudes that prevent freedom of expression. The interpersonal environment should offer the patient the experience of being accepted and respected as a person in his own right, with the freedom to talk out his problems and act out his conflicts — within the limits of safety and group living — without censure or sanction. Such an environment allows him to communicate his feelings, to examine his thoughts and actions, and to make choices and test out solutions to his problems. As communication is established with the patient, some understandings are possible, his needs can be recognized, and provisions to help him meet them can begin to be made.

Group Planning

Group planning by the psychiatric team is required to create a therapeutic environment and to work out a consistent approach that is in accord with the psychiatrist's goals in therapy. Close working relationships should be developed among all of the psychiatric workers who are in contact with the patient. Group participation serves several purposes: (a) workers have the opportunity to share observations and compare notes on the patient's responses to various situations; (b) cues to the patient's patterns of behavior and kinds of responses to people can be picked up from these shared observations that are useful in ascertaining the patient's needs; (c) the group can formulate ways to help meet the patient's needs and plan the learning experiences he might require for emotional growth; and (d) the workers can plan how their interpersonal relationships might be used to structure these experiences.

The group has another important function. Group meetings offer an opportunity for each member of the staff to discuss his relationship with the patient and possibly to gain insight into some of the interaction between himself and the patient that may be taking place outside of his awareness. Inferences can be made from these discussions on how the relationship is used by the patient and by the team member, and how the behavior of the team member might be changed or modified to effect a change in the patient's behavior. This kind of group work requires mutual respect and acceptance, and freedom to express feelings and ideas within the group.

Group planning might be developed in a variety of ways; the method chosen would depend on the type of ward unit in which the group works. The team membership also would vary according to the kinds of personnel working in the ward unit, and the kind of teamwork that is planned. Psychiatrists, nurses, social workers, psychologists, psychiatric aides, occupational and recreational therapists, and others who work with the patient might all be members of the team.

A system of interlocking teams may be useful. People who are working closely with the patient would be on the first team and would plan the therapeutic program. Members of this team would join allied teams to communicate information to and from personnel working in other divisions or on other shifts. In large units, it might be expedient to have ward group conferences for all workers, and to have the planning for small groups of patients or individual patients centered in small teams operating within the large group. If interlocking groups are used, it is important to have free communication between them.

There are many problems in establishing a group approach of this kind. It is not easy for people with different orientations and different kinds of training and competencies to work closely together. There has been much enthusiasm lately about the team approach, but it is hard to raise our concept of the team beyond the horse and buggy stage in which every team has a driver. Truly collaborative teamwork is difficult to achieve, but if we can approximate it on the psychiatric ward, we have a valuable therapeutic tool with which to shape changes in the social patterns of ward life. As a team develops, it is also a positive educational device for those taking part in it. It can be used as an inservice teaching group to help members who need further training.

The Nurse's Role

If the ward is to become a place in which the patient experiences therapeutic learning, the psychiatric nurse must have interpersonal skills that enable her to work with the patient in these learning experiences. In many units, the nurse is now expected to be mainly an observer who records and verbally reports her observations to the psychiatrist and others. She is expected to provide a safe living area for the patient and to give him things to do that help him socialize. Her focus is to encourage the patient to drop his symptoms and adopt the accepted patterns of behavior through conforming to the social patterns of the ward.

In fostering a change that involves experiential learning rather than mere conforming, the nurse's goal changes. She assumes a more active role of interaction with the patient. Hildegard Peplau outlines the nurse's function as that of a participant-observer who make inferences from her observations and who intervenes in behavior patterns (1). As the nurse works with the patient she questions: What is the patient saying with his behavior? What is he trying to communicate to me? What are his needs? How do my responses affect his behavior? What kinds of experiences with people does he need? How can I use my interpersonal relationship with him to help him learn? How can experiences in the ward life be used to help him?

With this approach, the nurse is still an observer and she still communicates her observations to other members of the therapeutic team, but she also uses her observations and makes judgments in determining how to help the patient use his relationship with her to foster emotional growth. Some of the judgments affecting her relationship with the patient may be made collaboratively with other team members, and some she makes alone. For example, she may observe that a patient repeatedly creates situations in which people will reject him. To change this pattern of behavior, he must repeatedly experience acceptance and inclusion by others. As a group, the psychiatric team may discuss ways in which team members may intervene in this behavior pattern through their individual contacts with the patient and how they may construct group situations in which he can feel accepted. The nurse must be able to recognize when the patient is creating such a situation with her, and she must decide how to respond to prevent him from feeling the rejection that he expects. She should also be able to detect how the patient reinforces this pattern with other patients, and she should learn ways to intervene in this behavior in group situations.

As a participant in an interpersonal relationship with a patient, the nurse observes not only the patient's behavior, but also her own, and she studies responses and learns to use the interpersonal experience constructively. Naturally, there are limitations in her ability to be aware of her behavior and to make inferences about what is going on in the relationship. Therefore, a collaborative relationship with the therapist and other team members is essential to the nurse. In her communication with others, she has the opportunity to clarify her role, validate her judgments and experiences, and use the group's formulations more effectively.

The nurse's functions in intervention include interrupting behavior patterns by her own response to the patient. For example, the patient who feels unworthy and disrespected may need the experience of learning personal worth. The nurse may convey a feeling of respect and an impression of his personal value as she carries out nursing procedures, such as dressing, feeding, or bathing. Through her manner, as well as through verbal communication in these contacts, she can provide the patient with the experience of being accepted. Many similar patterns of behavior may be changed when the patient repeatedly experiences a different kind of relationship than his beliefs have led him to expect. As psychiatric problems are worked with in the doctor-patient relationship, the therapist can plan with the nurse intervention techniques consistent with his therapeutic goals.

The nurse's role in intervention also involves setting necessary limits with the patient, and helping him to work within these limits. She must learn the skills of handling individual differences in groups so that each patient's needs are met. She learns to intervene in interaction between two patients in such a way that they may be able to talk out and accept each other's differences without either feeling that one has been favored over the other. She often becomes the strategic person who helps to coordinate team relationships and to clarify interrelationships of the various people in the ward society with the patient.

Defenses in Problem Situations

The nurse becomes more acutely aware of patterns or themes in behavior that interfere with relationships as she works with the problems that are involved in establishing therapeutic interpersonal relationships. These patterns often become social forces that affect both patient and staff, and, in the course of planning a therapeutic ward environment, many of them require intervention or modification. One such pattern is the tendencey to move away from situations that are uncomfortable. This is seen in a nurse's withdrawal from patients who are withdrawn when unresponsiveness makes her anxious (2). Avoidance of the patient whose behavior is erotic, bizarre, hostile, or overdependent is also common.

Milton Sapirstein says that we use three defenses against anxiety — we run away, we battle it out, or we go for help (3). If the nurse does not have the skills to handle an interpersonal problem, running away is one of the defenses readily available on the psychiatric ward. She may avoid the withdrawn patient and still feel useful because she spends her time with the more responsive patients, or she may find other useful tasks such as arranging the medicine closet or doing the book work. Some of the complicated procedures and routines of psychiatric wards seem to have been created out of a need to withdraw from patients. This defense may be used not only by nurses, but by any member of the psychiatric team.

The second defense — to approach the problem situation — presupposes that the person has certain skills, that she has some understanding of the meaning of the behavior she observes, and that she has learned ways to communicate with the patient. If such skills are lacking or if the attempt is unsuccessful, the approach may become hostile. Since overt hostility is rarely accepted, the nurse may make covert expressions of hostility without recognizing that she is hostile.

The third defense — to go for help — might be useful if constructive help were available when it is sought or if the help obtained is consistently not useful, attitudes of indifference or hopelessness may result.

These patterns of behavior alert us to the nurse's need to acquire techniques for handling interpersonal problems with the patient before changes in patterns of withdrawal, hostility, or indifference can be expected. If we find ways to decrease the "detail work" of nursing to give the nurse more time with her patients, and yet fail to teach her the skills she needs, the anxiety that is created in her because she does not know what to do only increases her need to use a variety of unprofitable defenses.

Another pattern of behavior or theme that may interfere with a therapeutic environment is control. This theme may promote inflexible regulations and rigid routines which seriously inhibit the freedom to express conflict. If the nurse has the notion that she must always have the situation under control, she sets limits on the patient's behavior if it is unmeaningful or upsetting to her, and thus interferes with her opportunity to learn what he is trying to communicate. For example, the patient who becomes disturbed may be immediately secluded or transferred to a ward for disturbed patients, without having an opportunity to talk about what is upsetting him, because his behavior interferes with the nurse's control of the situation.

In the carefully controlled setting, a pattern of efficient routine is often adopted. The expediency with which bathing, feeding, dressing, and other tasks may be done becomes more important than the patient who is involved in the procedure; his needs and feelings may be disregarded in the process, and the opportunity to use these tasks in communicating with him is lost. For example, on one ward, the admission routine included a shampoo. The shampoo was given to one patient even though she had spent the morning having her hair done.

An atmosphere of hurriedness may be a part of the nurse's concept of efficiency, and this interferes with the establishment of satisfactory interpersonal relationships with patients. The importance of being busy is so well ingrained in nursing that student nurses feel uncomfortable when they are just talking with patients during the first part of their psychiatric affiliation. In one well-staffed ward that I visited recently, patients prefixed every request with "Nurse, I know you are busy, but...." The nurses were far from busy, but the impression of business had been effectively established.

The theme of control is manifested also in the behavior of the nurse who always operates in an information-giving role. This interferes with her ability to listen and accept, and her patient may be denied the understanding he needs and the chance to communicate his feelings. This pattern stereotypes the nurse as "the uninformed." The role may be adopted by the nurse who needs to feel important, with the consequence that the patient is made to feel unimportant. The connotation that the patient does not understand and cannot understand may develop with this trend. The result is that attempts at conversation are reduced, or conversation may be carried on in the patient's presence, but without including him.

The theme of control is also reinforced when there is a pattern of set expectations on the part of the staff regarding the patient's behavior and a demand that he conform to these expectations. One operation in this pattern is the stereotyping of the patient's behavior by the staff. When the patient moves out of his stereotype, the staff becomes anxious and places restrictions upon him. Take, for example, the patient who has attempted suicide and whose every move may be taken to be a suicidal gesture. He is rigidly restricted in his activities far beyond the point of reasonable protection. Another stereotype is that an excited patient cannot communicate, so the opportunity for him to communicate with others is not provided. A common belief is that a "good" patient is a quiet patient and all behavior outside this stereotype must be restricted.

Real understanding of patients is not possible if the staff operates within set expectations of behavior. Patients learn to take on the fixed, expected behavior pattern to gain approval or to be left alone, or they learn to cross the limits of their stereotype so that they will be noticed. Thus, a patient may stay disturbed because it is expected, or because it is the only way he gets attention.

In some situations a patient needs merely to conform to our concept of proper adjustment to the ward life to be considered well enough to go home. This may be seen in wards where the emphasis is on short-term treatment. In one such unit which I visited, I was interested to see that there was very little "acting-out" behavior and very few verbal expressions of conflict from patients. They knew that if they were not able to show improvement within two weeks they would be committed to the state hospital, and they seemed to concentrate all their effort on gaining control and hiding their symptoms in order to be well-behaved patients. When so little time is allowed for working with complex problems, conformity seems to be the only chance for survival.

Some administrative policies develop from the theme of conformity. The methods of working with patients may be so predetermined that sensitive nurses who are aware of their patients' needs are unable to work effectively within the seriously limiting circumstances. For example, disapproval of dependence may be so great that dependence cannot be allowed even when it is therapeutic. Disapproval for neglecting to carry out a ward routine may be so marked that personnel will forfeit the patient's welfare. For example, a very anxious patient was forcefully stripped of her own clothing and dressed in hospital attire upon admission to a hospital. Nurses were aware that this was extremely disturbing to her, but the hospital policy was followed and the patient's feelings were ignored.

Patterns of conformity are usually enforced by fear of punishment or disapproval for the violation of limits. A nurse who expects blame or punishment from her teammates or the administration if something goes wrong in her interpersonal relationship with a patient will find it quite difficult to accept behavior that makes her feel that she has lost control. Thus, one of the basic premises of the therapeutic ward — freedom of expression — cannot be attained. It is difficult for the nurse to be accepting of patients when she does not experience acceptance in her working relationships, and to be permissive with patients when she works in a rigidly regulated setting. In one instance, a head nurse who was able to develop a permissive environment in a ward of a rigidly regimented hospital was regarded by the administrator as poor and inefficient, and was derogated by other head nurses.

The need to cling to these themes of control and conformity may be partially reduced when the nurse learns new techniques for meeting problems and has different kinds of experiences with patients as she tries out these techniques in clinical situations. For example, as she learns communication skills through which she can relate to disturbed patients, the impression that disturbed people cannot and do not want to communicate with others may be changed.

We have considered here only a few of the many themes in the ward life that concern us in creating a therapeutic environment; most of these themes present multifaceted problems as we seek methods to change them. We have been concerned with ways in which these themes influence the patient-nurse relationship, but they affect other team members similarly.

There are many sources from which these themes develop — cultural patterns, community patterns, the patterns of professional training, of hospital life, and individual patterns. To change well-established social patterns is a laborious process; however, it seems possible that one of the most effective tools for instigating social change in the ward environment is the psychiatric team whose members are constantly working with social forces in their interpersonal relationship with patients. As a part of the social group in the ward life of the patient, the team member is capable of increasing or reducing the influence of prevailing ward themes.

Summary

The psychiatric nurse's role, then, is to help extend the therapeutic process into the ward environment by creating nurse-patient relationships that promote emotional growth and that are consistent with the therapeutic plan of the doctor-patient relationship. She functions in interpersonal relationships with individuals and with groups of patients, and she collaborates with others to plan learning experiences and to discover and modify the social patterns or themes that influence the ward life of the patient.

Resources

1. Peplau, Hildegard. Lectures and discussions at Teachers College, Columbia University, Division of Nursing Education.

2. Tudor, Gwen E. A sociopsychiatric nursing approach to intervention in a problem of mutual withdrawal on a mental hospital ward. *Psychiatry* 15:193-217, May 1952.

3. Sapirstein, Milton R. *Emotional Security*. New York, Crown Publications, 1948.

4. Ruesch, Jurgen and Bateson, Gregory. *Communication: The Social Matrix of Psychiatry*. New York, W.W. Norton and Co., 1951.

5. Busse, Ewald W., Director, Department of Psychosomatic Medicine, University of Colorado School of Medicine. Personal communication.

6. Van Nuben, Betty J., Instructor in Psychiatric Nursing, University of Colorado School of Nursing. Personal communication.

Nursing Consultant for a State Mental Hospital Authority

Annie Laurie Crawford

Miss Crawford (Highland Hospital School of Nursing, Ashville, North Carolina, B.S., University of Washington, Seattle) is the Institutions' Nursing Supervisor of the Minnesota Department of Public Welfare.

Reprinted from *Nursing Outlook*, Vol. 2, No. 10, October 1954.

Approximately 87 percent of more than 600,000 hospitalized mentally ill patients in the United States are cared for in state mental hospitals. Slightly more than 9000 registered nurses and nearly 90,000 psychiatric aides and attendants are employed to provide nursing care for them. Relatively few of these patients receive direct nursing care from professional nurses. Many of the aides and attendants who give nursing care do not have supervision, guidance, or direction from professional nurses.

The professional staffs of the various units within a state hospital system vary considerably in their attitudes toward educational programs designed to increase the quantity and improve the quality of nursing care. A psychiatric nurse consultant employed by the state mental hospital authority is a catalyst and a coordinator. Her hospital visits constitute a "honey bee circuit," wherein she brings ideas and procedures found useful in one hospital to the attention of nurses and aides in others.

In November 1953 the Minnesota Department of Public Welfare surveyed mental hospital authorities throughout the country to get information about consultants in other states. We asked for the title used, date of first appointment, appointee's relationship and services to state mental hospitals, and other information concerning the appointment of the consultant.

Report of Survey

Fourteen states employ professional nurses on their state central mental hospital authority staffs; two states are considering appointing a nurse, and one state "hopes for" an appointment, according to information received from these agencies in the final quarter of 1953. Some of the central mental hospital agencies did not give the date of their first professional nurse appointments. Pennsylvania reported that it first appointed a nurse in 1924. Others reported appointments in the period from 1947 to 1953, indicating a relationship between current interest in state mental hospitals and the new emphasis on care, treatment, and research in such hospitals.

In response to my request for a statement concerning the factors and agencies which influence nursing appointments, the replies stressed the need to coordinate hospital nursing services, improve nursing education programs, and recruit more nursing personnel. An important factor mentioned was getting the mental health commissioner's recommendation for appointing such a consultant. One reply stressed the need for someone who could interpret and coordinate the services of nurses working in the public health department and those employed in institutions.

None of the replies mentioned getting help from professional nurses and nursing organizations in developing positions for nurse consultants. It is believed, however, that psychiatric nurses in many states — as individuals, and through their professional organizations — have played a decisive role in establishing the position and in assuming leadership in recruiting candidates for the appointment. This is certainly true in Minnesota. A temporary committee to explore psychiatric nursing conditions in the Minnesota state hospitals was appointed by the Minnesota Nurses Association in 1948. In 1949 the committee report, *Survey of Nursing in Minnesota State Mental Hospitals*, recommended:

> That a full-time nurse consultant to Minnesota state hospitals be appointed and be made directly responsible to either the Director of Public Institutions or Director of Professional Services in Public Institutions. That her responsibility and authority be sufficiently broad to cover both nursing services and educational programs in nursing (student, graduate, and aide or attendant) carried on in state hospitals.*

This report served as a basic guide to the state civil service department in preparing the job description. Shortly after the report was published the Governor's Advisory Council on Mental Health was formed, and a subcommittee on nursing was appointed to advise the council on nursing needs and nursing problems.

In 1948 the Council of State Governments, taking concerted action to improve the care and treatment of mentally ill patients in state hospitals, recommended that all states with more than a single

*Memo dated February 4, 1949 from the chairman to members of the Temporary Committee on Psychiatric Nursing Conditions in State Mental Hospitals, Minnesota.

mental hospital provide for a central mental hospital authority and employ a qualified psychiatrist to direct the medical care of state hospital patients.

The California Department of Mental Hygiene made a study of the titles, salaries, and duties of psychiatric nursing consultants employed by the various states. They released this data, in mimeographed form, in August 1952 (1). At the time of this survey, 11 states reported that one or more professional nurses were employed on the staffs of their central mental hospital authorities. Eight of the states reporting use the title "director" or "supervisor;" 3 used "consultant."

In Minnesota the title is "institutions' nursing supervisor," and the "class specifications" of the state's civil service act indicate that the position entails no direct line of authority. The announcement of open examination for applicants states:

> [The institutions' nursing supervisor] acts in an advisory capacity to the State Mental Health Commissioner and institutions (mental hospitals) superintendents . . . is responsible for planning, developing and co-ordinating a statewide program of nursing services. . .is also responsible for educational programs for psychiatric aides, affiliating student nurses, and graduate nursing staff within state hospitals.

Other duties assigned to her include reviewing staffing patterns; requests for nursing personnel prepared by hospitals for presentation to the state legislature, and consulting with architects about plans for hospital buildings and units.

In the California Department of Mental Hygiene the nursing consultant is called the "director of nursing services." Her work is designated as:

> . . .developing and supervising educational programs for all nursing personnel, planning and implementing conferences and institutes to assist directors of nursing and educational directors, visits to hospitals for the purpose of observing nursing care of patients, surveys of institutions upon request, preparation of annual reports, assistance with Civil Service examinations for nursing personnel, consultation to superintendents on professional qualifications of nurses in administrative and teaching positions, assisting with recruitment of personnel, interpretation of the nursing program to groups. . . .

These are pioneer jobs, which have been established because of a conviction that professional nursing can and will assume responsibility for providing nursing care, and for improving nursing education programs for all personnel who give nursing care to the mentally ill. The broad scope and general nature of these functions offer the nurse consultant an unlimited opportunity for service as a team leader.

But the tradition of autonomy which has characterized state mental hospitals for so many years does not disappear automatically with the enactment of legislation and the appointment of a central office staff. Creative imagination and the brand of intelligence characterized as "the ability to see the ultimate result of the present action" are called for. Assessing needs and evaluating resources to meet these needs come first. Certain definite goals must be set, but discriminating judgment is essential in choosing objectives. Some of the most pressing problems and apparent needs usually have been recognized. Others may be apparent to the "director" or "consultant," but remain unrecognized by those who, ultimately, must provide the means for meeting these needs. Resources may be readily available, or they may become available only as a gradual evolution in thinking and concerted action takes place. Major goals should be dictated by basic needs but they also should be established through group planning whenever possible.

Minnesota's Program

Since a large part of the care was provided by attendants, improvement in their socio-economic status and education became one of the major criteria of improvement. The title "attendant" was changed to "psychiatric aide." Salaries and other employment conditions were adjusted. Four of the state hospitals which had conducted diploma programs for nursing students dropped these programs in 1943, and accepted students only for affiliate programs in psychiatric nursing. Orientation and inservice training for psychiatric aides was relatively stable in these hospitals. Each of the state hospitals and the two institutions for mentally retarded and epileptic patients employed at least one nurse instructor.

One of the first goals in the improvement program was a "uniform" orientation and training program for psychiatric aides. The nursing supervisor arranged for a conference at one state hospital to consider the training program's content. All the other hospitals sent professional nurses and psychiatric aides, and some sent other members of the psychiatric team. Representatives also came from the state's civil service department, its vocational education department, the board of nurse examiners, and professional nursing organizations. Consultants from psychiatry, nursing education, social work, clinical psychology, and recreational therapy were invited to take part, and a full day was devoted to discussing the general knowledge and nursing skills the aide should possess to function as an effective member of the psychiatric team. The institution's nursing supervisor served as moderator at the discussions which were tape-recorded and used as a reference by the curriculum committee.

The curriculum committee — comprising professional nurses and aides attending the conference — and its psychiatrist and nurse-educator advisors worked out a 1-year course for aides. Copies of this were circulated to the mental health commissioner and state hospital superintendents. They were asked to present it for study to their staffs and faculties and to be ready to discuss it at the next superintendents' meeting, three weeks later. This group accepted the program, arranged for the facilities needed to carry it out, and met other related problems; they assumed the responsibility for introducing the program to their hospital staffs and agreed to the "achievement examination" which was to follow the study course. They also agreed to having uniform insignia provided for all aides who completed the course satisfactorily.

The medical superintendents continue to encourage psychiatric aides with several years of satisfactory work experience to attend selected classes, to take part in hospital and ward classes and supervised experiences, and to take the examination to qualify them for the achievement certificate and insignia.

The value of the program's official acceptance already has been tested. One hospital abandoned a plan to drastically reduce the course content when it was pointed out that such a modification would require consideration by all the superintendents before it could be approved.

Expanding and extending psychiatric aides' training brought into sharp focus the inadequate number of professional nurses available and prepared to do either classroom or ward teaching. To help meet this need, funds which had been appropriated for "training" were offered as educational stipends to graduate nurses for advanced preparation in psychiatric nursing, on the condition that they would accept employment in state hospitals following a year of study. Since the funds had not been appropriated for that specific purpose, extensive negotiations were necessary before it was possible to make this "offer" to graduate nurses. Wending one's way through mazes of officialdom — laws, rules, and tradition, sometimes the most formidable of all — requires an absolute conviction of the proposal's usefulness. Skill in communicating one's conviction also helps, as do a stout heart and tireless feet.

The existing law allowed the director of civil service discretionary power to approve "training" programs proposed by agencies of the state government. Administrative officers in the state government and hospital superintendents supported the proposal to use funds for stipends to graduate nurses. The proposal finally was approved, but so much time had gone into the process that little time was left for recruiting applicants. Only four stipends were awarded for the 1951-52 academic year. These nurses are now employed in three state hospitals, and they more than justify the hopes for the training project.

In 1953 the state legislature appropriated funds specifically to provide educational stipends for professional workers in the several disciplines. Enough money was granted to permit six nurses to receive stipends for the academic year 1953-54, and seven nurses applied for them. Six more stipends are available for use this September, and all have been requested. Significant, long-range gains in the quality of psychiatric nursing care for Minnesota's mentally ill should result from this program in the next few years.

Educational Programs

Educational programs for nursing personnel in Minnesota are classified by the Department of Public Welfare as "accredited" or "non-accredited." All programs having approval by accrediting agencies or approving authorities are listed for reference in the department's central office as "accredited."

The University of Minnesota approves and gives academic credit for field experience to graduate nurse students enrolled for the certificate in psychiatric nursing, master's degrees in education, nursing service administration, and mental health, and for extension courses offered on and off the campus.

The University of Minnesota requires a minimum enrollment of 25 students for off-campus extension courses. In order to make the extension courses in ward management, student counseling, and principles of teaching available to nurses who are employed by state hospitals, and are unable to take leave for full-time study, these courses are open also to nurses employed by general hospitals. Thus, two benefits are derived, opportunity for further study is provided to graduate nurses and a closer working relationship is provided between nurses employed in neighboring hospitals.

We classify programs which carry no academic or professional credit as "non-accredited." These include psychiatric aide training courses, institutes, departmental workshops and conferences, orientation conferences for the faculties and staffs of hospital schools of nursing, students' affiliate programs at state hospitals, and institutional assemblies. These non-accredited programs are reviewed and evaluated periodically to determine the progress being made in them. The institutions' nursing supervisor assumes responsibility for arranging institutes, conferences, and workshops.

Quarterly Institutes

The quarterly institutional assembly, to which each institution sends a representative from each of its departments for a 1-day meeting, is an interesting and vital force in the total mental health program. A program session for the whole group is held in the morning. Following lunch each group convenes for a separate session which lasts about two hours. The program content for the year is determined earlier by responses to a questionnaire survey. (As an example, the 1953 program included consideration of administrative problems and three clinical subjects.)

Nursing personnel from the hospitals elect a chairman, a vice-chairman, and a secretary, and appoint a program committee. General policies and problems related to the specific services of the group are considered, and a program is presented. The whole day's program usually is coordinated with the subject of the morning session. One program, for instance, was devoted to state hospital care for aged patients. In this session, the nursing education supervisor from one hospital reviewed nursing care as a part of the team approach in a special program of rehabilitation for aged patients who are being discharged. Her report was reproduced and copies were sent to each hospital. These were to be used as a basis for the report given to their co-workers by persons who attended the conference.

There is time during these assemblies for informal chats and an exchange of ideas. Best of all, perhaps, is the feeling of togetherness they offer, and the opportunity for group action in planning nursing care for the state's 12,000 mentally ill patients.

An important function of the institution's nursing supervisor is recruiting nursing personnel, and consulting with hospital superintendents and personnel officers about the qualifications which nurses need in order to fill certain positions. Professional isolation and lack of provision for organizing professional nursing services have kept many nurses who are genuinely interested in psychiatric nursing from accepting positions in state mental hospitals.

Many state hospitals make no provision for the type of nursing service organization which is considered essential in general and other special hospitals. The American Psychiatric Association strongly recommends that the nursing service in psychiatric institutions be directed by a competent, professional nurse to whom all nursing service personnel — including psychiatric aides and attendants — are responsible. In a survey published in 1950, the American Psychiatric Association reported that seven state mental hospitals did not have even one graduate nurse on their staffs (2). The survey did say that a trend toward the recommended pattern was observed, however.

Effective nursing service organization and the amount of assistance which can be offered to hospital superintendents often depend upon successful recruitment. The Minnesota institutions' nursing supervisor visits every nursing school in the state annually. She is accompanied by a member of the state civil service department, and they discuss the needs and opportunities for professional nurses in state mental hospitals and the program of educational stipends for graduate nurses. Many of the students have had their basic psychiatric nursing experience in state hospitals, and they have an opportunity to ask questions about such state hospital policies as planning for patients' care, budgets, staffing, and other items.

These visits also give the nursing supervisor an opportunity to interpret policies and programs associated with her duties and, since the position is still a relatively new one, to tell the students in effect that we are trying to provide the framework for them to continue building a program of better nursing care. We remind them, "If you are kept informed about how and why we make plans and decisions it should be easier for you."

Maintaining reports and records is an essential part of the program for improving nursing care. Nursing programs must be interpreted to other members of the health team, to departmental and hospital administrative officers, to legislators, and to pro-professional and citizen groups interested in the mental health program. In Minnesota, the form for the quarterly report of nursing services in state hospitals has been constructed to help directors of nursing and members of their staffs evaluate the hospital's nursing care and nursing education programs and thus serve as an educational tool. The nursing supervisor uses the reports to evaluate and interpret the total program of nursing care, and to point out those areas where special help and guidance is needed.

The nursing care on a ward can be evaluated by making regularly scheduled ward rounds and by observing activities which the patients appear to enjoy. The nurses and aides on a reception and treatment ward in one state hospital, and the patients' attitudes toward hospitalization, were heartily commended when only two of the 47 patients who were interviewed expressed doubt about getting well and going home.

Research as a function of the psychiatric nurse on the staff of the central mental hospital authority was not mentioned in either the California survey or the Minnesota job description, but promoting nursing research projects in state hospitals can be one of the nurse consultant's most important functions. Nursing functions studies sponsored and supported by the American Nurses' Association, investigations to determine the effectiveness of specific nursing care projects, experimentation leading to approved training for psychiatric aides, and the refinement and extensicn of educational programs for graduate nurses are urgently needed to assure expert nursing care for patients. To the statement made by a leader in the field of psychiatry that "a hospital building never cured a patient — that is done by dedicated personnel" — we would add, *trained as well as dedicated* (3).

References

1. CALIFORNIA STATE DEPARTMENT OF MENTAL HYGIENE. *Studies of Salaries and Duties of Psychiatric Nursing Consultant at State Level.* (mimeographed) Sacramento, Calif., 1952.
2. AMERICAN PSYCHIATRIC ASSOCIATION. *Psychiatric Nursing Personnel.* Washington, D.C., The Association, 1950, p. 4.
3. STEVENSON, GEORGE. Training in the psychiatric disciplines. *Mental Hygiene,* 34:29, Jan. 1953.

Reassurance

Dorothy Gregg

Miss Gregg (B.S., University of Colorado School of Nursing; M.A., Teachers College, Columbia) is coordinator of psychiatric nursing and mental hygiene at the University of Colorado School of Nursing.

Reprinted from *The American Journal of Nursing*, Vol. 55, February 1955.

A nurse walked into a patient's room and found her looking very forlorn and upset. This was their conversation.

> NURSE: Oh, come now, Mrs. Carson, nothing could be that bad! You look like you have lost your last friend!
>
> PATIENT: The doctor just told me that it will be impossible for me to get well if I don't have the operation. I'm so mixed up — I wish I knew what to do.
>
> NURSE: There is only one thing to do, and that is to have the surgery! You haven't a thing to worry about. You have the best surgeon in town. He has done hundreds of operations just like yours.
>
> PATIENT: You don't understand — I have confidence in my doctor's skill — it's — well — .
>
> NURSE: Most people are a little scared when they think about having an operation. Remember when you had your first baby several years ago while I was working on OB? You had the longest and hardest labor of anyone on the ward, and I never heard a whimper out of you! I was so proud of you! You were the best patient in the whole hospital! After what you went through, this operation should be a picnic, and this time you'll be completely unconscious from the anesthetic. You won't feel a thing.

During this conversation the nurse probably was sincere in her desire to reassure the patient, but she was not aware of what constitutes reassurance. She may not even discover that she has failed, but she will probably wonder why the patient talked more freely to someone else than she did to her. If we attempt to see how the patient felt in this conversation, maybe we can make some guesses about what she experienced.

Mrs. Carson's reaction to the nurse's first comment might have been: *I feel very upset, and she can see that I am upset. Why does she say, "nothing could be that bad?" How could she possibly know? And losing friends has nothing to do with how I feel. This is worse than losing friends — what a silly remark!*

Such cliches frequently are used socially to reduce the danger of an unwanted "scene" and to preserve social equanimity. What happens most often is that they reduce the importance of the other person's feelings. In this situation they failed to convey to the patient that the nurse understood the concern that she has perceived in the patient. Webster defines reassurance as a "restoration of confidence." There was little in this opening to the conversation that restored Mrs. Carson's confidence.

The patient's feelings about the nurse's second comment might have been: *I tried to tell her that I was mixed up. It is hard for me to explain to another person how I feel, and she didn't even let me finish! Maybe she doesn't care how I feel. Now she thinks I am frightened about the operation. I guess she wouldn't know what it's like to be afraid of something bigger than an operation! She tells me there is only one thing to do — if life were only that simple! Why does she have to tell me what to do? I didn't ask for that! What does she mean — "I haven't anything to worry about?" I wonder what she would do if she had my little boy? She doesn't even know what I'm worried about! Maybe that's it — maybe she doesn't want to know — maybe she is afraid to know. I guess I really shouldn't bother other people with this. No one could possibly understand how I feel. What is this about the surgeon? Does she think my doctor isn't good enough? Why else would she be so eager to tell me he is good? I have confidence in him — well — I think I have — .*

This is one possible outcome of jumping ahead of a patient's expression of her feelings and guessing at what she is trying to say. The guess can easily be wrong and, furthermore, it conveys that the patient is not important enough to the nurse for her to care what the patient has to say. A second error in the nurse's approach was that she immediately started telling the patient what to do. This action was based on the assumption that the patient couldn't make a decision for herself and that she wished the nurse to make it for her. Erroneously, the nurse believed that she was helping the patient when she told her what to do.

In addition, in an attempt to allay unknown fears, she made another guess that the patient was not sure of her doctor's skill, and in so doing, she was in danger of creating doubt. If the nurse is fortunate, the patient may be able to perceive that the nurse is anxious and has made a false assumption regarding her own fears, but there is the possibility that an anxiety-ridden patient may not be capable of such perception at the moment, so she takes the cue from the nurse to worry about her surgeon's skill.

Regarding the nurse's third response, the patient may have felt: *She didn't let me finish — she must think I am stupid because I can't talk without stumbling over my words. There she goes on about the operation again. She just can't understand! There is just no point in talking with her! What is this about the way I behaved at the birth of my baby? If she only knew — I was so scared I couldn't whimper — but she was proud of me! That very baby is my biggest problem! What is she saying? Does she mean good patients don't cry? I guess I'm supposed to be brave and silent, and here I am telling her about being so mixed up! Is she afraid I'll make a scene? Oh, what's the use? How could anyone understand about John? She says I won't feel a thing — maybe I won't — maybe I really won't!*

Twice the patient tried to express to the nurse how she felt and as she hesitated and searched for words, the nurse became anxious and guessed at her problem, thereby cutting off the patient's chance to talk about what was bothering her. The nurse further expressed her own anxiety when she unwittingly told the patient how she expected her to behave by holding her past performance up to her as an example of behaving as a "good" patient should. She also conveyed disrespect for the patient in her present disturbance by telling her that the coming episode would be "a picnic." The implication was that she blamed the patient for her present distressed behavior. It is rarely comforting to an anxiety-ridden person to be told that she will be unconscious, for in her apprehension, she may look upon this as simply another situation in which she will be "out of control."

Later in the day, another nurse entered the same patient's room to prepare her for the night. Mrs. Carson smiled a greeting, but initiated no further conversation. She seemed preoccupied, and her face was tearstained. The nurse began to rub her back.

NURSE: It seems hard for you to relax tonight. You must have had a difficult day.

PATIENT: Yes. (silence)

NURSE: Would you like to tell me about it?

PATIENT: It would seem silly to you. It's so hard to explain — . If I thought I could make it home, I would leave — . No one understands.

NURSE: I would like to try to understand if it will help you.

PATIENT: They say I have to have an operation, and I'm so scared and mixed up. They think it's the operation that scares me, but — oh, well — I don't know how you could understand. I'm such a mess! (silence)

NURSE: It's hard to talk about it.

PATIENT: Yes — if I weren't around maybe he could get someone who would really help John. I just don't have the patience any more — maybe I never did! (pause)

NURSE: Could you tell me who John is, and who could get someone else?

PATIENT: John is my oldest child. He has cerebral palsy. He is a sweet little boy but he needs so much care, and you have to be so patient with him, and I'm just not. Since I've been sick we haven't been able to send him to his special school. My medical bills stand in the way of his chances to get help, and when he is home all the time — well — I guess I get impatient with his troubles, and I'm always scolding when I know he can't help it. My husband has the burden of both of us. He is so kind to the boy, and so patient with me. They would both be better off without me. I shouldn't have the operation.

NURSE: Are you saying that you may not live if you don't have the operation and that this would be better for John and your husband?

PATIENT: The doctor said I can't expect to live long without surgery. (thoughtful silence) I guess I really am silly — that would be kind of like suicide, wouldn't it? (crying) Now you know how mixed up I am! I guess I am a little crazy — worrying about John and the money and everything. (sobbing)

NURSE (hands patient a handkerchief): It's such a tough problem that you would just like to escape from it.

PATIENT: Yes, but I don't really want to die. I can't really say that my husband would be better off if I died. He would be all alone with our little boy. What a coward I am. What would he do all alone? And Johnny — he needs me even if I'm not much of a mother. If I just knew what to do! If I could just be patient like other mothers!

NURSE: All mothers get angry and impatient with their children sometimes.

PATIENT: I do get angry at the other children, but I don't feel so bad when I jump on them.

NURSE: It's more difficult with John, because he has special problems.

PATIENT: Yes. I feel so helpless with John. I guess if I knew how to work with him better I wouldn't be so impatient.

NURSE: There is a specially trained person on our staff who works with children with cerebral palsy. She might be helpful to you and John, and if you feel you would like to talk with her, it can be arranged.

PATIENT: Yes, I would. I used to talk with John's teacher, and that helped a lot, but since he hasn't been in school I haven't seen her. We must get him back in school soon. We will have to borrow money for the operation; that is why his schooling has to wait. I wish there were some way to pay for both at the same time.

NURSE: There are also people on our staff who are trained to help with financial problems. Maybe one of them could help you make a payment plan for your operation so it would not be such a burden to you.

PATIENT: Could my husband and I both talk to them before I have the operation? I would want him to see the person with me.

In this conversation, the nurse recognized the patient's distress, as the nurse in the first episode did. Contrary to the way her colleague responded, however, she did not derogate the patient by making light of her feelings. She made an opening for the patient to communicate her distress, which the discouraged patient fenced off by a simple "Yes."

The nurse's next question, "Would you like to tell me about it?," opened further the opportunity for the patient to speak. To be helpful, this question would have to reflect the nurse's sincere interest and warmth for the patient. If it were a curious probe without real interest in understanding the patient better, the patient would probably be able to detect it as such. This is only one of several similar kinds of openings. For example, one might use, "Tell me what happened," or further identification of feelings might be attempted to encourage expression, such as, "It must have been pretty upsetting." The nurse observed that the patient had a need to talk with someone, but at this point she needed a little help to feel that the nurse would actually accept her.

Next, the nurse attempted to convey to the patient that she wanted to try to understand her, even though the patient thought that it was impossible. The patient gave three clues to the fact that it would be difficult for her to feel accepted enough to talk about her problem: (1) she expected nurses to think that her distress was silly; (2) she said that her feelings were hard to explain; and (3) she wished to escape the whole issue by going home. The nurse made the inference that the patient's confidence might begin to be restored if she could be assisted to work out her problem for herself. The nurse's second inference was that the patient might experience further distress, perhaps to the point of devastation, if she were allowed to escape from working with her difficulties.

The patient's first step in having a successful experience in problem-solving is to feel accepted and understood, so she can feel free to talk about all the facets of her problems in order to view them clearly in making her decisions. The nurse created a feeling of acceptance by what she said and did as she listened to her. By listening with sincere interest, by identifying the feelings that the patient was expressing and by seeking clarification when meanings were not clear to her, the nurse conveyed that she was trying to understand.

The nurse's statement, "It is hard to talk about it," was an attempt to identify and accept the patient's feeling of half-wanting and half-not-wanting to talk "it" over, and to show that she accepted the turmoil that the patient felt.

As the patient started to work with her problem, she made opening statements that were not quite clear. When the nurse sought clarification by asking, "Could you tell me who John is...?" she accomplished two things. First she conveyed that she was really interested in knowing exactly what was being said, and secondly, she helped the patient communicate more clearly. Issues sometimes can be perceived more adequately as they are described to another person. If the factors involved in a problem are clear, accurate identification of the problem is possible.

The nurse's question, "Are you saying that you may not live...?" was also a clarification maneuver, using a slightly different method. The nurse picked up something the patient said and tried to help her re-examine it to see if she really meant what she was saying. There are a variety of clarification-seeking responses that might have been used. For instance, "What do you mean?" or "Why shouldn't you have the operation?"

When one uses any "helping measure" there is the possibility that he is using it to serve his own purpose rather than that of the person he is helping. If the nurse uses a clarification maneuver to help the patient look at her meanings more clearly and use her own resources to reformulate her concepts, the patient experiences a feeling of confidence that comes when a problem is successfully resolved. However, if the nurse uses the clarification maneuver to achieve a sense of power in manipulating the patient and thus to raise her own feeling of prestige, her patient may feel foolish for approaching her difficulties as she did. She will not be reassured about her own strength, but she may feel more helpless and inadequate than she did before, and become more anxious and less able to solve her problems rationally.

Within an accepting relationship, a patient is able to take the next step in problem-solving. Mrs. Carson took a second look at what her death would mean. As she realized somewhat more clearly what she had been thinking, she became self-condemnatory. She expressed her feeling through crying and by saying that she was "mixed up" and "crazy." The nurse's behavior conveyed that it is all right for her to feel and act upset. She sympathetically realized with her that hers was a difficult situation. This acceptance made it possible for the patient to explore and express her feelings further, and perhaps to uncover more facets of the problem.

The nurse made several responses that identified the patient's feelings. This helped the patient look at the feeling herself and identify what she actually felt. Secondly, they helped her realize that the nurse saw the feelings too, and did not dislike her or blame her for having them. Thirdly, the nurse identified feelings that Mrs. Carson had in common with other mothers which helped her realize that she was not an unusual, bizarre, or bad person. In other words, these responses conveyed to the patient that the nurse could accept what she was saying and understand what she was feeling. This made it possible for the patient to look at her feelings more realistically and to express some of her other feelings that were difficult for her to accept.

The nurse would be of little value to her patient if her role stopped here. The purpose of exploring and examining feelings is to help the patient see how they relate to her problem and to make it possible for her to identify her problem. Mrs. Carson identified her problem as being an inadequate mother to a child with special needs. As she was helped to express and clarify her feelings, she replaced her nonrational thinking of death as a solution with a more constructive approach. She began to consider making plans for the care of her child with the assistance of someone else, and she began to take steps to work out her financial problems.

Talking things over is helpful only if new insights are gained, insights that were not present when the situation was being mulled over alone. The nurse uses techniques in her interpersonal relationship that convey acceptance, ask for clarification, and identify feelings and issues to help her patient get all of the parts of a problem examined. This examination includes a survey of the facets that make up the problem, identification of the problem, the choice of possible solutions, and the recognition of factors that are involved in possible outcomes. Whether a problem is great or small, the nurse's role is not to make choices for the patient, but to help him arrive at a solution after considering all the factors involved.

To return to Webster's definition that reassurance is "a restoration of confidence," a patient experiences this restoration when his "mixed-up" and indecisive feelings disappear and his thinking becomes clearer. He can then discard the nonrational solutions made in panic and begin to work toward a realistic outcome.

Frequently the patient will need the aid of specially trained persons to deal with certain problems or facets of problems. The nurse needs to know who is available on the health team and in what ways other services can be useful to patients. She also needs to interpret these services skillfully to the patient. Concrete help, such as finding a resource person to help with a financial problem, is not always a part of the reassuring process. Also, one cannot assume that simply referring a patient to a source of aid suffices as a reassuring experience, for it does not replace the necessary emotional reassurance.

Essentially, then, the technique of giving is very difficult to separate from the total interpersonal process of the nurse-patient relationship. In the examples we have cited of nurses' conversations with patients, we have suggested that patients feel reassured when they are helped to use their own skills to work with problems that seem overwhelming at the outset. Patients probably feel reassured when someone is willing to listen and to value them as persons, accepting what they say without condemning them for expressing what they feel. As a part of this, there is probably a feeling of reassurance when a patient feels that the nurse's actions, feelings, and words indicate her respect for him.

There are other elements in the problem of reassuring people that command our attention. There are times when a person is so anxious that reasonable problem-solving is not possible at the moment. Reassurance for this person requires a different approach. In moments of great apprehension it is usually comforting not to be left alone. A child is comforted by the calm presence of his mother when he runs to her terrified, and finds that the terror is not duplicated in her. As the mother comforts the child by holding him and saying she will not allow him to be hurt, his terror is reduced, and eventually he begins to talk about the experience that frightened him; thus the problem-solving process begins. This is similar to many situations with adult patients.

During labor or just before electrotherapy or surgery, for example, the adult experiences reassurance by having someone with him whom he knows and trusts. The reassuring person may be a member of the patient's family, a friend, or a churchman; in the hospital, this person is often one of the members of the health team — most frequently, the nurse.

Correcting a false expectation or a misconception by giving correct information can be a reassuring measure if the patient has an opportunity to discuss the issue adequately with someone he trusts. A patient's apparent efforts to seek information are not always an attempt to get the facts, however. For example, when a patient who is about to have an electrotherapy treatment asks the nurse, "How many patients die from this?" he is usually not seeking a factual answer. More likely, this is a "front" question that tests to see if the nurse will respond with understanding. Behind this "front" the patient may be feeling, "I'm afraid I am going to die, and I need to tell you how afraid I am!" If the nurse responds with a factual answer, she conveys that she does not understand his underlying fear, and the patient will usually refrain from pushing the matter further. She has not given the patient the opportunity to express his feeling, and what she expected to be reassuring has become a blocking measure. On the other hand, when information is needed but is withheld, a situation is produced that is far from reassuring. A patient experiences reassurance when he is given authentic information, by someone he trusts, when he needs it.

Reassurance is also experienced when a limit that is reasonable is set with fairness. There are always a few necessary limitations on one's behavior, at any age and in any situation. In illness, patients are sometimes unable to set their own limits without help. It is reassuring to a psychiatric patient when a nurse enforces a limit that prevents him from damaging himself or others. It is reassuring to a patient when the nurse sets some necessary limitations on the behavior of those around him as, for example, when she observes that visitors are disturbing to him, and tactfully helps them terminate their visit. It is also reassuring to a patient to be oriented to the limitations and the expectations of the hospital setting.

A patient is reassured by his trust in those who are in the "helping" role — trust in both their interpersonal and functional abilities. The patient observes the nurse's competence in administering technical procedures and hygienic measures, and when he perceives that these are done well, he is reassured. He is aware of the clinical and administrative judgments that concern him directly and indirectly. When he feels that competent people are making these judgments, he is reassured. Verbal reassurance cannot substitute for functional competence, nor for sincerity and warmth of feeling toward people.

It is not uncommon to hear professional people attempting to reassure patients with the social "bromides," such as, "Everything is going to be all right" and "There is no reason to worry." These are of little value to a person in trouble. They are false reassurance because they lack a rational operating principle and do not provide the opportunity for the person to experience reassurance. The urgings to "cheer up" or "buck up" are equally useless to the person in distress. Another kind of false reassurance, the frank falsification or lie, can be quite devastating when the patient discovers the falsehood.

A common misconception is that it helps to change the subject when a patient starts to talk about something that is disturbing, either to himself or to the listener. This maneuver only prevents the patient from working a problem through, and it betrays the listener's lack of acceptance. A similar measure is to stay away from, or leave, patients who are upset, in order to avoid a "scene." In this situation, the patient experiences isolation and loneliness; he is rarely reassured.

Reassurance involves all of nursing. It is an element of every procedure and every personal contact with patients. Its effectiveness depends on a basic philosophy of respect for another person. Reassurance is experienced by a patient when he finds that he is respected and understood by the nurse who assists him to recognize and develop his own resources and thereby restore his confidence in himself.

Research in Psychiatric Nursing

Alice M. Robinson, June Mellow, Phyllis Hurteau, and Marc A. Fried

The report of this project was prepared by Alice M. Robinson (Duke University School of Nursing; B.S., Catholic University; M.S., Boston University) who is director of nurses at Boston State Hospital and was director of the project described here; June Mellow (Salem Hospital School of Nursing; B.S., University of Rochester; M.S., Boston University) who was the research nurse on this project and has been working on her doctorate at Teachers College, Columbia; Phyllis Hurteau (St. Joseph's Lowell, Mass.) who was the apprentice-observer on the project and is now studying at Boston University; and Marc A. Fried, who is a psychologist at Boston Psychopathic Hospital.

Reprinted from *The Americal Journal of Nursing*, Vol. 55, No. 4, April 1955.

1. The Role of the Nurse-Therapist in a Large Public Mental Hospital

During the past several years, some nurses at the Boston State Hospital have been doing what has been termed therapy with both individual patients and groups of patients. This concentrated work with patients has been done with the approval of the administration, and under the supervision and direction of staff doctors.

The actual work with patients has been carried out in three major ways: (1) the nurse meets with a patient or patients for a specific number of hours per week, every week, or (2) the nurse spends some time every day on the ward with a specific patient or group of patients, or (3) the nurse draws on her general therapeutic orientation in all her work on the ward.

Nurses have not been required to have any special preparation for this kind of work but have, in a sense, been limited by the certain qualifications. The first and most important has been that the nurse must really want to assume the task of therapy with patients, and must be able to minimize her own fears in taking on such responsibility. In other words, no nurse has been asked to take on patients for individual work unless she has first expressed an interest in such a project. Nurses with less than one year of experience with psychiatric patients have been discouraged and asked to wait until sufficient experience has given them some knowledge about the dynamics of patients' behavior and some security in working with the problems involved.

Physicians have given their time willingly in guiding potential nurse-therapists in selecting a patient or patients, and also in helping the nurse to assess her own personality factors in her relationships with patients, and to deal with the dynamics of the interrelationships as they progress. Further, nurse-therapists are encouraged to study the literature on therapeutic process, to attend staff conferences and seminars regarding psychotherapy, and to become members of personnel groups. It is interesting to note that all but two of the nurse-therapists working at the Boston State Hospital during the past four years have had at least a bachelor of science degree, and have been in therapy or in analysis themselves.

Some measure of success had been observed as a result of these experimental ventures, and yet no specific study had been made of the potentialities of nursing therapy. The idea of a project to study the therapeutic functions of the nurse in a large public mental hospital originated in the early summer of 1952. The director of nurses, in preliminary conferences with the hospital superintendent, formulated plans for carrying out such a study without the aid of additional funds.

Plans, Personnel, and Problems

The first administrative problem to be solved was to select nurses to act as research workers; this was made doubly difficult by the fact that there already was a shortage of nursing personnel. In order to attract a nurse who was qualified by education and experience for the role of nurse-therapist, it was necessary to offer a salary of at least supervisory level. Plans also called for an assistant, foreseen in the dual role of apprentice-observer, who would be given a head nurse position. Although the research nurses would not be fulfilling the supervisor's or head nurse's role in a practical, full-time sense, the presumed results of the study seemed to justify the use of these ratings.

One of the implications of the project as it was originally conceived was its tremendous potentialities for teaching. Another implication was the possibility of redefining the role of the head nurse in a large psychiatric hospital as the ward leader who could be much more influential in creating a therapeutic ward atmosphere than had been perceived previously. For this reason, it was believed that the apprentice-observer should be a recently graduated nurse rather than one whose experience would have conditioned her to the head nurse's role as it exists.

All these points were kept in mind when the

personnel who would carry out the project were selected. The nurse who was selected to be the research nurse had previously worked at Boston State Hospital as a head nurse, and during that time had demonstrated the ability to work successfully with individual patients in a therapeutic relationship. Her educational background and her personal experience in analysis rounded out her qualifications for this position. The nurse who joined the project in the apprentice-observer's role had had no previous experience in a state hospital other than as an affiliate student, and she had demonstrated initiative and interest commensurate with the task she was going to undertake.

On October 1, 1952, the project was introduced in a specific ward situation — a 31-bed admitting unit for disturbed women patients. Two things were apparent immediately, one of which later became a serious problem. The first was the need to understand the role of the psychiatric head nurse in a large public mental hospital as it exists, in order to plan a different kind of orientation and training which would produce a new role — that of the therapeutic psychiatric head nurse. This would entail conferences with head nurses about their jobs, and time studies of their functions.

The general concept was that the head nurse is usually the only nurse on the ward, and thus becomes so involved with administrative details that she has little actual contact with patients. Such administrative details include ordering, receiving, and distributing supplies, writing reports and nurse's notes, making assignments, preparing time schedules, holding conferences with personnel, running errands, relieving on other wards and in the supervisor's office, and so on.

In the meantime, the psychiatric aides and student nurses are doing things with patients which provide the necessary contacts that can be therapeutic and which set the pace for the interpersonal atmosphere of the ward. We assumed that the head nurse could train a capable aide to take on these administrative responsibilities, thus freeing herself to establish contact with the patients, both individually and in groups. Under this plan, although the head nurse is still ultimately responsible for the administration of the ward, she is a leader and adviser, and not the actual doer. Because of her increased contact with patients, and because she works along with her students and personnel, she becomes much more valuable as a teacher, particularly in directing the care of patients, which would be one of her major functions.

The second thing which became apparent in the beginning was that the project nurses had to be relieved of all administrative responsibility and that they must be free to act in their therapeutic role wherever and whenever the need for such activity arose. This was the cause of major interpersonal problems which for the first two or three months seriously interfered with the progress of the study. Everyone who had been consulted about the study had been enthusiastic about it. Yet, when the project was begun, resistances developed, even though the type of work that the research nurses were doing had been done for years by good nurses. When this function was put into a research framework it became threatening.

With the chief of service, communication apparently had not been carried far enough. Previous to his appointment as chief of service, he had reviewed the first description of the study and found it acceptable. With his change in status and new responsibilities, he felt that further clarification was needed, and since it was not forthcoming, he was concerned as to where the research nurses fitted into the administrative hierarchy — to whom were they responsible? He instructed the research nurses to keep out of problems of ward administration; he also emphasized that when a patient became disturbed, regardless of whether that patient was directly involved in the project or not, the management of such a patient was his responsibility.

The head nurse, in her administrative role, was threatened by the research nurse who had previously worked as head nurse in the same ward. The aides were approaching the research nurse rather than the head nurse with patients' and ward problems. Although they favored the project, they caused a split in the ward personnel because they supported the research nurses rather than the head nurse. Other graduate nurses in the admitting building viewed the research nurses as special people with special privileges because they were not carrying administrative responsibilities. The nursing service personnel were continually checking the whereabouts of the two research nurses.

By December, concerted efforts were being made to solve these interpersonal problems. It was obvious that they were a result of failure to communicate the complete picture of the project thoroughly and clearly to all the personnel involved.

After a conference with the chief of service, the research nurses became more aware of their limits, and avoided interfering with the head nurse's job; they made it clear to the aides that the research nurse was no longer the head nurse, and that problems should be brought to the proper person. At this time, the research nurses themselves had become so overwhelmed by the various resistances that they withdrew to their office for about a week. Finally, feelings of guilt about not doing the job drove them back to the ward. The head nurse expressed her own feelings of guilt during their absence. This mutual expression of guilt, plus more frequent meetings with the head nurse, helped improve relationships. Increased awareness on the part of the research nurses made them more careful to avoid becoming involved in administrative situations which were clearly the head nurse's responsibility.

Subsequently, the first patient, who was taken for individual study on October 27, 1952, improved and was discharged on January 6, 1953. This had a good effect on the morale of both ward personnel and patients. It also was tangible evidence that the research nurses could be of value to the ward.

Thus, the solution to the resistance came through improved interpersonal relationships throughout the situation, and the research nurses could now settle down to work in earnest.

The Research Nurse's Work

During the 12 months allotted for the project, the senior research nurse worked with four individual patients. In each case the nursing therapy was adapted to the patient's needs and therefore a different approach was used to establish a positive therapeutic relationship.*

As the project progressed, the nursing therapy and the teaching of personnel became integrated functions. The personnel observed the research nurse's relationship with the patients and she discussed its elements with them, explaining the dynamics of the patients' psychotic behavior and pointing out how the personnel's behavior affected it. In teaching conferences, she encouraged them to talk out their own feelings toward their patients and helped them to make constructive changes in their attitudes. They began to see themselves as significant persons in the patients' life in the hospital, and their acceptance of what was not meaningful behavior was supportive to patients.

In the meantime, the apprentice-observer was carrying out her dual role. She was learning the value of the nurse's role in creating a therapeutic ward atmosphere and thus was preparing herself for the head nurse experiment. Her second objective was to record the therapeutic and instructional activities of the research nurse in order to validate them. She was expected to keep written notes, some verbatim, about everything that went on in the ward situation and to compile them in a report that was presented at the weekly project conference. At first, the notes were concerned with ward activities and were focused on attitudes. The verbatim notes were, of course, most valid. The assistant wrote down exactly what she saw and heard, and from these notes, material was extracted which was important and relevant to the purpose of the project.

The research assistant was not present when the research nurse was with individual patients. Thus, it was important for her to observe and record the climate of interaction surrounding each patient who was in individual therapy. This included the:

1. Attitude of the personnel toward the patient.
2. Patient's attitude toward the personnel.
3. Attitude of other patients toward the individual patient.
4. Attitude of the individual patient toward other patients.
5. Individual patient's attitude toward the research nurse.
6. Attitude of the research nurse toward the individual patient.
7. Attitude of personnel toward the research nurse.
8. Attitude of the research nurse toward personnel.

The notes which were made on the activities of the research nurse revealed that her functions were these:

1. She carefully observed patients and personnel and the situations which arose involving both.
2. She used these situations as focal points in her teaching, even during the early stages of the project, by incorporating the implications of each situation into all communication with personnel and student nurses.
3. She demonstrated skills in managing disturbed patients.
4. She guided the attitudes of personnel and students in an attempt to create a more therapeutic ward atmosphere.
5. She gave patients individual attention.
6. She taught personnel the dynamic aspects of psychiatric nursing, particularly in relation to her patients in individual therapy.

*The nursing therapy with these four patients will be described in detail in the next article in this series which will appear in a forthcoming issue of the *Journal*.

7. She included personnel when evaluating her interpretations of individual patients' behavior, so that they could assume a more constructive role in the patient's progress.
8. She made every attempt to maintain good interpersonal relations with personnel on all shifts, since effective communication among all personnel definitely affects patients.
9. She utilized every opportunity to teach the research assistant not only how to observe, but also how to gain something from each observation. This was accomplished through detailed discussion of the observations that were made.

The Research Assistant Learns

As time went on, the research assistant began to attend group meetings of patients as an observer. For three years, a nurse — the project director — had met with a group of ten chronically ill schizophrenic women. Observation of this group was greatly enhanced by the teaching conferences for the student nurse observers which immediately followed each session. At these conferences the observers were encouraged to offer their interpretations of significant behavior, and discussion was guided by the nurse-leader. This experience helped to increase the research assistant's ability to utilize observations, and it also enabled her to become more comfortable with very sick, disturbed, and potentially assaultive patients.

At about this same time, the research nurse and the project director suggested that the assistant choose one or two patients to whom she would give special attention. One patient was selected from the project ward, and one from the group of chronically ill patients. The assistant saw the first patient every day, and the latter twice a week. The patient from the project ward was a paranoid schizophrenic, generally disliked by both personnel and patients; her chief difficulty on the ward lay in her refusal to eat. Her response to the assistant was a constant effort to drive her away. This patient was eventually transferred to a large service for chronic patients where the assistant continued to see her, but much less frequently.

The patient who was selected from the project director's therapy group was a schizophrenic whose illness dated back some 20 years. The research assistant was able to establish a warm relationship with her, and from this experience learned much about the symbolic meaning of verbal and nonverbal activity. She was given guidance frequently by the project director and the senior physician on the service.

On the project ward, the research assistant observed still another group of patients. This group virtually formed itself — the assistant sat in the day hall each morning, and a group of patients gathered around for group discussion. This socialization type of group reinforced our knowledge that patients can and frequently do help one another. Patients who would not respond to the approaches of ward personnel responded easily to other patients, frequently "opened up" and seemed less anxious when they were with others whose problems were similar to theirs. Observing the research nurse's conferences with the student nurses who were assigned to the project ward provided still another learning experience for the assistant. Deftness in getting at students' reactions and opinions seemed to depend on ability to throw out a debatable issue and then listen. On one occasion, the research nurse was not present at the students' conference and the students voluntarily told the assistant about their feelings toward the research nurse, and their interest and approval of the project in general.

Probably the most valuable learning experiences that the research assistant had were her many conferences with the research nurse or the project director, or with both of them. The carefully guided interpretations of the problems inherent in the project, the greater understanding of mental patients, the valuable "on-the-spot" teaching, and the supervision, by experienced persons, of the assistant's work with individual patients combined to broaden her concept of a useful and therapeutic psychiatric head nurse.

Finally, gathering statistical data gave the research assistant experience in the more rigorous aspects of research and helped her to develop ability which was useful later.

As the action phase of the project drew to a close, the time came to test the supposition that training as a research assistant on this project would prepare this nurse to function more effectively and therapeutically as a psychiatric head nurse. Thus began the 3-month period during which the research assistant's work with patients supported our premise that a psychiatric head nurse, with certain personal qualifications, with training through observing, and with freedom from administrative responsibility can help to create a therapeutic ward atmosphere and can become an experienced teacher for personnel and students.*

**This part of the study will be discussed in another article in this series.*

Conclusions

There is little question that, with vast numbers of chronically ill mental patients still going without any sort of treatment other than custodial care, there is a role for nurses and aides in psychotherapy. A feasible method for training nurses and aides to deal therapeutically with groups of patients is needed, and the project reported here suggests such a method.

The first conclusion which became clear as the project advanced was a negative one. *Removing administrative responsibility entirely from the research nurses was actually an inhibiting factor. It aroused resentment on the part of the physician-in-charge and of other graduate nurses in the building; it created the problem of dual leadership between the head nurse and the research nurse; it allowed a permissiveness for the research nurses which they found difficult to handle.*

The success of the research nurse in her work with individual patients leads to the conclusion that *a nurse can develop a therapeutic relationship with a patient which is conducive to marked improvement.* Three of the four patients whom the research nurse took for individual therapy left the hospital during the 12-month period allotted for the entire project. The fourth subsequently left the hospital without permission. Only one of the four patients received any other treatment (electroshock therapy).

We can conclude that we had been right in believing that *there were many potentialities for teaching.* First, the nurse can use her work with individual patients as a base for teaching all categories of personnel, thus helping to change interrelationships of personnel and patients from non-therapeutic to therapeutic. Second, the research assistant observed the value of being with patients, leaving administrative ward routine to other personnel. Third, recognizing this, the research assistant was able, upon assuming her head nurse role, to teach student nurses the potential therapeutic value of being with patients not only during trying periods of their illness, but also during everyday ward activities.

Although the specific functions of the head nurse in a psychiatric ward unit have not been spelled out, we can conclude that *creative psychiatric nursing includes being with patients during the majority of time on duty, delegating administrative duties to a capable, nonprofessional assistant, and making a serious attempt to broaden concepts of psychiatric care through participation in seminars, staff conferences, and so on.*

We cannot say that any nurse, given the kind of training which the research assistant received during this project, will become a successful and creative psychiatric head nurse. Certain personal qualifications are necessary. We can conclude however, that *if a nurse is given a six-month period of training through observation, without accompanying responsibility, such as this project provided, she might prepare to function as an effective and therapeutically-minded head nurse,* provided she also possesses the necessary personal qualifications.

We recognize that this project is only a beginning. Further study is recommended in the following areas: exploration of the potentialities of the nurse's unique situation to prepare her for her leadership role in creating a therapeutic ward atmosphere; the training and use of nonprofessional personnel as ward managers in all types of psychiatric ward units; the application of the apprentice-observer technique of learning for field work in psychiatric nursing university programs; and the use of the prepared and experienced psychiatric nurse as a therapist for individuals and groups, particularly in the chronically ill patients' services, until such time as the role of the nurse-therapist can be clearly defined.

Many interesting sidelights emerged during the project. We are continuing to use capable nonprofessional personnel to manage some of the psychiatric wards at the Boston State Hospital. Although this has not yet enabled us to free our psychiatric nurses for more effective work in establishing a therapeutic ward atmosphere, we have learned from the project that it can be done, and we shall, in the future, assign our head nurses with this understanding.

Research in Psychiatric Nursing

June Mellow, Alice M. Robinson, Phyllis Hurteau, and Marc A. Fried

Reprinted from *The American Journal of Nursing*, Vol. 55, No. 5, May 1955.

2. Nursing Therapy with Individual Patients

A nurse's position on a ward is unique because she is able to be in direct contact with patients for long periods of time. Perhaps the most vital contribution she can make to the patient's recovery is the relationship she is able to establish with him.

The elements of such a relationship can be the basis for an excellent teaching situation for aides and students. Nursing therapy and the teaching of personnel become integrated functions. The ward personnel — through their observation of the nurse's relationship with the patient and through conferences in which the nurse discusses the patient's behavior and helps them to discuss their own feelings about it — become involved in the therapeutic process and begin to apply their own therapeutic skills.

A study of the role of the nurse therapist in a large public mental hospital was begun at Boston State Hospital in October 1952. The object of the study was to determine the potentialities of nursing therapy — its implications for the care of individual patients, for the education of personnel, and for the preparation of psychiatric head nurses.*

Two nurses were selected to carry out the action research of the study. One, who was called the research nurse, had been a head nurse at Boston State and had demonstrated her ability to work successfully with individual patients in a therapeutic relationship. The other, who was to be an apprentice-observer, had no experience in state mental hospitals and thus had no previous conditioning to affect her experimental work.

Although difficulties were encountered frequently throughout this project, many of the therapeutic and teaching potentialities were realized.

Ethel Popolus was the first of four patients whom the research nurse worked with during the course of the study. Ethel was a 29-year-old, single, white, second-generation Greek woman.** Her diagnosis was schizophrenic reaction, paranoid type.

While she was sick, she appeared extremely disheveled and ugly. She usually remained in the corner of her room; she would not look at anyone, and she talked continuously, keeping her face turned to the wall all the time. From her ramblings, one could assume that she was intelligent and well-read. Frequently, she banged on the wall and chanted in Greek. She hallucinated and had delusions of grandeur. The personnel left her alone, because they felt that she wanted to be left alone and they also believed that there was nothing they could do for her.

Her condition improved only slightly during her first month in the hospital. At the end of that time, she was placed on electroshock therapy. The request of the research nurse to take her for individual therapy and the decision to place her on shock therapy coincided. After six shock treatments there was a marked superficial improvement in the patient's condition. However, she denied that she was ill and would talk only on neutral subjects. At this time, the doctor decided to discontinue shock treatments on the supposition that the material she was repressing might now come into consciousness.

The research nurse saw Ethel once a day for about an hour in the ward office. Ethel said she had been upset over an unfortunate love affair and that she was all right now and would find a new man. Later, after she and the nurse came to know each other better and she seemed to want to confide in someone, the nurse asked Ethel if she was still confused about anything. She replied, "There are strange influences around here. The Greek police brought me to this place." This incident served as an opening for the nurse to establish a therapeutic relationship on the basis that she would like to help Ethel, and that they "could take a look at the strange influences together."

On several occasions Ethel mentioned that she was just a factory worker and the nurse was a college graduate. Many times they discussed Greek philosophy and literature, subjects which Ethel knew much more about than the nurse did. This helped to preserve her self-respect and gave her the opportunity to realize that the nurse saw her as an educated and intelligent woman.

Gradually, material came forth about her parents, and the hostility she felt toward them became apparent, although it was disguised. As she began to

*A detailed report of this project began on page 441 of the April *Journal*. The third article in this series, which describes the results of the apprentice-observer's assuming the role of psychiatric head nurse, will appear in a forthcoming issue.

**The patients' names used here are fictitious.

confide in the nurse, she also became frightened and anxious, especially when the nurse tried to make her face the fact that she was still sick. In two weeks time she again became actively psychotic. But the personnel expected this and were prepared for it.

For the next couple of weeks, no attempt was made to have Ethel come into the office; instead, the nurse went to her. The patient usually remained, by her own choice, in an unlocked seclusion room. She appeared much as she had before. She beat tom-toms, chanted in Greek, and talked continuously in a disjointed and at times incoherent way. But although the illness was going on, the patient was relating to someone, and she acknowledged the nurse's presence. The research nurse felt that in spite of her illness, Ethel wanted to have someone break through this self-imposed isolation. However, for a while, the patient directed much of her efforts toward driving the nurse away by warnings of what a dangerous and horrible person she was.

The important point in therapy at this time was not what the patient said, but that she wanted to drive the nurse away and convince the nurse and, thus, herself, that she was too horrible and dangerous a person to be liked and accepted by anyone. This had to be counteracted by the nurse's acceptance of her under any circumstance. The nurse also showed Ethel that, although she accepted her illness, she also expected something from her — that Ethel would be able to overcome her illness.

One morning Ethel began to beat her usual rhythm on the table in the kitchen after throwing her food around and refusing to eat her breakfast. The nurse said that she wished to join her and learn the rhythm.

After this incident, Ethel went into the day hall and was no longer a feeding problem. From then on, she often remained in the day hall and beat out her rhythms and sang Greek chants. It is interesting that the patients accepted this from her and did not act against her.

After about a 3-week period, Ethel calmed down enough to benefit from discussions in the office. She came in willingly but said that the nurse had caused her to become ill again. She expressed this by saying, "You hit me over the head with the black bag." Using her language, the nurse replied that she didn't want to "hit her over the head with the black bag," but felt it necessary for Ethel to realize that she was ill and that although this had to be done, she would not desert Ethel in her illness.

Ethel discussed her problems in a symbolic way, but they held a logic of their own. The things that the nurse understood she interpreted to Ethel; those that she did not understand, she made no issue of, and the focus was on the immediate nurse-patient relationship.

Shortly before Ethel was discharged, she voluntarily recapitulated many of the events of her psychosis. Her final sessions with the nurse were spent in discussing her feelings about going home and her anxiety over the prospect of not having anyone who understood her to talk to. She felt much less anxious about her discharge when she was reassured that she could come back to the hospital to see the nurse.

Ethel was discharged two and one-half months after individual nursing therapy began. She continued to see the nurse once a month for three months. She is now living with her family and has returned to her former job. She seems to have made an excellent adjustment.

The major highlights in nursing therapy with Ethel Popolus were the acceptance of — and at times participation in — her psychotic behavior and also a certain expectation that she would recover. It was possible, while dealing with her psychotic behavior, to work with the healthy aspect of her personality. During the early stages of the therapeutic process, it was extremely important for the nurse to not let herself be driven away, and thus permit Ethel to become isolated. Even though she was very disturbed, Ethel was relating to someone else during her illness; she could test her thinking and did not allow the psychotic ideas to settle into convictions. The nurse became someone with whom she could identify, and this, perhaps, helped to reintegrate her ego. She also placed great symbolic significance on the nurse's uniform, pin and sweater. "These were the only things I could hold on to," she said later.

The experience with Ethel provided a wealth of material for teaching the student nurse and aides. For example, it was possible to demonstrate that a feeding problem could be avoided by temporarily indulging the patient's need to play with her food rather than taking a punitive attitude toward this behavior. Also, the nurse was able to demonstrate to the personnel that Ethel was still sick, even though shock treatments had made her look well and the patient was able to relate to them as if she were well.

The probability that Ethel's psychosis would be reactivated when the shock treatments were discontinued was discussed thoroughly with the personnel. It was very important for them to realize this; otherwise they might have felt that the special attention caused the reactivation and they might have become hostile to the research nurse.

Throughout the therapeutic process, the personnel were kept up to date on the progress of the nurse-patient relationship, and the dynamics of Ethel's behavior were explained to them. Thus they gained some understanding of her illness. In addition, the research nurse's hopeful attitude toward the patient, the opportunity she had to point out the healthy aspects of the patient's personality, and the fact that Ethel herself was struggling to get well, all helped to create a therapeutic attitude toward the patient.

In teaching conferences the personnel were encouraged to assume a permissive, friendly attitude toward Ethel and not let her hostility drive them away. Perhaps the most important teaching opportunity with this patient stemmed from the experience the personnel had in realizing the great value of their friendly and supportive attitude. *The acutely ill psychotic patient can offer a healthy opposition to his illness if he has the security of a protective environment and is cared for by personnel who are interested in him and with whom good interpersonal relationships can be established.* These positive relationships that reach outside his illness may keep him from feeling that he is in a fearful state of isolation and can help to keep him in contact with reality. Although one cannot always understand a patient's behavior, if he is given the necessary and consistent support, he can struggle with the illness in his own particular way.

The second patient who was taken for individual therapy was Anna Markle. Anna was the most disliked patient on the ward. She was disliked by both patients and personnel. The research nurse had also rejected her and showed this by ignoring her as the rest of the personnel had done. She was taken for individual work about three weeks before Ethel was discharged.

Anna had been institutionalized twice before, at another hospital, for manic attacks with a large schizophrenic element. Anna was an obese girl, 24-years-old, but with a fairly attractive face. When she was first admitted, she was suffering from a manic attack with schizophrenic features. After this subsided, and at the time she was selected, her behavior appeared more rational. She was extremely annoying to the personnel, however, because of her superior attitude — such as bragging about her important job — and because of her demanding and condescending approach. She was extremely clever in instigating fights between patients and then stepping aside and blaming others for starting the conflicts. This resulted in total rejection by almost everyone in her environment and only aggravated her behavior. This kind of behavior kept her in the hospital, where she was thought of by personnel as a "pest" and a "goon."

Individual nursing therapy with Anna was directed toward understanding why her annoying behavior persisted when her psychotic episode had presumably passed and she appeared to be in a rational state. By expressing a special interest in her and seeing her daily, the research nurse was able to get at many of the reasons for her antisocial behavior.

Anna said that she felt no one liked her, no one paid any attention to her, and that she felt like a "big hunk of nothing," and "a nameless quantity" on the ward. In essence, she was being ignored and rejected here as she had been for many years at home. When the research nurse gave her the opportunity to express her feelings and showed her that someone cared and was interested in her, the patient's behavior and attitude changed. She stopped instigating fights and was helpful to other patients. The personnel began to change their attitude toward her. When Anna felt that she was liked by the personnel, she was not only able to discard her superior attitude but also to confide in them. It became apparent that the patient really felt that a constructive change had come about in their attitude toward her — that they liked her as much as they had previously disliked her.

In conference with the research nurse, the personnel were given an opportunity to frankly express their feelings about Anna. Then it was necessary to discuss the reasons for her behavior. They had objected most of all to her superior attitude and her attempts to impress them with her important background. At the same time, she had belittled them because they were "only aides." When they realized how she really felt, and that she was compensating for a deep-seated feeling of inferiority, they began to accept her behavior instead of ignoring her. They also came to realize that to be bold, to cause fights, and to demand as if she were a person of great importance was the only way Anna knew to get attention. She had to do this because she felt ignored and like a "big hunk of nothing." The simultaneous change in attitude by both the personnel and the patients resulted in Anna's discharge from the hospital about one month after the research nurse had begun individual work with her.

The third patient, Helen Maxwell, requested therapy with the research nurse. The patient's symptoms indicated that she was a severely neurotic person, and the research nurse felt she would not respond well to short-term nursing therapy. It seemed possible, however, that some improvement might occur. Helen was later diagnosed as "mixed neurotic with hysterical features and with some underlying schizophrenic elements."

Helen was 23-years-old, tall, and well-built; she was attractive when she was well-groomed. Her mother had died when she was seven and her father when she was 15. She had an older brother and sister, neither of whom cared for her. She had been brought up by two old-maid aunts, whom she disliked. She had no home or person to return to.

This was her first admission. She had been admitted because of a suicidal demonstration, and had been on the ward six months before the research project started. The ward personnel considered her lazy, not sick, sarcastic, haughty, and unwilling to make any effort to help herself. She remained aloof from other patients and seldom entered into any social activities on the ward.

During the course of nursing therapy, the research nurse kept trying to get across to Helen that her inferiority feelings about herself affected her relationships with others. She entered a social situation feeling inferior and rejected, and so, in turn, without being aware of it, she immediately rejected other people and then felt that they had rejected her. Usually, she tried to "save her pride" by being contemptuous and sarcastic; that is, she gave people something to be angry about or gave them grounds for rejecting her. She could not offer herself to people as herself for fear of what they would do. When things got particularly tough, she withdrew from a situation or could only express her anger indirectly through sarcasm.

The research nurse pointed out two of the main issues to Helen. One was that she had established a definite pattern of running away from situations and of feeling rejected by people and then giving them some reason for rejecting her. The other major issue was that because of her negative feelings toward herself she had overlooked many of her assets and could not apply herself well to work situations, nor could she express satisfaction in her social life.

Helen began to gain some insight into her illness but complained that it was extremely difficult for her to change. She revealed that she had made the suicidal demonstration because she wanted to show her anger toward her aunts, and she felt that no one really cared about her. Her main conflict seemed to have revolved around the wish to be dependent and the need to be independent. To her, dependency meant closeness and all the significant people in her life had always disappointed her. She became dependent on the research nurse, was able to express her hostility without running away, and began to confide in her. She also became more sociable on the ward, entered into various activities, and made friends with other patients.

Allowing Helen to be somewhat dependent on the research nurse, however, complicated matters. At the time the project ended, she was still in the hospital, and it appeared as if the nurse was deserting her. Actually, Helen has improved enough to leave the hospital but she has no place to go. The doctor feels she would do well if she had a home to go to and could, at the same time, receive psychotherapy in a clinic.

Teaching conferences revealed that, because of her rational behavior, Helen was not regarded as being sick. The personnel could see nothing wrong and treated her as if she were feigning illness. They thought she was lazy and could live outside the hospital if she would make the effort. Of all the patients selected for individual care, they found Helen most difficult to understand. But, after the research nurse explained her poor home life and her conflict with dependency and independency, their attitudes began to change. They then regarded her as someone in need of their help and sympathy. They were helped to realize that a patient can be ill without showing obvious symptoms.

The fourth patient, Sylvia Blum, was chronically ill and had been diagnosed as a paranoid schizophrenic. Sylvia had been transferred from another hospital with a guarded prognosis; she had been suffering from paranoid schizophrenia for 10 years. She was a voluptuous looking redhead and placed great stress on her sexual seductiveness and femininity. Her psychosis was fixed in a delusional system regarding a woman friend of hers called "Lottie."

According to Sylvia, "Lottie" had put her in the hospital and was trying to ruin her looks because "Lottie" was jealous of Sylvia's appeal to men. According to the patient, "Lottie" participated in perverse sexual activities which had ruined Sylvia's husband and also her boy friends. "Lottie" was "tuning up" the doctors and nurses to say and do bad things. "Lottie" hated all men and wanted to destroy them. Sylvia hallucinated frequently, received messages from cars and mysterious airways.

With the exception of her complicated delusional system, Sylvia acted quite rationally. She was actively disliked by the personnel and student nurses, because she continually spoke of her good looks. They felt that she was extremely vain about her looks and that she had "gone crazy" because she was overly interested in men. She spoke constantly about "Lottie" and accused the ward personnel of "taking sides" with her. She would not take part in ward activities nor socialize with other patients.

In spite of Sylvia's paranoid condition, it was possible to establish a warm, friendly relationship with her, although it was impossible to disrupt her delusional system. At first, she spoke of "Lottie" most of the time. She repeated many times how much she hated her, that she was filthy, evil, over-sexed, that she hated men and tried to destroy them, that she was extremely ugly although she thought she was glamorous, and that she spent most of her time "dolling herself up." When the research nurse tried to get Sylvia to realize that she was sick, she always denied this and said "Lottie" had put her into the hospital.

Whenever Sylvia spoke of "Lottie," the nurse told her that "Lottie" was very sick and needed help. After awhile, Sylvia would say that "Lottie" was sick. Sylvia then got to the point of talking about her real problems, her fear and loneliness when her mother died, her disappointment in her husband, and her concern about her only son. However, when she spoke of her real difficulties, it usually called forth so much anxiety that she would revert back to "Lottie" and would say, "That no good bum has caused me all this trouble."

Although Sylvia developed little insight into her illness, she did improve in the environmental situation. On the ward she talked less about "Lottie" and eventually was able to carry on a pleasant social conversation. She did not appear to hallucinate as frequently. She took part in social activities and was much friendlier with patients and personnel. Sylvia began to identify with the nurse; she would put the nurse's cap on and say that she could be a nurse. On two occasions when an aide yelled at her to leave the cafeteria, she reversed roles, playing the part of the aide, trying to console the aide, and actually bringing the aide out of the cafeteria.

Sylvia is still in the hospital and after the project was terminated, she began to hallucinate more frequently and to speak of "Lottie" almost constantly.

In teaching conferences the research nurse tried to help the personnel understand Sylvia's behavior and to learn how to distract her from her delusions by encouraging her to take part in ward activities.

Whenever Sylvia talked to the personnel about "Lottie" and what had been done to her, they were instructed to tell her that "Lottie" was "very sick and needed help." This was done with the hope that if "Lottie" represented everything that Sylvia hated about herself, then perhaps she could realize that "Lottie" was more sick than actually evil and she might be able to develop some sympathy for herself.

Through her relationship with Sylvia, the research nurse was able to learn that Sylvia wasn't sure whether she was male or female. Her excessive interest in her femininity and seductiveness with men was apparently a defense against more positive feelings toward women. She implied in her relationships with men that she felt extremely inferior and inadequate as a woman.

Sylvia used "Lottie" to project all her inadequacies, all her fears, her hatred for men, her jealousy of other women, her obscenity; in short, everything she hated in herself. She had to do this to minimize her inner anxiety. Unfortunately, she had been so successful in handling her anxiety in this way that it seemed obvious that it would take some form of prolonged and intensive psychotherapy to produce any significant improvement.

Conferences revealed that the personnel thought of Sylvia as someone in difficulty because she was "over-sexed," had a "dirty mind," and was overly concerned about her personal appearance. When it was pointed out to them that Sylvia actually felt extremely inferior and confused as to her sexuality, and that her seductiveness was a defense, they began to deal with her as a person with a mental illness. A marked constructive change in their attitude resulted, and they were quite successful in engaging Sylvia in various ward activities. One aide who had detested Sylvia became very fond of her, and Sylvia in turn developed a good relationship with the aide.

Throughout this project, the nursing therapy was adapted to the needs of the individual patients and ultimately involved a different type of therapeutic approach with each one. As had been foreseen, the nurse's work with patients had tremendous potentialities for use in teaching aides and students. Also, the students' and aides' experiences with these four patients helped them to achieve a more comprehensive understanding of other patients.

All the ward personnel began to realize that if one patient was relating to them as being significant to her life in the hospital, then other patients must be doing this, too, in varying degrees. They began to see other patients' behavior as meaningful, and to appreciate their own contributions to a therapeutic ward environment which, in turn, is conducive to the patients' recovery.

Research in Psychiatric Nursing

Alice M. Robinson, June Mellow, Phyllis Hurteau, and Marc A. Fried

Reprinted from *The American Journal of Nursing*, Vol. 55. No. 6, June 1955.

3. The Psychiatric Ward Head Nurse

How much influence could the head nurse in a psychiatric ward unit exert on the recovery of patients if she were free from some of the administrative details involved in running a ward, and could really devote her time and creative energy to her patients? Finding the answer to this question was one of the objects of a study recently carried out at the Boston State Hospital.*

Action research was the method chosen for the study; to carry it out, two nurses were selected carefully. One had worked previously at the hospital as a head nurse and had demonstrated her ability to work successfully with individual patients. She was to be the "research nurse." The plans for the project called for her to work with individual patients in a therapeutic relationship and to teach other personnel on the research unit — aides, attendants, students, and so on — what was involved in such a relationship and how they could make their relationships with patients therapeutic.**

The second nurse on the project was to work as an apprentice-observer. The nurse chosen for this role had had no previous experience in a state hospital other than as an affiliate student. Her inexperience was considered an asset — when the study had progressed to the point at which she could work as a therapeutically minded head nurse, she would take on this job without bringing to it the preconceived ideas she might have acquired in previous state hospital experience.

On October 1, 1952 the project was begun in a specific ward situation. During the next nine months, the research nurse worked with four individual patients. In each case the nursing therapy was adapted to the patient's needs, and so a different approach was used in each to establish a therapeutic relationship. Throughout this time the personnel observed the research nurse's relationship with the patients, and she discussed its elements with them, explaining the dynamics of the patients' psychotic behavior and pointing out how the personnel's behavior affected it. In frequent conferences, the personnel had the opportunity to discuss their feelings about the patients and to examine them, with the research nurse's help.

In the meantime, the apprentice-observer was carrying out her dual role. In observing the research nurse, she was learning how to create a therapeutic ward atmosphere, and thus was preparing herself for the head nurse experiment. Also, she was keeping written notes about everything that went on in the ward situation so that they could be compiled and reported. She also attended regular meetings of patients' groups as an observer. One of these was a group of schizophrenic women who for three years had been meeting with the nurse who directed the project. Immediately following each session, there were teaching conferences at which any observers were encouraged to offer their interpretation of significant behavior. Discussion was guided by the nurse-leader. This experience was valuable to the apprentice-observer, both in increasing her ability to utilize observations and in helping her to become more comfortable with very sick and disturbed patients.

As time went on, the apprentice-observer chose two patients with whom she worked intensively herself, under the guidance of the project director and the senior physician on the service. Frequent conferences with the research nurse and the project director were also valuable learning experiences for her and all of these experiences combined to broaden her concept of a useful and therapeutic psychiatric head nurse.

Finally the time came to test one of the original important premises of the study — that a psychiatric head nurse, with certain personal qualifications, with training through observing, and with freedom from administrative responsibility, could help to create a therapeutic ward atmosphere and could become an experienced teacher for personnel and students.

The apprentice-observer was placed on a ward and was given relative freedom to perform her job as a head nurse in the light of what she had learned. The 3-month experiment was under way.

The Head Nurse Orients Herself

In orienting herself to the ward, the new head nurse used a new approach. During the week *before*

*This project was described in detail in the April *Journal* (pp. 441-444).

**A report of this aspect of the research project appeared in the May *Journal* (pp. 572-575).

she actually started to work as head nurse, she saw each of the ward aides individually and posed the important question: "What do you expect of a head nurse?" She saw each one individually because she felt that they would be more comfortable that way, and also would feel freer to say what they thought. Because time was limited she met with the student nurses as a group, but she asked them the same question. Both groups were virtually unanimous in giving these four answers:

1. She should know her patients.
2. She should be with her patients.
3. She should support co-workers in any difficulty.
4. She should communicate information about ward matters to all personnel.

The head nurse's next move was to see each patient individually and informally in the ward office. Her purpose here was two-fold: (1) to learn names and faces, and (2) to note signs, symptoms, and degrees of illness. Patients who refused to come to the office (because of a greater degree of illness or for some other undetermined reason) were seen on the ward. For example, the new head nurse sat on the porch with a mute catatonic patient for 10 to 15 minutes. Although no conversation took place, there was ample opportunity for the nurse to observe the degree of the patient's illness, and, in turn, to be observed by the patient. Several times she talked through the observation window with a patient who was temporarily disturbed enough to be in seclusion, and thus she and the patient got to know each other's faces and voices.

The Administrative Plan

The final, important step in orientation was a conference with the aides concerning a new plan of ward administration which was in accordance with one of the theories inherent in the original project. This theory, essentially, was that a capable "charge aide" could assume responsibility for the administrative *details* of running a ward with the provision that the head nurse would be ultimately responsible for any major decisions.

In other words, the charge aide can check lists of patients for shock therapy, group activities, and privileges; he or she can count and issue linen, make ward housekeeping assignments, check patients' clothing and valuables; he can make appointments for such things as x-ray, laboratory and psychological tests, and can see that appointments are kept; he can write reports, check doctors' orders, assign lunch hours for personnel, and carry out many other administrative details which are usually taken care of by the head nurse.

This plan of ward organization relieves the head nurse of many tasks which keep her away from her patients. It leaves her relatively free to do psychiatric nursing — to talk with patients, take part in ward activities (group discussions, games, dances, and so on), to bathe and feed sick, disturbed patients, to make rounds with doctors, to accompany and observe patients who have off-ward therapy (occupational therapy, electroshock and so on) and to work with student nurses and help them in their relationships with patients. If she is an effective psychiatric nurse, the head nurse can utilize all of these activities in teaching by example.

When the aides were approached with this plan, they (including the charge aide) were willing to try it, but they seemed concerned that the head nurse wished to help in any way possible with disturbed or assaultive patients. They said that the head nurse who had previously been on the ward "stayed in the office all the time and was afraid of patients." Further, "Nurses shouldn't get into any fracas because they will get their uniforms soiled and rumpled!"

Work with Patients

The head nurse felt a distinct need to dispel this idea, and as soon as she became familiar enough with the patients on the ward, she set out to prove to the aides that it was her job to share behavior problems with them. She concentrated on being alert and getting to trouble spots as soon as possible, and, in fact, made an effort to get there first. She utilized every opportunity to convey the idea that seclusion is a treatment, not a punishment. "What good does it do to seclude a patient after an assaultive or destructive outburst?" she would ask. "If we are giving good nursing care, we can pick up hints or signs from the patient himself when he is becoming disturbed. One of our important responsibilities is to recognize these signs and give the patient the care he needs before the outburst occurs."

When the head nurse was on the ward, this suggestion usually was followed. Communication with the evening and night personnel apparently was inadequate, however; the record showed that patients were put in seclusion much more frequently during the evening and night than during the day time.

The aides became relaxed enough with the new

plan to allow the head nurse to make a reasonable attempt to work verbally with disturbed patients before they stepped in with the necessary physical restraint. For example, it was more or less routine for the aides to take a certain patient by physical force to the shock unit each day. Usually two aides from the ward and two aides from the men's service helped the patient downstairs. It seemed to the head nurse that this must be a very frightening experience for a paranoid person to undergo, (undoubtedly intensified by the patient's knowledge about the destination) and she asked the aides to let her try reasoning with the patient.

When she approached the patient, however, the head nurse ran into not only the paranoia, but also a delusional system of which she had not been aware. "God told me I didn't have to have these treatments. God will punish all of you if you make me have them." The head nurse said, "Carol, you must have them. You are sick and need them." Carol said, "It is you who are sick, not me." The head nurse then explained that if the patient did not go with her, the aides would have to take her down. She still refused, and so had to be taken down by several aides. This morning, however, no physical force was used, and she went quietly. She was accompanied throughout the treatment by the head nurse.

Mornings, after reading the night report, the head nurse would usually attempt to spend as much time as possible with the patient who appeared most likely to disrupt the normal routine on the ward. The aides appreciated this as an effort to have the ward run as smoothly as possible.

Frequently the head nurse asked not only which patient the aides and student nurses felt presented the greatest *problem*, but also which patient they felt was the most *neglected!* This helped them realize that sometimes the whole ward withdraws from such a patient, even taking her so for granted that her basic care is neglected. Discussing such a patient with the personnel prompted the head nurse to ask: "Would sending her to another ward be therapeutic?" (to doctor); "Would somebody here try to befriend her?" (to personnel and students); "Could someone take her for individual therapy?" (to doctor); "Could she have active treatment of some kind, such as occupational or recreational therapy or group therapy?" (to doctor and other department heads).

Ward Rounds

The head nurse made rounds as often as three or four times a day so that she could 1) let the patients know how important they were, as individuals, to the personnel; 2) note any requests from patients for future action by doctor, nurse, or aide; 3) observe the patients' physical as well as their emotional condition.

On the basis of her daily 8-hour observation of the patients, the head nurse was asked by the doctor on morning rounds what therapy she thought might be useful for certain patients. She was also asked many questions concerning patients' behavior. The charge aide accompanied the head nurse and the physician on morning rounds.

If patients were not already out of bed when rounds began, they were afterwards because the visit of head nurse stimulated activity. At least one student nurse was invited each day to accompany the head nurse on rounds. Innumerable teaching situations developed. For example, one morning the head nurse did not have her cap on. When she approached a patient who had been a nurse before she became ill, the patient, whose previous reaction had been totally hostile, received her in a friendly manner. This was an opportunity to discuss with students the problem of authority in relation to certain patients. During rounds, the head nurse also pointed out to the students the importance of observing physical signs and symptoms.

One day, an incident occurred which highlighted the vital need for complete communication. A patient who had always dreaded electric shock therapy was told by her doctor that her treatments would be discontinued. The doctor neglected to tell the ward personnel and did not write an order. The next morning, despite the patient's objection and insistence that the doctor had told her she would have no more treatments, she was taken downstairs to the shock unit. She had made these same statements many times before, and having nothing more to go on, the personnel had not considered that they might be valid. Upon reaching the shock unit the patient had to wait with other patients, and went through very real anguish. It was only when she was brought to the door of the shock room that the therapy nurse told the ward personnel that orders had been issued for her treatment to be discontinued. Exhausted and depressed, the patient was led back to the ward. She had suffered needlessly because of poor communication among those caring for her!

Promoting Harmony and Activity

The head nurse was very much concerned with making the ward a harmonious place for patients and personnel. Both the head nurse and the ward doctor assumed a permissive and democratic attitude and good interpersonal relations were the rule rather than the exception. This was particularly true after a ward meeting of personnel and students in which everyone expressed feelings about one another — including the head nurse. For example, the aides told the head nurse that she was having too many conferences, and that she sometimes "overinterpreted" patients' behavior. The students, on the other hand, voiced real appreciation for their conferences; they said that the head nurse seemed interested in them, and fitted pretty well into their concept of what a psychiatric head nurse should be. The head nurse, in turn, said that she felt the aides were "passing the buck" in the business of assuming responsibility for administrative details, that no one seemed to want the job, even though they had all, at first, expressed willingness and enthusiasm about the plan. After this meeting, feelings and work seemed to run more smoothly. Special attention was paid to those patients who were left on the ward after others had gone for various therapies. The head nurse, students, and aides tried to bring various activities to the ward. The charge aide played the piano and sang for the patients. The head nurse and students also sang and encouraged the patients in Ping-pong, whist, and handball. The aides encouraged the patients to help keep the ward clean and attractive.

The climax of the drive for activity on the ward came at a painting party. Doctors, nurses, students, and both men and women patients painted the entire dayroom in one evening. One of the patients played the piano, and when all the work had been finished, refreshments were served. The cohesiveness of that entire group was a source of real satisfaction to the head nurse, who had initiated the project by suggesting that the patients paint the beds and furniture in the ward. This minor painting project stimulated the patients themselves to organize the "dayroom painting party."

Teaching Opportunities

The ward doctor had established a therapy group in the ward setting, through which he had gotten to know all the patients better and had been able to give them more help. Later, because of an increase in his duties off the ward, the doctor asked the head nurse to take the group twice a week, since it had become customary for the patients to come to the dayroom after breakfast every day for the meeting. She reported what went on in these meetings to the doctor during conferences which the student nurses also attended. This gave students an opportunity to learn from both the head nurse and the doctor.

The opportunities available to the head nurse for teaching student nurses and aides were innumerable. For example, she felt that there were some misunderstandings between the ward personnel and the members of other departments — occupational therapy, psychology, rehabilitation, and so on — which were primarily due to a lack of knowledge about each person's job in relation to patients. To correct these misunderstandings it was necessary for both the aides and the personnel on the ancillary services to learn to appreciate each other's jobs, to cooperate with one another, and to use each other's services properly.

In order to bring this three-way understanding about, the head nurse asked a member of each ancillary service to come to the ward for a conference concerning their departments and treatment plans for the patients. Why does a patient have a particular therapy? What happens to her while she is getting it? What are the objectives of the therapy? These three questions were discussed. After the conference there was better understanding and everyone realized that all were working to help patients get well.

Evaluation

It became obvious to the head nurse during this 3-month experimental period on the ward that the key to good teaching lay in her knowledge of her patient. She gained this knowledge by delegating administrative details to others and spending the greater part of her allotted time on duty with her patients (see table). By constantly doing things with patients, she was able to utilize all kinds of different experiences as teaching situations, and to set a useful example for students who might later enter the psychiatric nursing field.

In an attempt to gauge the effectiveness of the research assistant in her role of head nurse, the influence of this head nurse on student nurses was compared with the influence of two other head nurses.

After they had been on the wards for several weeks, twelve students were interviewed — four who had worked on the experimental ward and four from each of two other wards. They were asked: "What are the three main things you would do if you were head nurse on a psychiatric ward?" The responses to this question were grouped into four broad categories: 1) patient-therapy orientation (time spent with patients in some type of therapeutic relationship); 2) interpersonnel orientation (concern with relation-

Five-day Time Study of Three Head Nurses' Activities on Similar Psychiatric Wards

Head Nurse's Activities	Distribution of Hours Spent By:					
	Head Nurse A (Men's Ward)		Head Nurse B (Women's Ward)		Research Assistant — Head Nurse (Women's Ward)	
	Number	Percentage	Number	Percentage	Number	Percentage
Activities in which she spent time with:						
Patients	10.2	26.6	13.8	36.5	17.6	50.3
Administrative duties in office	9.5	24.7	6.6	17.4	1.5	4.3
Administrative duties out of office	3.5	9.1	3.6	9.5	0.7	2.0
Students (directly concerning patients)	2.9	7.5	1.7	4.5	3.3	9.4
Students (not directly concerning patients)	0.7	1.8	0.4	1.1	0.1	0.3
Aides (directly concerning patients)	2.5	6.5	2.1	5.6	3.5	10.0
Aides (not directly concerning patients)	2.1	5.5	2.1	5.6	0.5	1.4
Administrators: supervisors, director of nurses, and so forth	2.1	5.5	1.4	3.7	1.1	3.1
Doctors	0.5	1.3	2.1	5.6	2.5	7.2
Nonadministrative duties, in office	0.3	0.8	0.3	0.8	0.1	0.3
Off-ward activities	4.1	10.7	3.7	9.7	4.1	11.7
Total*	38.4	100.0	37.8	100.0	35.0	100.0

*Totals for numbers of hours are not the same since the nurses sometimes worked overtime or undertime. Hours spent attending seminars, conferences, and so forth are not included.

ships among personnel); 3) traditional administration (concern with status relationships, administrative duties); 4) traditional activities (concern with cleanliness of ward, activity of patients *per se*). The most marked differences in their replies were in the areas of interpersonnel orientation and traditional activities. Students from the experimental ward were far more conscious of the need for fostering good relationships among personnel than the others were. And the students from the experimental ward relied on traditional activities to a much smaller extent.

Another relevant observation from the interviews with students concerned the extent to which they found the head nurse helpful. All of the student nurses from the experimental ward indicated that the head nurse had been thoroughly helpful while *none* of the students from either of the control wards believed that the head nurses on those wards had helped the students as much as possible. Furthermore, all of the students on the experimental ward indicated that their experience on this ward was different from their experiences on other wards. This finding is more meaningful when we consider that all of these responses — both of students who felt that the head nurse was helpful and those who felt she was not — are concerned with one issue: the extent to which the head nurse clarified the dynamics of the problems with which the students had to deal and the extent to which she guided them in their approach to patients. Thus, it would appear that while the students from the experimental ward were not more conscious of the need for a therapeutic relationship with patients than the other students were, their actual experience indicates that there probably was a more therapeutic atmosphere on the experimental ward than there was on other wards of the hospital. Moreover, this situation, according to their replies, helped them in developing an understanding of patients and greater ease in approaching them.

Conclusion

Certain general conclusions have evolved from this experimental project. Although it provides no specific solutions, it offers challenging evidence which should stimulate thinking and promote further study in two areas: 1) the education of psychiatric head nurses, and 2) psychiatric nursing therapy with individual patients and groups of patients.

The Nurse and the Dying Patient

Catherine M. Norris

Miss Norris (Massachusetts General, Boston; B.S., Boston University; M.A., Teachers College, Columbia University) is assistant professor of psychiatric nursing at the University of Colorado School of Nursing.

Reprinted from *The American Journal of Nursing*, Vol. 55, October 1955.

In an attempt to help students handle some of the problems they encounter in caring for dying patients and for bodies after death, we planned for conferences in which the students could meet as a group and talk together about this aspect of their nursing experience.

Thirty sophomores, in a four-year collegiate program, met for this discussion. They had had the nursing care procedures that are associated with the care of the dying patient and the care of the body after death. In addition, they had talked with chaplains of various religious denominations.

Our purpose in planning the conference was to help the students become aware of their problems and to help them understand some of the dynamics that are involved in these problems. We felt that real learning would result from the students' thinking and study outside of class. The use to which the students put their class experience then could be measured by observing, first, how they used the experience to work through their own problems, and, as a result, how they were able to help patients and patients' families.

Since we are all products of the culture in which we live, the teacher approached the discussion of the dying patient from this point of view. She began by pointing out to the students that nearly all that they knew about dying and death they had learned before they came to the university. She suggested that it might be helpful for them to look at some of the ideas that people in their communities have about dying, as shown by the expressions they use to describe it.

As the students volunteered the expressions they had heard, she listed them on the blackboard. The list included the following expressions:

Passed away
Croaked
He's through
He's gone to his reward
He's gone to eternal rest
He's gone to God
He's left this life
He's left this world
He's gone to rest
He went to sleep
He was released from his suffering
They are going to lay him six feet deep
He went out feet first
He knocked off
He died
He was killed
Passed out
He's finished
He's gone to his Maker
He's joined his Maker
He's gone for a while
He's passed on
God took him away
God called him away
He departed this life
He kicked off
He kicked the bucket
He's pushing up daisies
He's kissing angels
He's gone to the happy hunting ground
Expired

The discussion then continued:

TEACHER: If we look at all these expressions can we see any difference in the way people describe dying?

STUDENT: Some people are facetious.

TEACHER: Can we make any guesses about why people are facetious in talking about death?

STUDENT: Some people aren't afraid.

STUDENT: I think some people don't want to talk about it so they make a joke of it.

STUDENT: That's what I think; I think they *are* afraid.

STUDENT: Why would you joke if you're afraid?

STUDENT: Maybe it's nervousness. I feel like giggling right now.

TEACHER: Are there others who feel like giggling?

STUDENTS: Yes.

TEACHER: Why?

STUDENT: I feel funny inside.

STUDENT: I guess I get nervous. (Some giggling among the students)

TEACHER: Do we sometimes use laughter as a way of feeling easier or of getting more comfortable?

STUDENT: Some people do, I guess, but I just

want to run away.

TEACHER: Yes, that's another way to get more comfortable. What are some of the other kinds of thoughts about death that we hear expressed?

STUDENT: Some people think that you go to another life.

TEACHER: What kind of a life?

STUDENT: A better life than this one.

STUDENT: Some of those answers look to me as if some people just think you die — as if that were the end.

TEACHER: Would you be willing to make some guesses about how this might affect the way different people feel when they look at dying as one of the experiences of life?

STUDENT: Well, people don't talk about death much unless someone they know is dying or has just died.

STUDENT: I never gave it much thought. I can't imagine it happening to me.

STUDENT: I don't like to think about it. A patient the other day just floored me. I was giving him a bath and the conversation was pretty general. Then out of the clear blue sky he asked me if he was going to die. My jaw dropped to the floor; I was just paralyzed.

TEACHER: Do you think you will have to think about death and its meaning in the life process before you can be helpful to patients when they ask you such a question?

STUDENT: I think we do have to think about it.

STUDENT: I just never came face to face with it before.

TEACHER: Maybe this has something to do with America as a young country symbolizing youth, beauty, health, and growth. I wonder if old people represent the old country that should have been left behind. Is this one of the reasons that we don't give much thought to it or why we apologize for the aged and dying instead of accepting this aspect of the life process?

STUDENT: I don't feel that way about my grandparents and I hate to think of losing them but I don't think I really like old patients. Their skin is loose and wrinkled and most of them look unattractive. They can't remember anything, some of them, and they are so helpless and useless, I get the feeling that it would be a blessing for them to die. I suppose I shouldn't feel that way, but I do sometimes.

STUDENT: I don't like to think about getting old or dying. There are too many nice things to think about. I've got my whole future ahead of me, and I like to think about that and not about dying.

STUDENT: I think we've got to think about it if we're going to take care of dying patients without becoming nervous wrecks.

STUDENT: It says in this book (reading from the book) "All conversation in the room should be in a natural tone of voice. . . . The room should be light and cheerful. . . . The nurse's calm manner and natural voice and her reassuring presence will help overcome fear." I don't think I'll ever be able to act that way.

STUDENT: That is saying for us to act like everything is all right, nothing's wrong, nothing's going to happen. . . .

STUDENT: When all the time it's a crisis for the patient.

TEACHER: Do you think the book is asking you to deny that there is something very serious going on for the patient?

STUDENT: It's very serious for us too. (Class laughs)

TEACHER: Yes, it's hard for you too. It is my opinion — and you may not agree with me — that when the nurse acts as if it's not going to happen and the relatives act as if it's not going to happen, and the patient does too, then the patient is left alone to handle his fears and worries by himself. I think it is very hard on the patient and everyone else, but particularly on the patient.

STUDENT: But how can we help a patient who asks if he is dying? We can't tell him he's dying, no matter how much he asks.

TEACHER: It is true that a nurse does not tell a patient he is dying, but is there something that she can do when he asks?

STUDENT: I think it's a nurse's job to feel that where there is life there is hope.

STUDENT: I do, too.

STUDENT: I do, up to a point, but there are some patients who realize that they are going from bad to worse and the doctors, with all the tests they do, know there is no hope for them. So, why shouldn't we use what they tell us and face the problem instead of expecting a miracle to happen?

STUDENT: But miracles can happen.

STUDENT: I suppose they can, but how can we work as a team if we don't take the doctor's word for the condition of the patient?

STUDENT: Doctors can be wrong.

STUDENT: Maybe so; anybody can make mistakes. But we have to start somewhere in finding out what is happening to the patient. We have to fit into the whole plan for the patient.

STUDENT: I don't see why you can't be hopeful and still recognize that the patient is worried about dying.

STUDENT: I still want to know what you say when a patient says, "Nurse, am I dying?" (Silence)

TEACHER: If you don't feel too uncomfortable, could you start out by trying to identify how he feels and talk with him about how hard it is to stand the idea that one is going to die?

STUDENT: Supposing it isn't hard for the patient to think about. If he is very religious, maybe he is looking forward to joining God.

TEACHER: If you can't tell whether the patient is distressed, do you think you might find out how he does feel as a first step?

STUDENT: I can usually get that far, but I don't know what to do when a patient pours out all his feelings.

STUDENT: A patient said to me, "If I'm going to die I want to know; I've got things to do, and I want to have a few more good times."

STUDENT: That's why I can't ask a patient to tell me about how he feels. They tell you that they don't want to die, that they are afraid to die.

STUDENT: If a patient is really religious he won't be afraid or have as many problems.

STUDENT: I don't think that follows.

STUDENT: If you really trust in God you shouldn't be afraid.

STUDENT: I think you can really have faith in God but when you go into something you don't know anything about and leave everything behind, you're afraid. It doesn't mean you don't have faith in a life after death. Haven't you ever been afraid — for example, that first day we went on the wards?

STUDENT: That is different; that didn't have anything to do with religion or dying.

STUDENT: I don't think it's different. It's normal to be afraid when you don't know the score.

TEACHER: What happens to the patient if the nurse does believe that he shouldn't be afraid?

STUDENT: He won't tell the nurse — he won't talk to her.

TEACHER: Why not?

STUDENT: Because she'll make him feel ashamed that he's afraid.

TEACHER: We may not agree on this point, but I think that regardless of the degree of the patient's spiritual well-being and religious faith, one might expect him to express some degree of anxiety and fear. Death is a new experience for the patient. The future is completely unknown as to its dimensions. We don't know whether people will exist in the same form, whether the physical world will be similar in any way, whether time, day and night, the seasons, or any of the other things with which we are familiar will be the same. Couldn't one have faith in God and a life after death and still have tremendous concern over leaving this life experience and one's loved ones for an experience that is unknown? Haven't we been expressing our own anxieties about our role in this experience for patients? If we get this tense over just helping someone else, is it not understandable that we would be very concerned if we found ourselves in the patient's place?

STUDENT: Now, I don't know what to think. All these ideas confuse me. I have to go home and think about them.

TEACHER: It is difficult for us to think this out for ourselves. But once you do it, you may find that you are much more comfortable when you must deal with this problem in your role as nurse. Let's consider now how you are going to feel and what you are going to do when you come to the point where you must be with the patient when he dies and must take care of his body after death.

STUDENT: I might feel sad.

STUDENT: I'm afraid.

STUDENT: I think we're all afraid.

STUDENT: I'm afraid that I'll be imagining what the patient was like when he was alive and I might not be able to really believe he's dead.

STUDENT: One of my patients died unexpectedly last week and I couldn't help crying.

STUDENT: I know I'll want to run away.

STUDENT: Are we ever left alone with a dead patient?

TEACHER: How do you feel about being left alone with a body?

STUDENT: I'd want to get out of there.

STUDENT: I'd feel much worse.

TEACHER: At first you'll have someone with you all the time. It really takes two people to care for the body. However, since we cannot always anticipate when death will occur you may be alone while caring for a patient who is close to death. What will happen if you do cry when a patient expires?

STUDENT: I guess I'd feel like a sissy.

STUDENT: It's really wrong. Nurses should learn to control their feelings.

STUDENT: (directed to teacher) Do you think we should be able to keep our feelings out of it?

TEACHER: Crying might not be the most useful thing you could do at this particular time, but we expect that you will be troubled and upset and if you do cry we know that you are expressing feelings that you cannot express in any other way. Crying might have constructive aspects. I can remember hearing about a mother who said some time after the death of her son, "Everybody loved Johnny, even the nurse cried." It's rather a shock to realize that people think of nurses as unfeeling. How does it sound to you, "even the nurse cried?"

STUDENT: I'm afraid they might make fun of me if I get upset.

TEACHER: To some degree this is probably true, and it represents the way nurses used to think about it. Today, I think you'll find that many nurses realize that there is considerable tension involved when a patient dies.

STUDENT: What if we laugh or get giggling?

TEACHER: Even then it doesn't help to blame yourself, but we would hope that you would be able to recognize mounting tension in yourself and try to get away from the situation until you felt more comfortable. When you blame yourself and say, "I should have done this, I should have been able," it keeps you from asking, "What happened? What feelings did I have that might have warned me about what I would do next?"

STUDENT: Isn't that just running away from the problem?

TEACHER: It does look like it, doesn't it? But sometimes when tension is great we have to do something to get comfortable before we can ask ourselves the questions that help us solve the problem. I think that getting away for a little while is more useful than laughing or joking or getting the jitters because it is hard for the family to understand what is going on when the nurse's behavior seems to them to be inappropriate.

STUDENT: I still want to know what to say when a patient talks about death.

TEACHER: I don't know that anyone can ever really tell you what to say. Maybe we could identify the functions of the nurse with the dying patient and then each nurse can create in her own way the experience for the patient. What do you think the functions of the nurse might be?

STUDENT: To let the patient talk about how he feels and not make him feel ashamed if he is afraid.

STUDENT: I would like to let the patient know that I am sharing with him, or maybe I mean that I feel for him.

STUDENT: That he's not alone in his trouble. If you can feel that you're not all alone with your troubles you feel better.

TEACHER: What you are saying implies that one of the first functions of the nurse is to get comfortable herself so that she can talk with the patient and share these experiences with him. How long do you think this might take?

STUDENT: It might take a while. I don't know if I can ever do it.

TEACHER: For most of us it does take time. You can't just think you should and then be able to go in there and function with the patient. We all make many mistakes too before we develop any degree of skill. Don't get too impatient with yourself if your attempts with your patient don't seem to be useful to him. It takes time.

Do you think we have any responsibility to help the patient be able to get close to his family, or to help the family handle the problems that patient may try to discuss with them?

STUDENT: I think it would be good but I think it will take me a long time.

TEACHER: Would it be hard for you if you saw a patient and members of his family all crying together?

SEVERAL STUDENTS: Yes.

STUDENT: When I see anybody cry I want to say, "Don't cry." I want to make them stop.

STUDENT: I always feel guilty when I see a patient cry. I feel that if I were a good nurse I should have prevented it.

STUDENT: I get uneasy too.

TEACHER: Then it would be hard for you to view this as one aspect of the patient's and his family's developing a closer relationship — a relationship in which not only the lighter moments but also the more difficult ones are shared.

STUDENT: It's so new for me to think about.

TEACHER: In our culture where there is so much loneliness can you visualize this experience for the patient as having worth?

STUDENT: I think it would be better for us all to keep our dignity and keep our problems to ourselves. It's true, if you laugh the world laughs with you and if you cry you cry alone.

STUDENT: Does that have to be true? I don't agree with all that's been said today but I'm going to think about it.

STUDENT: If everybody acts as if everything is just as usual and nobody helps the patient and the family — I don't think that's good, but I don't rightly know what is best.

STUDENT: About the only thing I'm sure of is

that if the patient wants to talk about his worries about dying or if he knows he's going to die, he should have somebody to talk with and if the family can't do it then I guess the nurse has to.

STUDENT: What about getting the minister or a priest to help the patient?

STUDENT: If a patient says to you, "Am I going to die, nurse?" are you going to say, "Who is your minister?" The minister might live a long way away.

STUDENT: And it might be in the night when it would be hard to get the minister.

STUDENT: If you did that, the patient might think he's really going to die, and maybe he isn't or maybe he really doesn't want to know.

STUDENT: How can you tell if a patient really wants to know?

STUDENT: You can't tell him anyway.

STUDENT: I know it but I wondered if you could really tell.

TEACHER: You can guess that if he finds out who the one person is who can tell him — the doctor — and then asks that person, maybe he really does want to know. I think that sometimes when the patient asks the nurse, he is just toying with the idea and looking for clues in the nurse's response to his question and is not really ready to hear something as final as the verdict the doctor might pronounce.

Could we talk for a moment about how the nurse can be useful to the family at the time of death. What do you expect those who love the patient to do at the time he expires?

STUDENT: I heard one woman screaming and crying — everbody heard her.

STUDENT: I think I'd be in a daze.

STUDENT: I feel like fainting myself, so I can see relatives feeling that way too.

TEACHER: Why do people act like that in a crisis?

STUDENT: They are desperate.

STUDENT: They don't know what to do.

TEACHER: There is a feeling that one is helpless to do anything about the situation or to handle the surge of feeling that comes over one in such a crisis. The body protects us when we faint. Fainting gives one a short period of oblivion from something pretty unbearable. Another way the body protects us is to not let us feel it all immediately, so there is a blunted or dazed feeling. Screaming helps us to expend the energy that comes with the surge of emotions. Would you say that the screaming and crying person was not in control of himself?

STUDENT: The woman I saw didn't even seem to hear when they asked her to be quiet so the patients wouldn't be upset. I don't think she was in control of herself.

TEACHER: I think it is true that when a problem is very great, an individual may not be able to control what he does and at this time he doesn't hear much and doesn't see much either. How can you help someone in these circumstances?

STUDENT: I felt like putting my arms around the woman I saw, but I thought the others would think...

TEACHER: Think what?

STUDENT: That I wasn't professional or that I was getting too involved. I can't really say, I guess, but I didn't do what I wanted anyway.

TEACHER: It seems to me that when a person is not accessible to reason and is out of control, the feeling of firmness and warmth and strength from the touch or clasp of another person might provide the strength he needs to move toward controlling himself. I think also that as nurses, we have nothing more valuable to offer people than the spontaneous expression of our own warm feelings and the demonstration of our concern for them. By the same token if the nurse can help members of the family communicate their concern and warm feelings to the patient, she is helpful to both the patient and his family.

We have no more time today but we need more time to discuss death and still more time to discuss anxiety or tension and to discuss the meaning of crying.

In summarizing this discussion I would like first to emphasize that the part of life experience concerned with death is one of the most difficult for people to think about and take part in. It is more difficult than the other big events in life like birth, coming of age, or marriage. This may be true because in our culture we put tremendous value on youth and to a considerable extent ignore aging and dying as important experiences in the life process. If nurses are to be useful to patients in these experiences, they must give some consideration to what death means to them as individuals and to others. They have to consider the meaning of fear, of crying, of anxiety and panic. They also have to consider the nursing skills they must develop if they are to be able to work with patients on these problems.

With the way most families now handle the dying patient, some consideration must also be given to loneliness, and whether movement in the direction of closeness would be useful. If it is useful, nurses must consider how one moves closer and how one helps others develop close relationships.

It is well known that it is not the nurse's function to tell a patient that he is going to die, but it is possible for her to share certain aspects of his experience with dying so that he does not feel alone with his problems. The nurse can also help him alleviate his guilt about his fears.

Most important is the nurse's need to work through her own feelings and tensions about death and bereavement, so that she will not be limited by tension when she attempts to be helpful to the dying patient and his family.

Loneliness

Hildegard E. Peplau

Miss Peplau (Pottstown, Pa., Hospital School of Nursing; B.A., Bennington College; M.A., Ed.D., Teachers College, Columbia) is assistant professor in nursing and director of the advanced program in psychiatric nursing at Rutgers University. She has a certificate in "psychoanalysis applied for teachers" from the William Alanson White Institute for Psychiatry. In this paper, Miss Peplau has included data which she drew from her experience with patients in private practice.

Reprinted from *The American Journal of Nursing,* Vol. 55, December 1955.

Being alone in a situation may be a pleasant state, or an unpleasant one — or it may be unbearable. True loneliness — which is unbearable — is a clinical problem in psychiatric nursing practice, but it has received very little attention as such.

Before discussing the feelings of the person who is without company, it may be helpful for us to consider the differences between lonesomeness, aloneness, and loneliness.

Lonesomeness is a common experience. It implies being without the company of others but recognizing a wish to be with others. Lonesomeness can occur when an individual is isolated or it can be felt despite proximity to others in a group. The lonesome individual recognizes his desire to feel closer to others and, more often than not, he is able to state it as a feeling. Also he can usually express specific wishes, and take steps to relieve the feeling of lonesomeness.

Aloneness also implies being without company. It may signify a singular position, such as being alone in making certain kinds of decisions which affect living. Erich Fromm, for example, speaks of man's "moral aloneness" in reaching decisions of ethical significance. An individual is alone when he casts his vote in an election. Individuals can choose to be alone — to retreat temporarily from the activities with other people which customarily go on in the social stream. Being alone offers an opportunity for concentration, for focusing on and working through particular kinds of problems. Scientists, for example, often court aloneness. They find that it improves their productivity; it is a way to avoid distractions which would impede or delay their accomplishment. It is possible to be alone without being lonesome or lonely, when retreat, seclusion, or protected isolation are recognized and chosen as desirable or essential for accomplishing specific purposes for which plans can be made and acted upon.

Loneliness, however, is not a chosen state. Often the lonely person is not aware of the reason why he does what he does when he experiences loneliness. It is an experience somewhat different in character and in intensity from either aloneness or lonesomeness. Loneliness can be defined as an unnoticed inability to do anything while alone.

Often loneliness is not felt; instead the person has a feeling of unexplained dread, of desperation, or of extreme restlessness. These feelings are so intense, so unbearable, that automatic actions are precipitated. These automatic actions force other persons to come into contact with the lonely individual. Although he is not aware that loneliness is one of the feelings which govern him, his automatic responses recur and become patterns of living which may seem senseless to other people. One psychiatric patient referred to her pattern of response to loneliness as her "trapadaptation."

The Roots of Loneliness

Loneliness is the result of early life experiences in which remoteness, indifference, and emptiness were the principal themes that characterized the child's relationships with others. Because it is an unbearable experience, loneliness is always hidden, disguised, defended against, and expressed in other forms. It may be expressed quite simply as homesickness, or it may appear as severe agitation, or in the form of alcoholism or drug addiction, and it is an important aspect of the schizophrenic pattern of living. In nursing situations, therefore, nurses do not deal directly with the patient's loneliness but rather with his defenses against experiencing the pain of loneliness — the plausible structure he has erected to cover up the problem and hide it from himself and from others.

Some general cues to the needs of lonely patients are available in the generic roots of the problem. When nurses can understand how loneliness has evolved, they can anticipate what kinds of relationships between the nurse and the patient would be similarly traumatic, and they can avoid acting in ways that might reinforce the problem.

Sullivan discusses loneliness as an acquired outcome of childhood situations.[1] He points out that during early childhood each child makes an effort to secure the attention of adults — as active participants or at least as spectators — in activities which interest the child and stimulate his curiosity. However, these efforts are too often met with indifference, misinterpretation, or punishment which the child interprets as being due to failure on his part. Adults often interpret the child's attention-getting behavior as merely a device to distract and delay, and this interpretation serves as justification for their feelings of annoyance with the child.

The actual purposes of these initial efforts on the part of the child are varied. He seeks an audience so that he can see himself in relation to another person. This is how he first experiences the feeling of being related to others. He also needs an opportunity to exercise his growing ability to communicate what is meaningful to him during an experience. He seeks to check the meanings of his current observations and experiences with another person. Thus, he is exercising an important and much needed capacity which will serve, later on, to limit the importance which he attaches to his fantasies and to his autistic interpretations which are highly subjective and which are based on his fantasies, rather than on reality. Autistic thinking serves to gratify unfulfilled longings.

Childhood is a time when autistic invention — the capacity to invent and assign highly personal meaning to events — is most active. The child who seeks the attentive participation of adults but meets with indifference, remoteness, or even punishment instead, must somehow fill the gap. Otherwise, life seems empty of meaning, of skill, and of the feeling that he is related to others.

Alone, he has to find plausible explanations for what is happening to him. Feelings of smallness, helplessness, and longing for closeness give way to defenses against loneliness. The wish for the cooperation of adults in interpreting events is replaced by the use of fantasies and autistic invention. Later on, these cause enormous difficulty when the individual attempts to maintain a distinction between what is real and what is fanciful. One patient put it this way: "For me it is always a struggle to think clearly." The nurse asked, "You know when you are thinking clearly?" and the patient answered, "You feel that you are."

Without help and without skill, the child must resort to fantasies to explain current experiences. To adults, the new set of interpretations which the child makes seem to be falsifications and misinterpretations, and they are not appreciated for what they are any more than the initial efforts to secure active, direct interest were. To the child, the expansive distortions serve only to explain experience, but to adults, they become proof that the child should be viewed as unmanageable, as a "liar," or as delinquent. The problem deepens and the child's sense of failure looms larger and larger.

This arrest in the socializing process at home does not prepare the child for contacts with peers in the next phase in development. Peers tend to poke fun at his ineptness, errors, and misinterpretations of the meanings of events. Not only the rebuffs of adults but now those of children, too, become a real and anticipated source of humiliation, punishment, and anxiety. Real or imagined threats, supported by the fear of error, deepen the sense of social isolation. The evolving need to be right, to be able, coupled with feelings of failure and of isolation from others, all help to nourish the developing loneliness.

Patterns of Defense

Sullivan tells us, however, that loneliness is so dreaded and so painful that it must be disguised; it is therefore dissociated, not noticed; instead, defenses against observation of it determine the individual's behavior. The patterns of defense are automatic and while the patient frequently can offer plausible explanations of what he is doing, the obvious purpose of the behavior escapes his notice. For example, a patient who drinks and then needs nurses to care for him during an alcoholic bout may offer many reasons for needing to have nurses to care for him. But he misses the obvious interpretation — that he is sorely in need of attention and contact with others, and that this need has erupted as a momentary experiencing of loneliness and has thus brought on the episode of drinking.

Recognizing what the behavior of an individual who is defending himself from bitter loneliness means may take sensitive observation, over a long period of time, but there are certain clues that nurses can watch for.

Time-oriented complaints are often observed. The patient may experience the "endlessness" of each day, even though he may carry out and complete his routine. He may have an aura of waiting, of enduring, of "putting in time," so to speak. In considering events in the future, the patient often observes aspects of the beginning and also the goals or ends relating to the event, but he does not anticipate the intervening steps — the transition points in the duration of the event. For example, a patient who is planning to move may recognize that the time to move has arrived and may consider the advantages of the new location, but he has no concept of what is involved in the preparation for moving and in the moving process itself.

With some patients, it often appears as if time were telescoped — past events and present experiences are considered and lived as if they were identical, fused together. While the person seems always to wait for something to happen, when the thing he has been waiting for is about to occur, he becomes impatient because he has to wait. For example, one patient put it directly by saying, over and over again, "I have to wait for the doctor and I can't." Another patient could not say directly, but indicated through her dreams, that the nurse was not noticing or attending to her needs in a complete way — it was as if, by this means, she was trying to indicate the remoteness of both her mother and the nurse by distorting time and telescoping the mother-situation and nurse-situation into one.

The feeling of *familiarity* seems to be time-related and can be observed in patients who are fighting loneliness. The familiarity is with things rather than with people and its seems more apparent when the patient is experiencing great anxiety. One patient, for example, would occasionally state with conviction that she had heard, read, or seen something before, although she was observing it in a newly purchased book or a freshly published newspaper. Further inquiry revealed that what was familiar was the feeling she had at being in that situation with the nurse, a feeling which she had experienced in an earlier situation. Another patient who was vomiting a good deal asked for a prescribed medication which was expected to relieve the vomiting and the discomfort associated with it. She was given the medication, but each dose was also vomited. As the patient became more anxious, a feeling of "everything seems familiar" developed and was expressed, in this instance, in relation to material in a newspaper she was reading. She then asked to test this feeling by having the nurse read from a new book which she was certain she had not read nor heard about, but here too "everything seemed familiar." The nurse wondered whether it was something in the nurse-patient situation which was being expressed indirectly in this way. Further discussion revealed that this patient had had a tonsillectomy at a very early age. During her hospitalization, her mother had brought her some lemonade, saying, "This will make your throat better." However, the tartness had increased the pain and discomfort, and now the medication for relief of vomiting had also failed to work. This indicated what was familiar: an unfulfilled expectation that a trusted mothering person would bring relief from discomfort.

There is also a sense in which lonely patients seem to feel familiar with people; but on further inspection the chief characteristic of this feeling is that they view all other persons as *anonymous* beings. One patient may treat everyone as a welcome and known stranger; another automatically dislikes everyone except in rare instances when he finds one person he can like. However, in both patterns — anonymity-of-all and the rare-approval-of-one — the common factor seems to be the focus on the "weaknesses of others." In the first instance, all individuals are disrespected, indeed often feared and held suspect. In the situation where one person who is liked seems to be accepted, this acceptance is followed by a search for the familiar — the ever-present weaknesses in others. Then when a so-called weakness is located, the patient can feel threatened, anxious, and thus can automatically keep his own familiar pathology going. It is as if he had a continuing need to see himself as powerless, mistrusting, lonely — to feel this familiar, accustomed self and to feel more lonely and more threatened at the thought of change, of seeing himself differently.

Difficulties related to making plans are also observable. Some patients hesitate, vacillate, and are indecisive, not knowing whether to continue living with marked planlessness or to use exaggerated overplanning in the hope of improving their pattern of living.

With *planlessness* it is as though life were viewed and lived as one continual accident, based upon an expectation that something is going to happen, sometime; the person responds automatically to minor details that actually do occur, but does nothing to prevent or produce them. He endures the "long, empty, time-crawling days," as one person described them, and never contemplates making any effort to change the situation.

On the other hand, *overplanning* may also be observed. It may involve making extensive lists of things to be done — letters to be written, shopping to be completed, or clothing to be packed. It is as if the patient couldn't remember to carry out even the basic functions of living without something tangible, like a list, to remind him of what to do and when to do it. Or he may feel the directionless drift of his living and set up projects and deadlines to be met in order to avoid feeling frantic about the emptiness and disorder which surround him. His reasons for wanting direction are obscure to the patient.

Occasionally, overplanning can be observed as an emphasis on personal dressing for social appearances. It is as if the patient were arranging a carefully guarded and rarely displayed picture of himself — the social self — to present to some potentially humiliating, disapproving spectator. Usually such great care in dress is in contrast to a more careless, casual daily appearance.

Efforts to Establish Contact with Others

To the lonely person, the opposite of loneliness — closeness and relatedness to people — always appears to hold potential threat. People — adults who did not respond to him when he was a child and then, later, his peers — have been a continual source of possible humiliation and therefore of anxiety. But he continues to make efforts, often dramatic ones, to have contact with adults — that is, the more mature persons in his psychosocial situation. These efforts, however, can suggest many pitfalls for nurses.

Efforts to establish contact or proximity can be complicated by an inclination toward *worshiping others*. As I have already pointed out, occasionally one person may be selected by the lonely individual and invested with all the potential qualities for meeting his so-far-unmet wishes and needs. This presents little difficulty if the "worshiped one" has the skill and training to understand the situation. If a nurse who does not have such training is selected, however, or if she needs this kind of interest from patients — perhaps on the basis of her own loneliness — then the patient will soon come to recognize and exploit this, unwittingly, and to the discomfort of the nurse. Worshiping others is very often an obligating maneuver; it is a way by which, in the long run, the patient gets attention on his terms; it is a subtle way of establishing nonrational dependence on another person.

I have noticed that lonely patients tend either to lump nurses together — viewing all nurses as identical — or to identify one nurse whom they establish as being "different, better than the others." Often the relationship with the latter nurse develops so that the patient comes to make more and more demands, as if to test the genuineness of her interest. These maneuvers are also a way for him to test whether he actually can incur her disapproval. Often the patient will go to almost any lengths to do this, as if to make open and apparent the very deeply felt need for disapproval which he has acquired. When the worshiped person does show marked disapproval, then the patient mobilizes his anxiety as anger or hatred, often taking active steps to cut himself off from the relationship. It is as if proof of the worshiped person's not caring has at last been secured, and further effort on the part of the patient is unnecessary. In this situation the lonely individual must have helped if he is to do anything to prevent the destruction of the relationship; he cannot do it by himself. It is up to the nurse to recognize what is going on and to sustain the patient's struggle with the problem, so that both he and she can clearly understand it.

Another kind of effort which these patients make at establishing contact, particularly in relationships with nurses, can be termed *role-reversal* — with the patient taking on the role-actions of the nurse while the nurse takes on some of the role-actions of the patient. An example of this was a situation in which the nurse became ill while caring for a psychiatric patient at home and, instead of signing off the case, permitted the patient to take over her nursing care — bringing meals, watching over her while she slept, and the like.

The patient talked about the feeling of worth and strength which she associated with helping the sick nurse; the feeling of interest and well-being that came to her when the nurse discussed her own problems. This no doubt is less apt to become a problem in hospitals, because the hospital system has too many checks on the actions of individual nurses to allow much reversal of roles. In private practice, however, where the nurse and the patient are together for many hours, it is much more common to observe the patient questioning the nurse about her personal affairs. There is, of course, a point at which this becomes one way in which the patient seeks to validate what he is emphasizing from the nurse — testing to see whether she really understands. But what we are referring to here is unwitting behavior on the nurse's part, in which she chats about herself in response to the patient's questioning.

When role-reversal occurs, it can sometimes be used to begin a new and more useful type of relationship. The skillful nurse can observe when the patient is purposefully shifting the focus from his needs to hers. She can be quite direct with patients, asking "Are you interested in switching the conversation to a discussion of my personal living?" Often, this type of comment may be needed when the patient becomes quite repetitious in asking about the nurse's food intake, the comfort offered by the chair or the room she is using, the temperature of the room, and so on. The patient often uses these diversionary conversations to find out whether the nurse's needs can supersede his own. When the nurse can demonstrate that she is well able to look after her own needs and can assist the patient to do likewise, then something favorable may happen in the nurse-patient relationship.

A third type of effort to secure the contact with nurses to avoid loneliness may be called *somatic participation* and is based on the expression of bodily needs. A hypersensitivity to noise or to stuffiness in a closed room may lead the patient to open and then to close the windows innumerable times in one day. Or he may make frequent requests for snacks between meals but beg off eating at mealtime. Or he may complain of pain in an arm, his head, his stomach, or any other organ that can be called into service to indicate the "pain of loneliness." Minor illnesses, such as colds and sprains, seem to occur just in time to bring contact, protection, and nurture. One patient phrased it directly, saying "I'm hungry but not for food. I don't know what I am hungry for." Vomiting and belching often occur when the patient perceives the nurse as rejecting him, lacking concern and interest; or they may occur as a way of demonstrating the desire to "get rid of" directions from others when the nurse has given the patient some advice.

The lonely patient often has great concern about strength, frequently expressing its absence in such ways as: "I feel I have no strength today," "the treatment weakens me — it takes a lot of strength," "I can't talk much today, I am too tired," or "I have to save up my strength today because I may go out tomorrow." This dwelling on the conservation of strength may indicate great fear of bankruptcy — powerlessness and feelings of failure — as the outcome of its use.

"Being well" may be equated with being active and good, as for example, "I'm all worn out; I wish I was better; I guess I am not good any more." The patient often requires and insists on a great deal of rest. This is a valid demand — it is well known that conflict can incur even more fatigue and exhaustion than physical exertion. It is easier, of course, to talk about the strength one lacks than to put it directly and talk about the weakness one feels.

Avoiding the Pain of Loneliness

Several patients have discussed what they call their "low tolerance of pain." Their whole living pattern reflects the great care they exert to avoid risk of any further injury, humiliation, and pain. Their familiar patterns of living — even though they are pathological, nonproductive, and essentially self-destructive in the long run — seem to carry less pain than new experiences do. A relationship to a nurse who is a mature person — and who is interested and able to help the patient look at peripheral expressions of deeper problems which require psychotherapeutic intervention — may well be a new and painful experience. The old patterns are better known and thus more comforting for the moment than new ones are.

One form of ineptness that stands out in lonely individuals is their inability to observe themselves in action. Even though they function more as spectators — watching, waiting, hoping — than as organizers of their life experiences, they protect themselves by not recognizing their own failures. They may work hard to offer plausible explanations for a particular pattern of action but they always seem to miss the obvious meaning of what they are saying. For instance, these comments which one patient made indicate how an obvious meaning may not be noticed: "I certainly can get myself sick in a million different places. You think this is bad — the last time I had four nurses. They were so good to me; they never left me alone. All kinds of attention I have to have — so much attention I think I must be a queen. What did I have to get sick for? Anytime anything happens in the family, anytime they look at me crooked, I get sick."

The basis of this problem — the individual's inability to see himself in action — lies in his distortion of the self-concept. The patient may be unable to see himself as a clearly defined entity, separate from his environment, just as a baby cannot differentiate himself from his surroundings. The baby sees the mother as part of himself; the lonely patient retains this illusion. For example, one patient repeatedly apologized when I dropped my notebook — as if we were so "attached" that she felt that she had dropped it and I was the observer.

The problem may also be based on the limitation of the patient's self-concept — his concept being too shallow to embrace the whole self and to discriminate the borders clearly. Along with this lack of self-definition go such general attitudes as worthlessness, powerlessness, and uselessness. Typical comments from these patients are: "Life doesn't mean anything," "I guess I have no use for myself," "I have such wonderful children but they have no use for me," or "There is nothing I can do."

In some situations, the patient's emphasis is on proving points — mostly proving what is not true rather than indicating what he is actually experiencing. It is as if he could ward off loneliness by proving that he is not dependent on others. This seems inherent in role-reversal — with the patient intuitively using the nurse to prove himself independent, powerful, worth something. Every one of these patients seems to have spent his whole life in activities calculated to prove the falsity of what is real — that he is a dependent lonely individual who has missed some vital experiences in the process of growing up.

Sullivan indicates that one outcome of arrest in a child's socializing process is the extensive effort that he must always make thereafter to maintain distinctions between the real and the unreal, between the actual and the fantasied, between the experienced and the imagined. Sometimes the nature of a patient's problems readily reveal this difficulty. For example, insomnia and intense interest in sleeping are usually observed together. Sleep symbolizes relief from loneliness; it is the one form of relief that the patient can achieve alone — if he can get to sleep. When he cannot, a longing for contact emerges and with it great anxiety which, in turn, insures his keeping awake. The patient may try sedation to get relief but sleep induced by sedation often brings with it terrorizing dreams which may repeatedly spell out the wish for closeness and interest from others.

We might speculate that loneliness is a *felt* component of a larger problem — emptiness. Emptiness might well be an over-all concept embracing a constellation of interrelated experiences. Emptiness must be so devastating that no one actually can experience it — it is nothingness, barrenness. Aspects of it can be observed, however, in patients whose life is barren of friends, who have sustained no role in the world of work, and who have been unable to fill any such social role as wife, husband, mother, friend, neighbor. The fixed points in the patient's sphere are all things — money, property, possessions — rather than persons. An ethical or philosophical frame of reference is lacking. As one patient put it, "There is no one and nothing to tell." Eventually, the patient may even restrict his movements to one room. He seems to feel tremendous need to keep feelings in a "deep freeze." It is not possible to feel such total emptiness; only the defenses against its variations — of which loneliness is one — can be endured.

Some lonely patients seem to have made early efforts to ward off the evolving pathology of loneliness. They have tried to forestall the consequences by substituting non-personalized transactions with knowledge, or with things, for relations with people. Reading copiously is one way of reducing autistic — or overly subjective and unreal — thinking; it is one way to "fill up" with the least risk of humiliation, failure, and disapproval. One patient recalled this when he said, "In college I think I felt that I was leading a life quite alone. I didn't have anyone to discuss anything with. I hated my teachers and the subjects but this didn't interest the family. They were like dead weight and I was in a hurry to get a degree. I wanted to compel my family to be interested. They encouraged the idea of college but they didn't encourage me."

The Nursing Care of Lonely Patients

The care of lonely patients requires the nurse to understand the generic development of the problem, its variations in the clinical situation, and its relation to the social structure of the ward situation. Reisman explores some of the shifting elements in our social structure which drive the individual to desperate pursuits as a "lonely member of a crowd."[2] He points out that the present generation is different from earlier ones in one important respect. The modes of conformity that individuals use and the qualities of feeling they have are developed in response to the evaluations of their peers rather than to concepts of authority which they acquired in the mother-child relationship. The earlier generation placed less emphasis on the individual's identification with a group, so the individual experienced loneliness more in relation to "internalized or illusory figures" than to his peers. The individual's relationships with his peers and their evaluations play a very large part in contemporary loneliness, however. Yet the need to conform, to be like others, to distort and destroy or deny human differences, is one of the leveling factors in both generations, and therefore it is a basic factor in loneliness. The hope of autonomy, of self-directed constructive use of capacities, lies beyond conformity. The realization of this hope is impeded for the earlier generation by internalized authority figures; for the present generation, it is obstructed by the need for status and approval in the peer group.

When a patient in a hospital has the underlying problem of loneliness, he tends to think of his fellow patients as his peers. Each patient, being more or less trapped by a need to belong, tends to form relationships with other patients. These relationships are based on "mutual loneliness" — pathological pull of the familiar — rather than on conscious choice. Caudill reports findings regarding the structure of closely knit groups of patients and its effect upon them.[3,4,5] We are greatly in need of data to help us determine whether nurses could render these situations more favorable for patients' emotional growth.

In private practice, where the patient does not have a peer group available to him, dependence on the nurse develops quickly. This dependence can have the qualities of a mother-child relationship or of a peer relationship. Since loneliness implies an early developmental arrest, dependence is to be expected and accepted, and the patient should be helped to use it as a step toward independence and interdependence.

It is useful to specify the limits of the relationship. A clear statement of fixed points helps the patient to recognize the necessary boundaries of a useful relationship. These limits need to be specific and to be stated simply, and they need to be adhered to because the patient will test them over and over again to check and recheck the sincerity, honesty, and integrity of the nurse.

In addition to providing contact and constant limits, each nurse ought to be able to offer the patient a procedure for working on the problems that arise in relation to the nursing situation. The nurse who spends eight hours with a patient will hear a good deal about his difficulties, hopes, and dreams. She cannot sit silently without responding in a human way. Her responses to the patient, verbal and otherwise, will therefore have a great deal to do with the alleviation or intensification of his problems. Procedure cannot be discussed adequately in a paper of this length, but I can say that there are opportunities to give constructive help to patients in all that goes on in a nursing situation: in the management of the situation; in the use of such customary nursing activities as bathing, feeding, dressing, and the like; in such socializing activities as conversing, card-playing, and the like; and in the therapeutic handling of terror, desperation, nightmares, hallucinations, and so on.

An understanding of the problem of loneliness suggests that what the patient needs is:

1. To experience and, therefore, to come to feel and know the active interest of mature persons and their attentive participation in his activities.
2. To secure the assistance of persons who are more mature and skillful than he is as he learns how to struggle with his problems.
3. To have a variety of opportunities to describe, interpret, and validate what is happening to him in a current situation.
4. To have contact with persons who can help him get in touch with other human beings, feel related to them, and work collaboratively and live productively with them.

References

1. Sullivan, H.S. *The Interpersonal Theory of Psychiatry,* edited by Helen S. Perry and Mary L. Gawel. New York, W.W. Norton and Co., 1953.
2. Riesman, David, and Others. *The Lonely Crowd: a Study of the Changing American Character.* New Haven, Conn., Yale University Press, 1950.
3. Caudill, William. Applied anthropology in medicine. In *Anthropology Today,* edited by A.L. Kroeber. Chicago, University of Chicago Press, 1953, pp. 771-806.
4. ____ and Others. Social structure and interaction processes on a psychiatric ward. *Am. J. Orthopsychiat.* 22:314-334, April 1952.
5. ____ and Stainbrook, Edward. Some covert effects of communication difficulties in a psychiatric hospital. *Psychiatry* 17:27-43, Feb. 1954.
6. Barnes, Djuna. *Nightwood.* New York, Harcourt Brace and Co., 1937.
7. Parsons, Talcott. *The Social System.* Chicago, Free Press, 1951.
8. Roth, Lillian. *I'll Cry Tomorrow.* New York, Frederick Fell, Inc., 1954.
9. Ruesch, Jurgen and Bateson, Gregory. *Communication: the Social Matrix of Psychiatry.* New York, W.W. Norton and Co., 1951.

Research in Nursing Therapy*

June Mellow

Reprinted from *The Improvement of Nursing Through Research*, The Catholic University of America Press, Washington, D.C., 1958.

For the past five years, I have been engaged in exploring and developing treatment techniques which are possible for nurses to use in working with schizophrenic patients. I have called this body of techniques nursing therapy. Since this term has gained some general usage in the field of psychiatric nursing, I would like to take this opportunity to explain how I use the concept and what some of its implications and ramifications are for the nurse's approach to the psychotic patient.

The psychotic patient, particularly the schizophrenic, may be viewed as someone who, among other things, has been deprived of some fundamental interpersonal experiences. As a result of these interpersonal deprivations, a state of emotional isolation develops in which the patient's ego is overwhelmed and the normal defense patterns are shattered. As a result, unconscious forces become the main determinants of the patient's thoughts and actions. In the acute phase of the psychotic breakdown, the patient urgently feels the need to reestablish his ego integrity and control. On the other hand, he feels terror-stricken that others will not understand the importance of his feelings or the reasons for his inability to control them. For this reason, much of the patient's speech and behavior is symbolic, so that his message can only be understood by those who are secure enough to accept and tolerate the force of his feelings.

It is my belief that the psychiatric nurse has an opportunity to assume certain well-defined therapeutic responsibilities for the patient. I feel that it is necessary to clarify and explore the use of the nurse as an active therapeutic agent.

Nursing therapy is a term used to describe a specific approach to the acutely ill schizophrenic patient when he is considered more or less unavailable to psychotherapy, with the treatment focusing on the nurse-patient relationship. During this critical phase of his illness, the patient may be likened to someone who has fallen into a strange and turbulent body of water; he urgently needs immediate help in his struggle to keep from drowning and to return to solid ground.

During this period, nursing therapy does not attempt to deal with the reasons for the patient's predicament but rather concentrates on the establishment of a corrective emotional relationship to enable him to rebuild his ego and reintegrate his personality. If his experiences in the acute phase of the illness are such that he is not able to build his ego by establishing meaningful contacts with another human being, the patient will often cease his struggle for return to reality and will surrender to the equilibrium of the chronic phase, which in itself provides relief from the turmoil of the acute stages. Thus, the intensive nurse-patient relationship attempts to provide for the patient a bridge to reality; a borrowed ego with roots that exist outside his illness. Essentially, the patient is overwhelmed; his ego shattered by his intense feelings of ambivalence — particularly of love and hate, independence and dependence towards the significant person or persons in his life. Usually, at the time when the ego is overwhelmed, there is a heightening, a skyrocketing of angry feelings towards the important people in his life. The angrier he gets at those he needs and is dependent upon, the more worthless he feels and the more emotionally isolated he becomes. There is a vicious circle here of anger, guilt, and worthlessness, and the patient wonders — how can anyone care about someone who has such angry thoughts and feelings? The anger is of such magnitude that it takes on magical omnipotence. The patient fears that his awful wishes to have something dreadful happen have caused it to happen. Frequently, we hear patients say they are to blame for many things that have happened or will happen, i.e., if we are out sick, they caused it.

One patient was angry at her family and felt they were in danger of dying. She said, "I hope my family is all right and hasn't been killed in an auto crash." Another, angry at a sister who had been a mother-substitute and who married and had children of her own, was very upset because this sister had gone to the movies. She told of her fear that the sister might be killed on the way to the movies and that her babies would burn to death at home. Another patient warned of how dangerous her anger was by saying that she was a black panther that stalked in the night.

It would seem likely that a person experiencing such feelings with such intensity, and with none of the usual defenses to handle them, is going to be in turmoil and is certainly going to be both frightened of people and frightening to people. All this leads to

*This work has been supported by the United States Public Health Service, #GN-4507 (C2) for the past two and a half years and has been conducted at the Massachusetts Mental Health Center, Boston, Massachusetts.

a terrifying sense of emotional isolation. Although he has few defenses to handle his feelings, he has plenty of psychotic defenses to keep us from getting close to him. Psychotic behavior and defenses are disturbing enough in themselves. They violate our esthetic sensibilities; they transgress many of our moral and social codes of conduct. Even more disturbing is the force and intent of his feelings that are so frequently upsetting to our own unconscious lives. There are many reasons, both in him and in us, that force him to keep us at a distance. Emotionally isolated as he is, disturbed as he is, and difficult as it is for us to reach him, contact can still be made with him. He brings to any therapeutic situation extreme problems of interpersonal relationships; but he also brings with him many possibilities and certainly an intense need for — as well as a fear of — a meaningful relationship. So it is in this realm of the problems and possibilities of interpersonal relationships as they are expressed in everyday living, in the continued contact of the on-going nursing situation, that nursing therapy takes place.

The nursing role affords many opportunities for the nurse to develop a close relationship with the patient. She sees that the patient is fed, dressed, bathed; she has the opportunity to satisfy regressive and dependency needs, provide controls and set limits. She is there to share in any crisis situation. These things can be done in such a way as to provide for the patient a new experience in interpersonal relationships that does not conform to the old patterns or to his psychotic concept of himself. Unfortunately, these things can also be done in such a way that he feels more frightened, more angry, more guilty, and more isolated.

What has been said here certainly is of concern to psychiatric nursing in general. The nurse wants the patient to feel accepted; she attempts to handle crisis situations with him so that he feels more comfortable, and so forth. So we might ask ourselves what the difference is between psychiatric nursing and nursing therapy. Primarily, the answer lies not in terms of differences of kind, neither in functions nor activities, but rather as a matter of differences of degree. Nursing therapy involves a greater amount of emotional commitment and responsibility to the patient; more struggling to understand the patient and to perceive his needs, and furthermore, a greater striving to understand one's own feelings in relation to the patient. The issue of heightened responsibility and emotional commitment to the patient — what the nurse feels towards the patient — is a crucial one, producing many anxieties in the nurse, especially when she has taken the patient with a long-range goal in mind. This is quite different from the way one feels when one is responsible for handling immediate situations on a day-to-day basis, but where one does not feel directly involved in the outcome of the patient's illness.

A number of problems arise for the nurse therapist because of her increased emotional commitment to the patient. Some of these arise from within herself and some are inherent in using this type of approach to a mentally sick patient. In supervising a number of trainees in nursing therapy, the following problems have appeared with considerable frequency:

1. *"The rescue phantasy."* A desire for a quick and immediate improvement or cure. When this does not occur, it is followed by feelings of inadequacy and guilt. At such times, the supervisor must give considerable support while pointing out the realities of the slow course of treatment;
2. *Over-identification with the patient.* A fusion of the trainee's feelings with the patient's feelings so that there is a loss of perspective and ego control and a feeling that the patient's emotions are the dominant force in the relationship. Going along with this, there is an inability on the trainee's part to separate her own feelings from the patient's feelings, and a sudden awareness of the similarity of some of her own dynamics and the patient's illness. At such times, the trainee's anxiety level is high and she will concentrate on her own needs or strive to sever the relationship;
3. *Fear of responsibility.* A concern that this new type of relationship will bring with it a greater responsibility than the trainee has ever experienced before. In past nursing relationships, no matter how giving or therapeutic a nurse might be, there were still many self-determined defensive mechanisms against a too close relationship which were socially sanctioned on the ward and by her fellow nurses. One of the commitments of this type of relationship which the trainee is entering into is the development of the ability to face these anxieties so the proper perspective can be maintained about one's own feelings and behavior in relation to the patient. Going along with these anxieties are the stresses that the new role involves in relation to the outcome of the patient's illness. In past nursing relationships, the interaction was limited to

actual physical and social interaction between patient and nurse. In this new relationship, the nurse feels a responsibility for the outcome of the patient's illness, even perhaps to the extent of continuing the relationship after the patient's discharge from the hospital; and

4. *Fear of aggression.* The trainee usually wishes to feel that the patient likes her and wants help. When hostilities are expressed, it is often difficult for the trainee to recognize or handle them.

The problems that arise from the nature of the therapeutic task which the nurse therapist is doing can best be discussed in terms of the three phases of the nurse-patient relationship.

The first of these is establishing contact and building a relationship; the second is handling the problems of the relationship once established; the third is resolving the dependency needs and handling the separation anxieties.

In the first phase, that of establishing contact and building a relationship, one of the biggest problems is that of communication. Somehow, the nurse must find a way to reach the patient. Frequently, during initial contacts, she may have to rely on nonverbal, disguised, and symbolic communication and try to communicate with him on the level of which he is capable. For example, Cathy, an acutely disturbed catatonic patient whom I worked with, was in seclusion. She would not talk when I first met her; I stayed in seclusion with her. After some time, she rather vaguely reached out her hand and I took hold of it. She held my hand and smiled very warmly; suddenly her eyes grew very cold and she twisted my hand before dropping it. She repeated this a few times. Then I took her role in this little game. I smiled; I reached out my hand; I looked at her coldly and then twisted her hand. I told her that two could play at this game; that it seemed she was trying to drive me away but I was not going to go. Then she began talking, wanting to know where she was and who I was.

Sometimes, in trying to establish contact with a very withdrawn and isolated person, when just the presence of another person is anxiety-provoking, one has to move very slowly in order to reach the patient. Jean, a young paranoid schizophrenic girl with somatic delusions, used to sit alone, hallucinating, giggling, and talking to the voices. She would not acknowledge my presence in any way other than to turn her head and talk more incoherently to the voices. I visited the ward each day just to sit with her — never too close — nor did I look at her directly. Sometimes, I made casual remarks such as, "It must be kind of lonely sitting there talking to people nobody can see but yourself." When she continued talking to the voices, I would say, "Well, I guess I have a lot of competition to get to talk to you, but I'll be back." After a few weeks, I asked her if she would like to get out of the ward and go with me to the occupational therapy department. She nodded in response. I took her through the department and showed her a few of the projects — painting, etc. I talked with her as if she were talking with me, that is, I made no demands on her for conversation nor did I let her non-participation affect my conversation. Then, for the first time in about four weeks, she spoke to me coherently. She said, "The pictures are very nice up here."

During this phase of the relationship, the nurse therapist tries to see if she can perceive the immediate emotional needs of the patient rather than exploring and investigating the clinical pathology. For example, Andrea, an acutely disturbed schizophrenic girl who was brought into the hospital by the police, said that she was fighting Communists; that they had discovered that she knew about one of their spy rings and she had been sent to the hospital as punishment. Andrea said that the hospital was a white slavery house; that I was the madame working for the chief of service who was keeping all these women in the hospital for his pleasure; that we were trying to feed her marijuana, and so forth. I paid no attention to these delusions other than to say that this was a hospital — although she had a right to her own opinion — but that it certainly must be frightening if she felt this way. Regarding her idea about marijuana in cigarettes — I would smoke one and say that it tasted all right to me but it was up to her whether she smoked or not. In general, I handled her delusional material in this manner. Her behavior was like that of an angry and rebellious child. I tried to satisfy some of these needs, but also set very definite limits. I remember when I first met her — I had taken her out of seclusion to eat breakfast. She threw all the food around the room. I gave her a tray and fed her. She screamed, kicked, and spit the food out. I told her to go ahead and spit it out — which she did. Then I gave Andrea another tray and she ate all of the food. She would be well behaved on the ward but several times caused riots in the cafeteria. We stopped her going there. After a while, we gave her the opportunity to use her own judgment and said, "If you feel you can handle the situation, you may go to the cafeteria; if not, we'll bring your tray to the ward." Usually, Andrea would use fairly good judgment and would say, "I'm too upset, I can't go upstairs." When she did go to the cafeteria, she behaved quite well.

There are many interesting facts about this case, but I will only touch on them lightly. One of the various roles in which she saw me was that of a madame. Then, she put me on the good side of her delusional system and said that I was a friendly spy investigating the slavery racket. (When I had all the information needed, we would escape together.) Andrea also saw me as her close girl friend. In actuality, the friend had become psychotic and committed suicide. This was one of the precipitating factors of Andrea's psychosis. She had never cried or grieved over this loss, and this is one of the things she did very intensely in our relationship. As she began to feel close to me, she feared that I would die or that I would go crazy. I think that one of the important factors in Andrea's recovery was her realization that she could be close without destroying me or herself.

This case illustrates very clearly how important it is for the nurse therapist to focus on the emotional needs of the patient rather than on the clinical pathology. When she was well, Andrea told me that she had reached a point in the relationship where she had to give up either me or her delusions. She gave up the delusions, and, although I did not know it, she thought she was giving me a great gift. Andrea said she had been able to do this because she felt that I was concerned about her, that she was important to me, and important to the ward. She explained her delusions by saying that she had felt she was a failure, and, being unable to handle this, she had made herself an important figure — someone crusading and fighting against Communism.

The second phase of the nurse-patient relationship consists of handling the problems in the relationship once it has been established — the problems the patient has in experiencing a close relationship, particularly his or her fears about it. In the early stages of the relationship, we try to reach the patient, to convey our acceptance of him, to satisfy some of his needs in such a way that he can move on, to set limits, and so forth. In other words, get across to him that we accept him, are concerned about him, and want to be helpful. Through these various experiences together the patient feels close to the nurse. It is at this point that the interpersonal difficulties he is having in living come into direct focus in the nurse-patient relationship.

For example, before this time, he might have expressed anger towards the nurse — but this would not have specific meaning in the relationship and, therefore, would be difficult to deal with. In the earlier phase of the relationship, the patient is angry at the whole world. In other words, much of the patient's behavior begins to take on meaning and can be worked on in the context of the relationship. How the nurse therapist deals with this behavior depends on the stage of the relationship. Let us take incontinence as an example, and see how it would be handled in various stages of the relationship. When I first met Cathy she was incontinent. She would sit and play in a puddle of urine. I tried to get her to take a bath but she would not budge. One day I said, "Sit there and play for ten minutes and then I'll be back. In ten minutes, you'll have had enough of this and can take a bath." When I returned and said, "Time's up, let's take a bath," Cathy came with me and I bathed her. Much later in the relationship, after not having been incontinent for some time, she became angry at me because I was seeing less of her. She acted out her anger towards me in this way. This time I did not bathe Cathy. I told her to change her clothes and then we would talk about it. She did, and when she returned said, "When I get angry at you there are a thousand things I do. I take other people's things, I wet the floor." We discussed this and decided that when she was angry, it would be much better if she could tell me directly rather than wetting the floor.

By allowing himself to get close to you, the patient is getting some of the things he needs from you. At the same time, the patient's fears are also increased as he thinks that he will be disappointed in this relationship as he has been in others. He fears most what he needs most. He begins to experience the intense feelings of love and hate towards you that he experienced towards other people who were important to him. One of the nurse's major therapeutic tasks is to help the patient with his overwhelming and conflicting feelings of love and hate towards her. This can be seen very dramatically, again with the patient Cathy. One day she was sitting quietly staring out the window. (This was in a later stage of the relationship.) She had put green paint around her eyes and looked very much like a ballet dancer made up to dance the part of death. She turned quietly and very matter-of-factly said, "I see you every day and I love you, but you must die." Then, she turned away and would not discuss it further. It seemed as if this were fact — that it would happen. The next day when I went to the ward, she was ranting and raving in seclusion. She said that I had killed her; that she had killed me; that I had turned her into a bedbug, a whore; that I had raped her, and so forth. I told Cathy that I did not think sex was the issue, but that she was afraid of getting close to me. She said, "I've always been afraid of getting close to you." Then she shouted, "Love is destruction! I am destruction! I destroy everything!" I think this patient was particularly afraid of getting close to anyone as she had lost two brothers and a sister who had all become mentally ill and had never returned from the hospital.

I think that any help the nurse can give the patient in working out these intense and contradictory feelings he has towards her, especially as they relate to getting close to the nurse, can be very useful in helping to restore and rebuild his ego. When the patient has the security of being able to master some of these feelings towards one person, he is better prepared to relate to others; to start exploring and understanding some of the reasons he became ill; to look at himself in view of how he relates to others and see some of the things he himself does to ruin his interpersonal relationships. When he reaches this point, we can say that he is ready to withstand some of the anxieties of psychotherapy.

The third or terminal phase of the nurse-patient relationship consists of dealing with dependency feelings and separation anxieties. All along, the nurse therapist has tried to help the patient with dependency by (1) allowing him to be dependent on her in areas where he felt that he must be, and (2) by trying, at the same time, to prepare him to take over some of these functions himself. At the same time, she supports the patient in every way in those things that he can do for himself. This may sometimes be done in very small ways. For example, if the nurse feeds the patient and the next time he reaches for the spoon himself, then the nurse would encourage the patient to feed himself. This can be done through other tasks such as dressing, going to occupational therapy by himself, and through helping him relate to others. She always tries to find and support what is healthy or adult in the patient. The nurse has to watch, particularly in this kind of situation, that she does not encourage the patient's dependency; otherwise, it can become a very hostile kind of dependency.

The patient is gradually prepared for separation. The amount of time the nurse spends with him depends on his need and the realities of the situation. When the patient is acutely ill, the nurse may see him three or four hours a day; as he improves, it may be as little as twenty minutes a day. After his discharge, the nurse may continue to see the patient in order to help him in his adjustment to family and community life. Here, it is wise for the nurse to continue in a supportive role, helping the patient with such things as reality testing rather than opening up the whole area of personality structure and questioning why he is the way he is, as this is in the realm of psychotherapy. As the patient begins to repeat the experience of gaining mastery over himself in the community as he did in the hospital, he will no longer have need of the nurse.

I have tried to present a rough sketch of an approach to the treatment of acutely ill schizophrenic patients which I am currently studying as a nurse. Many research questions remain to be solved, but the results to date indicate that this is a promising avenue of investigation.

Let's Talk It Over

Theresa G. Muller, R.N., M.A.

Ms. Muller is Director of Nurses, Sheppard and Enoch Pratt Hospital, Towson, Maryland.

Reprinted from *The Dynamics of Human Relationships*, Vol. 133, No. 12, December 1959.

You will readily acknowledge the difficulties encountered in acquiring satisfactory understanding of the available concepts on the dynamics of human relationships which foster or hinder effective communications in nursing. However, you might be reminded of similar feelings about other nursing subjects also requiring considerable effort and time before they are properly assimilated and further translated into appropriate action. For instance, you may remember the very slight degree of familiarity you had with human anatomy before going into nursing where you were required to learn the specific identification of innumerable anatomical parts — parts which had always been there but came into existence for you when you became aware of them. However, even then you found yourself unable to recall readily the knowledge necessary to understanding further the living functions of the parts as interrelated bodily systems affected by disease or emotional disturbances. Your introduction to anatomical terms was merely a foundation for a never-ending series of applications in better understanding the nursing needs of patients with varying disabilities.

Just so, you will find your study of the dynamics of human relationships and communications. I have frequently been told about the difficulties experienced by those who find the subject interesting but not readily understood and therefore voice their concern over the need for clearer presentations. In this connection I well remember the time when an instructor of obstetrical nursing had asked me to read and comment on a book presented to her while on an assignment in China, *The Secret of the Golden Flower*. It gave a common basis for psychological understanding in the teaching of oriental Taoism and the occidental similarities of Carl G. Jung. Though written in English the book to me was like a foreign language. However, I was intrigued by the beauty of the shadowy possibilities and wanted to know more about these. As time passed I found myself attuned to many helpful sources for clarification, and herein lies the secret of any continuing growth in understanding hitherto unknown matters. We are privileged to go no further when faced with the painful necessity to become involved in order to learn a difficult subject. On the other hand we may accept as a challenge opportunities to work on nebulous new concepts until they are crystallized into some meaningful form, thereby becoming available for practical application.

We might consider a singular human tendency — the one which urges us to seek an authority to free us from inevitable feelings of inadequacy. Here we must be on guard against intense dependency needs which are likely to blind us and thus make it difficult for us to distinguish authoritativeness arising from superior skill and knowledge from an imposed authoritarianism stifling our individual right or freedom. Unless we give some thought to these distinctions we may find ourselves succumbing to the influence which promises to save us from the pain of self-involvement only to find ourselves becoming less and less adequate as individuals secure enough in our human relationships to communicate spontaneously with patients and associates.

It seems as though our professional education has relied far too much on didactic teaching unrelated to practice. But even when the two are brought together we may not be attuned to assimilate the implications unless the knowledge and skill of an authority are related to the acknowledged need of the learner. Without a two-way process words are exchanged without relevant meanings and skills are acquired as mechanical imitations of observed performance. This will explain why our reliance on spokesmen from other fields fails to provide the important identifications with the practice which these spokesmen have never performed in a nursing capacity. When we come to realize this we might then be encouraged to communicate with our professional associates as a shared experience with respect for what each is trying to do. Faith in our effective experiences thereby establishes true professional competence.

Need for Objective Appraisal

Our nursing practice is founded on associations relevant to what we see, hear, smell, taste, and touch. These associations depend not only upon the soundness of our eyes, ears, nose, tongue, and skin as sensory avenues for the reception of stimuli but also on the functional readiness of each of these senses to select appropriate stimuli at any given time. Our communications with each other then will be affected by the different ways in which we shut out or distort the present with barriers of the past or any current unrealistic expectations.

Sometimes we tend to make common observations similar to the way we look at a picture in two dimensions without realizing the possibility of a three-dimensional perspective. Unfortunately, such a two-dimensional plane of flatness may be erroneously maintained as desirable objectivity. By way of illustration, I am reminded of the report given at a scientific meeting where the discussion centered on the site of facial herpetic lesions following an operation for trigeminal neuralgia. Medical students had learned to expect unilateral lesions and thereby failed to see any lesions on the other side until they were specifically pointed out to them. All of us tend to have similar experiences. I recall a social evening where one of the games involved a search for fifteen plainly observable objects in the room. The silver thimble on the chrome-finished light fixture, the white button in a white dish, the toothpick on the natural wood frame of a picture, the brown-handled kitchen knife blending in with a similarly colored edge of the rug were invisible to all of us until specifically noted and, in most instances, until we received help from one another.

Further illustrations may be cited of a study on the placebo effect of the personalities of the dispensers of drugs. In one instance the drug had been generally considered effective by comparison with the effects of a placebo given to a control group. However, on the placement of a renewal order for the drug it was disclosed that by error the placebo had been sent first. Thus the favorable results obtained by the placebo had come from the confidence generated by the favorable expectations of the personnel administering it rather than from the drug itself. Another possibility of the distortion of the observable phenomena was revealed in an experimental study where the physiological effects of a drug had been considered fairly constant, but were eventually affected by changes in the psychological climate of the ward, fostered by the anxiety-provoking conflict among the nursing personnel when they were asked to make a preferential rating of patients according to a scale of likes and dislikes. Here the nurses were confronted with an ethical concern about admitting distinctive preferences with regard to any patient. This stereotype of the good or fair nurse then stands in the way of realistic appraisals based on our feelings toward others.

Thus we see the necessity for becoming more fully aware about how our feelings distort the reality of conditions, people, and things. However, we also need to acknowledge those feelings which are true indicators of existence and thereby give proper nuances to sensory impressions. This will keep us from denying the existence of a shadow as a distorted reflection of something and thereby help us in distinguishing between the shadow and its substance. As we become aware of how our mind's eye tends to invest the immediate impression with past experiences, we no longer maintain a flat view of sameness when conditions have changed. An extreme illustration to show the effects of an incorrect assessment of nursing practice came to my attention when a procedure for shock therapy included as routine equipment a step-stool for a short physician, and its unsuitability for a tall physician was not readily noted.

Dangers of Didactic Approach

In similar ways we will find our communications with one another about the dynamics of human relationships in nursing maintained on a didactic level instead of associated with enlivening human values. We then need to become aware of our facility to lull ourselves into a false sense of accomplishment by giving attention to minute details of mechanical performance without a corresponding concern about human values. This becomes understandable when we realize that a meaningful application of the subject of human behavior to our own selves inevitably reveals unwelcome insights and arouses negative feelings.

Any by-passing of the painful task of facing up to ourselves imposes a greater discomfort in a continuing sense of inadequacy. We can, however, make the necessary effort to accept the challenge of stepping into the unfamiliar territory of new concepts. Even then, we do not readily note our defenses against a difficulty in learning about a complex subject. These defenses are generally voiced as resistances to elusive meanings and a plea for an easier way. Such protective concern about exercising our mental faculties will continue to keep us from comprehending the significance of a communication. All of us have had experiences which put us in touch with a source of information beyond our immediate grasp only to find at a later time that its meaning is revealed through thoughtful reflection on an appropriate relationship.

We see then that the subject of human behavior is part of our everyday concern and is never learned once and for all time. By giving due thought to this, our nursing tasks take on greater significance as creative experiences which vary according to our contacts with an infinite variety of human beings who differ also in degrees and kinds of physical and mental abilities and disabilities.

Aspects of Communication

Our interprofessional relationships are founded largely on verbal communication. A common meeting ground then needs to be identified, for each profession has a distinctive vocabulary of its own. It is not enough for nurses to be able to communicate with each other by using terminology which is understandable chiefly because of its context in nursing. Genuine satisfactions are derived in proportion to the time and effort expended in learning how to communicate with members of related professional groups.

We acknowledge that nursing practice is founded on our ability to make relevant observations and understand the implications for prescribed treatment. We also find that a surface manifestation reveals only part of the basis of any behavior. The less apparent aspects stem from our basic needs for survival and significance when interplay of these driving forces moves us into ever-changing kinds and degrees of negative and positive reactions with each other, and has become identified as mental dynamisms normally expressed as identification substitution, compensation, sublimation, compromise, and rationalization. Those with pathological connotation are known as fixation, projection, displacement, and regression. Such areas of behavior dynamics are only partially disclosed by the behavior of a person.

So we need to acknowledge that effective communications are not established on the basis of set responses. Our daily contacts are ever-changing and unpredictable and therefore have to be assessed anew before we react to them. Nevertheless we do draw on what we have previously learned and do make relevant associations to the new situation in proportion to our creative abilities. Such abilities depend on our own experiences but the experiences of another can also be vicariously shared as sources of understanding.

Subsequent articles will continue by illustrating these concepts by specific applications to our personal and professional lives.

Self-Concept and the Schizophrenic Patient

Shirley Smoyak, R.N., M.S.

Reprinted from *Nursing World*, Vol. 133, No. 7, July 1959.

Two factors in parental behavior, nondirectness and the switch phenomenon, contributed to the development of schizophrenia in John, a young patient in a mental hospital.

When this boy was dealing with the task of constructing his self-concept, his parents' attitudes and actions interfered seriously with his arriving at a healthy picture of himself. In this article will be discussed how these factors operated to disturb John so seriously that, at the age of 14, he tried to commit suicide. Verbatim data from the psychiatric interview will be used. At the time this article was written, John had been visited by the author for 2 one-hour sessions weekly over a period of seven months.

The child develops his concept of self from reflected appraisals of his parents and others in his environment. The parental appraisals of the child are of primary importance in the construction of the self-concept. From the rewards and punishments which his parents give, the child begins to see himself as a person who at times is good, and at other times, bad. Sullivan describes the *good-me* as "the beginning personification which organizes experience in which satisfactions have been enhanced by rewarding increments of tenderness, which come to the infant because the mothering one is pleased with the way things are going. . . ."[1]

Bad-me, on the other hand, states Sullivan, is "beginning personification which organizes experience in which increasing degrees of anxiety are associated with behavior involving the mothering one. . . ."[2]

John, now 24 years old, has been a patient in a state mental hospital for the past 10 years. He describes his childhood this way: "I wasn't ever punished; I was gently, subtly, verbally criticized. My mother babied me — she would always smile that way. I don't know if I'm a babied brat or just human nature. I never knew if that smile meant 'You're a nice baby.' Maybe she meant it just as a pleasant, normal reaction. Maybe not. Maybe it was an appreciative smile, but it could have been a babying smile."

The outstanding characteristics of John's mother were vagueness and subtlety. Her responses to the child could not be categorized as meaning good or bad. As the boy puts it: "I never knew just where I stood." He recalls an incident with his mother which further illustrates this nondirectness.

"I can remember the park where she used to take me," he states. "It was nice and we used to play cards. I would win every time and she would smile as if I were a very good player. But I never knew if I was really good or if she was letting me win. There's a scientific reason for card winning — the other person, wittingly or unwittingly, lets you win. I don't know what the case was with her."

This situation of never knowing, or not being able to formulate a self-concept, is extremely anxiety-provoking. It is a terrifying, panic-producing experience not to know who or what you are. In discussing the subject of playing cards, the nurse said, "John, what would happen if you lost?" His anxiety rose rapidly, and he shouted, "I'd go to pieces! I wouldn't know who I was!"

John's father also participated in this nondirect, vague pattern of relating to his son. The patient describes how he used to play checkers with his father, again winning every time, and again not knowing exactly how good or bad he was at the game.

In addition to this nondirectness, however, the patient's father used another, more confusing pattern: the switch phenomenon. At one time he would make one appraisal or take one course of action; but another time he switched to the opposite side. For example, his father would tell John that he was intelligent, a good scholar, and possessed brains. A few minutes later he might tell John he was "a stupid boy and just a good-for-nothing." The father would tell the boy that to succeed he had to work hard and long, and do what he was told. On the other hand, he would also tell John that all he needed was to be intelligent and outsmart others in order to succeed.

At times John's father became openly angry, using harsh, loud speech in his rage. When John tried this outlet for anger, he was told to shut up, that such behavior was insolent. The patient remembers his father having strict rules about what was "manly" and what was not. Yet the father participated in such unmanly actions as rubbing the patient's back when he was ill and using "very kind, syrupy-soft words."

Smoking was considered manly or masculine, but John's smoking was frowned upon. He describes the smoking this way: "My father never said, 'Don't smoke,' but on the other hand, he never said I should. He doesn't smoke at all, and I have the feeling that he doesn't want me to. I've asked him to bring me cigarettes and he always says he will bring them, but never does. I can't figure it out."

This switch phenomenon has prevented John from developing a clear concept of self. As soon as he had categorized some trait or behavior under *good-me,* the switch occurred and the trait or behavior was characterized as belonging under *bad-me.* Possessing brains and being intelligent was at one moment desirable, at the next moment undesirable.

He was not permitted to validate his actions, gestures, and words. In the absence of validation, John used autistic invention to explain what was going on. Being an alert and bright boy, he had to use his mental capacity to explain the situations in which he found himself. When he attempted from time to time to explain what he meant, his father would cut him off, and his mother would give him no answer. Not being able to validate would leave him helpless. Rather than be helpless, John employed autism to make himself comfortable and provide explanations.

During one visit, the nurse remarked, "It seemed as though you had to do a lot of figuring out by yourself as to what was meant." John's reply was, "Either that, or take if for granted. He told me not to give him any of my 'lip.' My reaction was to be quiet, as if I knew I was wrong. I would become more wrong if I questioned his statement. To be honest, I didn't know what to reply. He had the upper hand."

During a previous discussion, the patient had stated, "If I couldn't figure out something, I would make up an explanation. Then I would say it over and over and over until I really believed it thoroughly. Like I told myself that my mother loved me and that's why she smiled. The trouble is, when I talk to you, I wonder if it's that easy."

When John's efforts to seek explanations by means of consensual validation failed, he turned to autistic invention as a tool in finding answers. The nurse, in talking with the patient, is trying to reverse the process. Over the months, more and more autistic thinking has been replaced by validation. At present John is confronting his father with the request that he make a definite stand on smoking. So far, his father has not done so, and still is evading the issue. John's comment about this is, "I'm beginning to wonder who's sick around here."

References

1. H.S. Sullivan, *The Interpersonal Theory of Psychiatry* (New York, W.W. Norton and Company, 1953), pp. 161-2.
2. *Ibid.*, p. 162.

A Therapeutic Milieu for Borderline Patients

Estelle I. Carleton and Joan Canatsy Johnson

Miss Carleton (Kansas City, Mo., General Hospital of Nursing; B.S., M.S., University of Colorado) is director of nursing services at the Mental Health Center of America. Mrs. Johnson (St. Luke's School of Nursing, Denver; B.S., University of Denver) was formerly head nurse at the Center. She is now at the University of Washington in Seattle working for her masters degree.

Reprinted from *The American Journal of Nursing*, Vol. 61, January 1961.

The Mental Health Center of America, believed to be the first free, private, psychiatric hospital in the United States, was opened in Denver, Colorado on July 1, 1958. The Center is on the grounds of the Ex-Patient's Sanatorium, a hospital which served for 50 years as a rehabilitation center for patients with tuberculosis and chronic disease. When medical advancements and improved care reduced the number of beds needed for these patients, the board of trustees decided to convert the extra buildings for use in the badly needed area of treatment of the mentally ill.

Although sponsored by a Jewish organization, the hospital accepts, from anywhere in the country, patients who fit the criteria for admission. Every part of the patient's hospitalization is free, including room, meals, and treatment. The hospital is supported by donations from groups and individuals all over the United States.

This hospital is unique also in that only a particular kind of patient is treated here — the "borderline" patient. Borderline is a designation for that group of illnesses which fall between the psychoneurotic and the psychotic. These are often referred to as pre-psychotic, ambulatory or latent schizophrenias, severe neurotic, and pseudoneurotic schizophrenias.

Borderline patients may appear psychoneurotic, presenting obsessive-compulsive, hysterical, or psychosomatic defenses. But they can also manifest paranoid states and depressive reactions. Both neurotic and psychotic symptoms are present and can be demonstrated by careful clinical evaluation. Sometimes the psychotic symptoms can be observed in a diagnostic interview, but often they are not apparent except on psychological testing.

The outstanding characteristic of the borderline patient is a weak ego, and treatment goals are centered on strengthening the ego. Knight has described three attitudes which a healthy person must maintain: "(1) self-esteem, (2) a sense of responsibility for his behavior, and (3) a feeling of maintaining inner controls over himself."[1] The loss of any of these is a realistic danger for the borderline patient. Knight believes that a therapeutic, open-hospital setting is important in helping the borderline patient regain or strengthen these attitudes.

It was to meet such a need that the Mental Health Center of America was established as a small, open-door hospital offering a type of milieu therapy. Its milieu offers the patient a therapeutic environment and therapeutic relationships 24 hours a day. The treatment program includes individual psychoanalytically oriented psychotherapy, group psychotherapy, occupational therapy, recreational therapy, and intensive contact with all staff personnel. The amount of time each patient devotes to each part of the program is individually determined, according to the patient's tolerance and needs. Tranquilizers are used as adjunctive therapy, but we have no electric shock, no insulin therapy, no hydrotherapy, and no locked wards.

Physical Facilities

Patients' rooms and staff offices are on the first floor of a remodeled building. Occupational therapy and recreational facilities are in the basement. An auditorium and other recreational facilities are in an adjacent building, and spacious grounds allow for other kinds of recreation including vegetable and flower gardens initiated and cared for by some of the patients. Administrative offices, kitchen, and dining room facilities are in yet another building and are shared with patients in the Ex-Patient's Sanatorium building.

About half the patients' rooms are single and half are double. They are furnished with modern, hotel-type furniture rather than conventional hospital furniture, and patients are encouraged to add pictures, draperies, bookcases, and the like, of their own choosing. The hospital atmosphere has some of the flavor of a college dormitory.

The staff includes two psychiatrists, one part-time clinical psychologist, one part-time psychiatric social worker, one occupational therapist, four nurses, and two nursing assistants. This size staff is considered the very minimum necessary to provide adequate treatment for the 14 patients in the hospital. The team concept is in effect here and there is frequent sharing of roles. For example, one of the group therapy groups is led by a psychiatrist and a staff nurse; the other is led by the head nurse and the psychiatric social worker who also does casework with the patients' families. The clinical psychologist does the testing, but also has some patients in therapy.

For patients to be admitted to this hospital, they must meet certain definite criteria. They must be (1) referred by a physician, (2) between 21 and 50 years of age, (3) ambulatory, (4) in the borderline category, (5) able to function in an open-hospital setting, and (6) able to profit from treatment on an inpatient basis in six to eighteen months.

Although the five men and nine women who are patients here now are from nine different states and vary in age from 21 to 38 years, they make up a fairly homogeneous group. Nearly all of them fall into the "above average to superior" range of intellectual functioning and most of them have had education beyond high school. All have shown signs of illness for several years and many of them have had previous psychiatric treatment including hospitalization and shock therapy. A few of these patients have had an acute schizophrenic episode, but have reconstituted so that they again fall into the borderline category.

Nursing Role in the Milieu

Some of the nursing functions are quite conventional and include observation and recording, passing medications, and carrying out treatments. But these functions take up a relatively small amount of the nurses' time on each shift. During the patients' waking hours, each nurse has from four to six hours which she spends with the patients.

An important function of the nurse in this milieu — one which is generally accepted as a nursing function but is not yet carried out in many psychiatric hospitals — is using herself in a therapeutic relationship with the patients.

Since the borderline patient has a weak ego, many of the ego functions — such as reality testing, mediating between the superego and the id, and utilizing healthy defense mechanisms — are impaired, sometimes grossly. The relationships these patients have with other people are rigid and inadequate, and their own self-concepts are narcissistic and depreciatory. Through her relationships with patients, the nurse tries to create for them new learning experiences which will help them learn to trust other people, acquire self-confidence and self-esteem, and progress from dependence to interdependence. The nurse also helps patients identify and work through the practical aspects of what they learn in psychotherapy, for example, learning to work or play with a group of peers.

Another function of the nurse is connected quite directly to relating therapeutically with the patients — enforcing the hospital structure. Since the hospital is unlocked, there are few rules and few restrictions on the patients' activities. The staff has attempted to keep the structure at a minimum. However, there are some rules which patients need to abide by, such as getting up on time and being present for required activities. As with all contacts with patients, enforcing rules can be done therapeutically or punitively, and the way in which it is done can have an important effect on the patients' treatment.

Problems in Nursing Care

Having a very small hospital with a selected borderline population has presented a variety of problems which affect the nursing care of the patients. The ward structure is such that there is rather close contact between patients and staff over a long period of time. This close contact in such a small group appears to intensify the transference situation. The nurses are quite obviously seen as mother figures, and patients view each other as siblings competing against one another. Numerous situations arise in which the nurse uses herself and her relationship with a patient in order to help him learn to share her with others, or to be less dependent. The nurse must constantly guard against favoritism which would cause more problems.

Connected with the transference situation is the ambivalence which most of the borderline patients feel toward relationships with others. Although they need and long for close, giving relationships, they resist attempts by other people to form relationships with them and they express a great deal of suspicion and hostility toward those who make such attempts. Obviously, this strong admixture of negative and positive feelings makes it very difficult for a therapist to establish lasting, positive transference. The ambivalence that the patient may express toward the nurse therapist as a mother figure is trying and often quite discouraging.

These patients have difficulty believing that someone is really interested in them and cares about them. They do not accept this as a matter of course and the people who are involved in their treatment must do more than go out of their way to prove their interest. To lessen the distance between staff and patients, the nursing staff encourages informality. Nurses do not wear caps, and both nurses and patients are called by their first names. We have found that this does not endanger therapeutic effectiveness and seems much more natural in these long-term relationships.

One of the characteristics of a borderline patient is a tendency to regress. Many of them would like to go to bed and be cared for. Just being in a hospital often encourages regression and active steps must be taken to counteract it. Anti-regressive measures focus on encouraging patients to assume responsibility for their own treatment; however, these patients do show a definite reluctance to assume much of the responsibility. This reluctance is a byproduct of their regression, passivity, and withdrawal. We have some specific methods which we use to discourage regression — having the patients keep their own rooms and persons neat, making them get up by a specified hour in the morning, get to their own milieu activities on time, and pick up their own medications from the office at specified times. Some of the patients are encouraged to hold part-time jobs in the community.

One of the major roles of the nurse is to encourage group activities. Although these patients have many things in common — their illness, their common backgrounds, interpersonal problems, and feelings — they resist identification with each other, are very intolerant of one another's problems and characteristics, and do not readily support or try to help each other with their problems. To the staff, they often appear as little islands. A nurse may go from one to another, hearing identical fears and problems. Yet she will be unable to get them to share these with each other or even believe that anyone else could be having any of the same problems. Among the few times the patients function as a group is when they are united against the staff or hospital structure, or at a time of crisis such as the early discharge of another patient who cannot benefit from further treatment at the hospital.

Almost all the group activities, such as picnics or skiing trips, which are initiated by the staff are met with resistance, but the patients are unable to organize or agree on anything themselves. They are much better able to join spontaneous group activities.

Group therapy and ward meetings are structured ways to encourage group participation. Around the hospital, the patients often use the nurse as a focus for group participation and will join a group where she is present. Although she may try not to take too active a part, it is almost impossible for her to remain very inactive, for the patients direct much of the conversation to her or to others by way of her, and constantly look to her for approval and support. Increased ability to participate in groups is a sign of improvement in most of the patients.

Although the general tone of the hospital is permissive, in the time it has been open the staff has found that they cannot be as permissive as they would like to be. Limit-setting, or enforcing the hospital structure as we call it, has been found to be an important part of the milieu. The patients need consistent, reasonable limits; and although they resist being made to follow rules, they respond favorably to them, showing increased movement in therapy and more confidence in the staff. The structure is emphasized to a greater extent with patients who tend to be more disorganized, such as those who have had acute psychotic episodes.

Staff Problems

Those who work closely with patients of any kind are aware of the dangers of overidentification. It is not too infrequent for a nurse who spends several hours a day with a patient to become so involved that she is unable to participate objectively in the patient's treatment. She may, for instance, take the patient's side against the doctor for a seeming injustice. The patients are prone to manipulate and will play any and all staff members against each other if they can. Nurses may fall into the trap of helping a patient act out in a neurotic way against authority if they are not alert or if they do not understand the reason for particular restrictions or treatment plans.

Even with such a small hospital and staff, adequate communication is a problem. Consistency is an important aspect of every patient's treatment and this means that each staff member must be aware of all plans and changes in the general structure and in each patient's treatment plan.

Realizing these problems, the staff tries to minimize them by frequent sharing of ideas and problems at team meetings, staff conferences, and informal contacts during the day. The doctors share information freely with the nursing staff and listen to what the nurses have to offer.

We found very little published material about borderline patients and much of what we know about them now has been gained through our own experiences. During the first year, we had to differentiate between problems which came up because the hospital was new and the staff unaccustomed to working together, and those which were related to the milieu and the kind of patient we were treating.

The Mental Health Center of America was set up as a pilot project for the first year. Statistics about admissions and discharges are still too meager to be meaningful, but the hospital has proved its worth to the people involved in it.

References

1. Knight, R.P. Management and psychotherapy of the borderline schizophrenic patient. In *Psychoanalytic Psychiatry and Psychology*, ed. by Robert P. Knight and Cyrus R. Friedman. (Austen Riggs Center, Publications, Vol. 1) New York, International Universities Press, 1954, p. 115.

Coping with Chronic Helpfulness*

Sheila Rouslin, M.S.

Ms. Rouslin is Clinical Specialist in Psychiatric Nursing, Rutgers University, New Brunswick, New Jersey.

Reprinted from *Mental Hospitals*, October 1961.

"For years a mental patient who gave his orders in Polish drove a horse around the grounds to pick up trash," read a recent short newspaper story. "Recently, the patient was transferred. Now, officials say, they can't find anyone the horse can understand."

Nobody even remotely familiar with public mental hospitals will find that story unlikely. The quiet, cooperative, "helpful" patient is a fixture in hospitals which are all too short of paid staff. A typical example is an "indispensable" woman patient who, for 20 our of her 22 years of hospitalization, had been on the same ward — an admission ward. She did ward work from the day of her admission and soon took over the kitchen, saying that it was hers. Through the years, staff records speak of her as "assuming responsibility," "ambitious," "cooperative," "industrious," "dependable," and "very helpful."

Such patients become very useful in meeting the work needs of the hospital, an observation made by Greenblatt[1] and others. For instance, a psychiatric nurse wanted to have a series of therapeutic interviews with a patient who worked in the laundry. Said the charge attendant, "That patient will have to come off your list...it will cause too much trouble with Mr. X, the business manager, who is in charge of the laundry." The patient, it turned out, was an integral part of the laundry operation; he was well enough to assume a good deal of responsibility — yet he remained a patient.

It is not that the psychiatric hospital gives tacit approval to a pathological pattern because of its economic needs. What does happen is that the hospital, failing to recognize the behavior pattern as pathological, unwittingly reinforces the very problem which originally caused the patient to be hospitalized.

After conducting studies of patients who were considered valuable workers, we characterized this behavior pattern as "chronic helpfulness." It was found to exist in a substantial number of such patients. The initial uncontrolled clinical observations were confirmed by two systematic investigations.[2]

*Revised version of a paper read at the 117th Annual Meeting of the APA, May 1961, Chicago, Ill.

The Chronic Helper's Behavior Pattern

Operationally, the behavior pattern works as follows: the person has an unmet goal — to be liked — and this produces anxiety; he constantly does things for others in order to be liked; people expect him to be helpful and seek his help, which he gives. At this point, he changes his pattern. He may relax his helpfulness and seek a more mutual relationship, even exhibiting dependence on somebody else; or he may feel rejected because he is "being taken for granted;" or he may expect special privileges or favors in return for the help he gives. The other person, made anxious by the changed behavior pattern, rejects the chronic helper, who becomes anxious again and "feels used."

(We must distinguish here between chronic helpfulness and spontaneous assistance to others. The latter lacks the "demand" quality and is prompted by "wanting to do" rather than by "must do" motivation. The person who offers spontaneous assistance usually feels some satisfaction, whereas the end point for the chronic helper is to "feel used.")

Persons exhibiting this behavior pattern hold themselves in low self-regard. Sullivan[3] defined a person's low self-regard as a "...personification (which) is not very estimable by comparison with his personification of significant other people." It is accompanied by uncomfortable anxiety, which the person tries to minimize by camouflaging his low self-regard through indirect operations. Thus the chronic helper seems self-assured in that he takes on huge responsiblities on behalf of other people, while his unconscious purpose is to increase his self-regard.

To quote Sullivan again:

> "...there is a large number of people who appear to go to rather extraordinary lengths to get themselves imposed on, abused, humiliated, and what not; but as you get further data, you discover that this quite often pays — in other words, they get things they want. And the things everybody wants are satisfaction and security from anxiety. Thus these people who get themselves abused and so on are indirectly getting other people involved in doing something useful in exchange."

Quite often, however, it does not pay. The time comes when this compensating pattern no longer works, and repeated rejections lead to unbearable helplessness and anxiety. At this point, the chronic helper becomes a hospital patient.

The Problem Exemplified

One such patient entered the hospital after the death of her aunt — the only person with whom she "could be helpless" — and a series of rejections from the man with whom she had been living. Of her man, she said, "I did everything for him. He tells me a story; I believe him, then he does the opposite. And I say, 'What a fool I am.'" About her family and friends she said, "Nobody wants me for anything but service." Describing her anxiety following the death of her aunt (which occurred during a period when she had temporarily given up her boy friend), she said, "I punish myself for seeing and doing for other people when they don't see me and don't do for me. The hospital is a sanctuary for me," she said, adding that it gave her somebody to talk to.

It was obvious, however, that this was not the only thing the hospital provided. This chronic helper, who had been rejected in her private life, became exceedingly helpful to the patients and the ward personnel. She was always the one who set the tables for meals, did the dishes, cleaned the dayroom, listened to and advised other patients about their problems. The ward personnel unwittingly reinforced her pattern. When she did not volunteer for ward work, she was always assigned. She was asked to do special chores; ward personnel depended on her, and labelled her a "good," a "cooperative," and a "helpful" patient. In using the service she so willingly offered, they supported her pathology. Her central problem was finally formulated through group and individual counseling with the psychiatric nurse.

Another patient, with a similar pattern of chronic helpfulness, began to feel "used" when the ward personnel either rejected her help or rejected her as soon as she made overtures toward dependence. She would become fulminatingly self-abusive and self-destructive, saying, "I don't really want to kill myself, but I can't stop" — in the same sense that she could not stop herself from being chronically helpful. This dependent condition forced the staff to support her. Ward personnel then would solicit and accept her help to appease her, thus reactivating and nourishing her helpfulness pattern until again driven to reject her. This staff-patient interaction resembled a treadmill, turning in the continuous, unbroken line of a circle.

The Two Sides of Work Therapy

This illustrates that although work has a therapeutic potential, it may have an untherapeutic potential as well if used with the wrong patient, as noted by Greenblatt and others.[4] Which potential will be realized depends on the nature of the patient's problem. For the patient with a pattern of chronic helpfulness, the performance of and praise for hospital duties reinforces the pattern, thereby thwarting the opportunity to explore the source of his difficulties.

Because of the widely accepted therapeutic potential of work and the hospital's own need for assistance, the problem of the chronically helpful patient and the problem of the hospital merge in a symbiotic relationship under the guise of therapy. Both problems remain unsolved because the patient, at last in a situation where his pathology is partly successful, has no incentive to get out of the hospital or even to recognize the nature of his difficulty, and the hospital, because the patient remains institutionalized, has an increased financial burden.

The existence of this pattern in a substantial number of patients who are considered to be valuable workers implies that there is a reason why a patient becomes a valuable worker. His behavior has purpose and meaning and can be understood. Since chronic helpfulness is used to compensate for the underlying low self-regard, there is concomitant anxiety. These patients use work to reduce their anxiety and by doing so prevent investigation of its source. There is a strong possibility that they will remain chronically helpful — and hospitalized. The triangle of low self-regard, anxiety, and chronic helpfulness will remain.

The therapeutic plan with such patients would be to remove all opportunities for ward work, and thus allow the underlying anxiety to come forth. Its source, the patient's low self-regard, then could be explored. According to our findings, length of hospitalization and the number of admissions have no bearing on the initial (prehospital) existence of the pattern. This means that the hospital staff has an obligation to become aware of this pathological pattern in newly admitted patients before they become too comfortable in their sick role.

Comfort, for the chronically helpful patient, yields to chronic illness — another example of the "institutionalization" of patients. This happens because of the widely held view of work as "therapeutic" coupled with the hospital's own financial difficulties in employment of personnel. Ward and administrative staffs must be able to meet their own employment needs and fulfill their work roles so that the patient will not be forced to meet the needs of his purported healers as a pathological means of gaining satisfaction for himself. His real need is to have his low estimation of himself changed by experience, which can only be provided through a therapist and staff who do not reinforce his chronically helpful pattern.

References

1. Greenblatt, Milton; York, Richard H.; and Brown, Esther Lucille: From Custodial to Therapeutic Patient Care in Mental Hospitals, New York, Russell Sage Foundation, 1955, p. 9.

2. One systematic investigation is available on interlibrary loan from the Rutgers University Library, New Brunswick, New Jersey. Rouslin, Sheila: An Empirical Investigation of Chronic Helpfulness, M.A. thesis, Rutgers University.

3. Sullivan, Harry S.: The Interpersonal Theory of Psychiatry, New York, W.W. Norton & Co., 1953, p. 350.

4. Greenblatt, York, and Brown: op cit., pp. 7-9.

Regression — Some Implications for Nurses in Large Public Psychiatric Hospitals

Lillian R. Goodman

Miss Goodman (Peter Bent Brigham Hospital School of Nursing, Boston; M.S., Boston University) is director of nursing, Boston State Hospital, and associate clinical professor at Boston University School of Nursing.

Reprinted from *Nursing Outlook*, Vol. 10, No. 4, April 1962.

Nursing is concerned with helping patients get well. Nurses expect their patients to get better, to improve, to be able to leave the hospital. This expectation is borne out in the general hospital where nurses prefer assignments on the acute medical-surgical wards or the intensive care unit. Here, there is a concentration of professional and technical workers whose knowledge, skills, and resources are focused on one objective — to cure the patient of his illness.

Yet, if the nature of the illness does not allow for the patient's complete recovery — in the light of present medical and scientific knowledge — nursing is concerned with helping him make the best possible adjustment to his illness. Even as more nurses are recruited to work in large public psychiatric hospitals, however, they indicate a preference for assignments on the acute psychiatric wards. This has its merits, for we have learned that the sooner effective psychiatric and nursing resources can be employed in the treatment of acute mental illness, the sooner these people can be helped, and the fewer will be the number of patients in the continued treatment or chronic services.

It is in the latter type of service that nursing personnel encounter consistent problems of regression which are both heartbreaking and backbreaking. When we think of regression, we usually associate it with schizophrenic patients, who comprise nearly 50 percent of the patient population in our large institutions. This confronts us with the problem of what we can do to help the regressed patient loosen his hold on withdrawal and on infantile objects of attachment. How can we help this patient adjust to his illness?

A recent article in the *American Journal of Nursing** suggests that the schizophrenic patient holds a unique and baffling power over the staff, and that the nurse who is truly able to love the patient can help him communicate meaningfully with others. This requires a concerted and personal investment from the nurses, not only of time and patience but, most important, of themselves. Perhaps this is why so few nurses are able to work with regressed patients for a long period of time. Another reason might be that, all too often, these patients live under the most overcrowded conditions — on wards numbering from 50 to 100 or more patients, with one or two attendants assigned to care for them.

Some of our experiences with the problem of caring for large numbers of regressed patients at Boston State Hospital may be helpful. Approximately six years ago one of the buildings in the men's continued service had the worst reputation of all of the units in the hospital. Over 200 chronically ill men patients lived on four wards, one of which was the maximum security ward for the male service. Destruction of property, clothing, and furnishings was so rampant as to cause the maintenance and business divisions to avoid contact with the personnel in the building, and to criticize the medical and nursing management of the patients.

The men aides who worked there were very chauvinistic. They believed that only physically strong men could deal with the patients, and they were most resistive to the women nurses who were assigned there.

A supervisor who had demonstrated unusual capacity for giving to patients and staff, as well as endless patience and therapeutic orientation, was asked to accept the challenge this unit offered. Within a few months there were evidences that her intervention was yielding small but worthwhile benefits. She made herself available to both the staff and the patients. She made it her business to listen and to talk to patients who were upset. She showed the staff that she respected their masculinity, but that there were better ways of dealing with upset patients than to put them in seclusion. She was able to draw the personnel out — to get them to talk with her and each other about ways of improving the care given to the patients.

Two other staff nurses became interested in what was being accomplished in this building, and asked to be assigned there. This was done, and as they worked in close collaboration with the doctor and social worker, destructiveness gradually diminished

*Robinson, Alice M. Communicating with schizophrenic patients. *Amer. J. Nurs.* 60:1120-1123, Aug. 1960.

and a foundation was created for establishing a more therapeutic environment.

When Mother Is a Problem

One of the problems which the personnel brought to the attention of the supervisor was the manner in which the regressed patients' mothers dealt with their offspring. The staff noted that some of the gains they were making with regressed patients were lost after visiting days. The mothers came in heavily laden with food and clothing, and treated their sons like infants as they (the mothers) satisfied their own need to feed and clothe.

After discussing this with the administrator and the senior physician, the supervisor decided to start a mothers group with the mothers of the most regressed patients. This group met weekly for three years, and although no miracles took place, there were many obvious changes. One mother had always caused her son to become so anxious during her visit that he was incontinent of urine, and then she chastised him for this. The staff had taken particular pains to toilet train him so that his control was well established — on all days except visiting days. In the group meetings his mother was able to express her feelings about him and through the nurse leader's gentle support came to realize her part in this behavior. The first visiting day when the patient was not incontinent was truly a day of achievement for the patient, his mother, and the staff.

This episode encouraged the staff to persist in their work with both the patients and their visitors. Many of the latter had been regarded as necessary nuisances heretofore, but now the aides became increasingly aware of how the visitors related to the patients. They noted that the greeting used by many visitors was not the general "Hello, how are you?" but rather, "Your shirt is unbuttoned" or "You need a haircut." Certainly, remarks such as these were very rejecting, and served to compound the patient's feelings of being unwanted. These observations were reported to the nurses who then took painstaking efforts to help the relatives see what they were doing to the sick person.

Help from Administration

While the nursing personnel and the doctor were working toward the establishment of a more therapeutic climate in this unit, administrative action was taken to reduce the patient census and to eliminate the maximum security ward. These were realistic issues which had to be faced in order to facilitate the implementation of the treatment program, and we were fortunate to have administrative backing.

Not all continued treatment units for regressed patients are so favored as to have a full-time physician and nurse take leadership in instituting positive change. In some situations one cannot help wonder who causes whom to regress. Do the regressed patients cause the nursing staff to regress, or does the nursing staff, because of feelings of hopelessness and inadequacy, cause the patients to regress?

In other instances, the aides attend an excellent inservice education program which motivates them highly, then, they are assigned to wards of 75 or more regressed patients — and become immobilized by work pressure. All too often, they can do no more than see to it that the patients are fed, bathed, clothed, and the ward kept clean. Frequently, they identify more with the patients than with the professional staff which is attempting to carry out treatment programs. This develops into a circular reaction in which the patients, by having no good examples to identify with, become more regressed, while staff develop more hopeless attitudes.

Identification is a potent force in learning, in growing up, and in achieving independence. We are familiar with the psychological need each person has to find his own identity, and how this is (or is not) accomplished. The regressed patient has very great needs for identification with someone who can help him take some steps toward this objective. The aide needs someone with whom to identify so that he may more readily give to his patients.

Although not all of our chronically ill, regressed patients may be expected to attain self-realization and recovery, the proper use of drugs and other treatment techniques has taught us that many patients who had been "labeled" as incurable or unreachable, have become more capable of establishing relationships with the staff. The staff must be able to set up a "good" ideal for such relationship.

All too often, however, the hospital system has tended to foster regression. Not all of it is due to the staff, of course. For example, it has been common practice to concentrate regressed patients in one or more wards or buildings. In such a crowded ward of such patients, what incentive can they have to want to change? Many hospitals still keep men and women patients in separate areas for all activities.

If women patients are cared for only by women employees, and men patients are cared for only by men employees, what incentive do they have to try to change, to act more "normal" socially?

Several years ago, we experimented with assigning a carefully selected man aide to a women's ward of chronically ill patients whose living habits had deteriorated to a low level. At meal time, most of them crouched on the floor with their trays and shoveled the food into their mouths with their hands or a spoon. During the day, they lay on the floor or benches on the ward. Many of them kept taking off their clothes, and remained nude. We thought it reasonable to expect more acceptable behavior when a man joined the full-time staff.

At the start of his assignment, he worked closely with the women attendants in doing the required ward duties, and showed the patients that he wanted to help care for them. Gradually, they raised their standards of daily living and tried to live up to *his* expectations of them. The first noticeable change was seen in the cafeteria where, bit by bit, he encouraged them to sit at the tables. The next step was to interest them in using a full set of silverware.

Several months later the night shift personnel noted that the patients took more pains with their morning care. They wanted to "look good" and be properly dressed when Mr. C came on duty at 6:45 a.m. This was an obvious gain which the staff recognized, and they used it as the basis for their next step — group responsibility for the daily upkeep and improvements in the ward living situation. As this began to happen, the next step was taken — planning social activities with men patients, inviting them to a dance, party, or picnic.

From Nursing Personnel

These are very simple illustrations of how nursing personnel can attempt to deal with the problem of regression in patients. From psychology, psychiatry, and psychoanalysis, we have learned much about the dynamics of growth and development and the basic elements of regression. The patient who experiences anxiety over a lack of affection denies his anxiety, and moves from an "I don't care" kind of defense to the extreme reaction of catatonia or hebephrenia. The nursing care plan for such a person is obvious — he needs to feel cared *for* and *about* for a long, long time. He needs such simple demonstrations of caring as a touch on the hand or shoulder, a friendly smile.

The patient who has been overwhelmed by his anxiety and his hostile inclinations tries to project his feelings onto others. He needs someone to share the responsibility for what is happening to him. The patient who develops paranoia needs a helping person to sit down with him and say "I want to help you work this out," rather than to say "You're sick and I will help you."

The patient who has turned to delusions and hallucinations because of anxiety over his unsatisfactory experiences in living obviously needs help in making his hospital living experiences as satisfying as possible. He has to "get something" from them which will make him feel more worthwhile and important.

Nurses have a major role to play in teaching, motivating, and encouraging regressed patients to move toward reconstructing their daily patterns of adjustment. Nurses who are able to function effectively in this role have a great capacity to give to others, and to love. It is not likely that there will be enough psychiatrists or psychiatric nurses to meet the enormous need which such patients present. The burden of responsibility rests with those nurses who are willing to invest the time and energy, and who are creative.

The pattern of nursing care of the regressed patient needs to be changed. Nurses and aides tend to keep patients regressed because of their need to do *for* them. The more that is done for patients, the more dependent they become, and the less able to do for themselves. Nurses are in a hurry to get the work done and to do what is necessary for others. It is easier and quicker to bathe and dress a patient than to help him do for himself.

Nurses need patience to give the patient the opportunity and freedom to do for himself — to button his own trousers, comb his hair, shave, and carry out the numerous other small tasks of daily living. Nurses have to help the patient consistently to try to do for himself. Over and over again, he needs to be encouraged to get up off the floor, to sit on a chair, to comb his hair, to care for himself.

It has been routine in most large hospitals for the nurse to carry matches and light the patients' cigarettes. This was done, even when it was common knowledge that many patients had their own matches. Recently, at Boston State Hospital, matches were installed in the cigarette machines in patient areas. As more and more patients received "ground" and "off ground" privileges, they were obtaining their own matches, anyhow. Now carrying their own matches is accepted policy. The patient who might try to start a fire or to harm himself is the exception, the one who has to be closely observed, rather than the large group who can handle the privilege of lighting their own cigarettes.

Billions of dollars are spent annually to house and provide care for the chronically ill, regressed patients in our large public hospitals. This major problem, which concerns hospital administrators and legislative groups, is beginning to concern the national community. Additional funds, if they were available, would not solve the problems of lack of professional staff and treatment facilities.

Perhaps we can involve the families of the regressed patients to a greater extent than we have in the effort to rehabilitate such patients. Dr. Schweitzer's method of having the entire family participate in the care of the sick member has implications for nursing. If nurses invested more thought and energy in devising techniques of helping family members find ways of assuming some of the responsibility for the patient, we would do much to reduce chronicity.

There are no ready solutions to the problems of regression. Each institution has its own unique methods of functioning, and what might work in one might be a failure in another. Yet, the needs of people are the same — in New England or in the Far West. As nurses, it behooves us to understand why a patient is regressed, and then to help him work diligently, steadily, and patiently toward greater self-realization.

Does the Psychiatric Nurse Have Independent Functions?

Elizabeth Maloney

Miss Maloney (St. Elizabeth Hospital, Utica, N.Y.; B.S., M.A., Teachers College, Columbia University, New York) is an instructor in nursing education at Teachers College where she is a candidate for a doctoral degree. She has practiced psychiatric nursing as a head nurse, supervisor, and assistant director of nursing.

Reprinted from *The American Journal of Nursing*, Vol. 62, No. 6, June 1962.

The problem of who is to "do therapy," what kind, where, and how much, hangs over the psychiatric field like a fog. It is a controversial and potentially explosive subject.

In many educational programs and hospitals, interdisciplinary efforts to clarify the situation are being made. Occasionally, doing therapy becomes a status symbol. When it does, inevitably, the patient gets trapped in the ensuing scramble for power. In such situations, the overt and covert disagreements among established therapists and aspirants to doing therapy, actually create a more pathological situation for the patient. Making patients sicker is hardly the goal of any health worker, be he psychiatrist, social worker, nurse, or psychologist, but it is fair to state that role confusion appears to retard the therapeutic effort to some degree.

It would seem that if nursing were reasonably clear on its role in the matter of psychotherapy, the patient would benefit at his everyday living level, the psychiatric ward. Let us look at the current psychiatric nursing attempts to formulate a psychotherapeutic role but from the viewpoint of how this relates to nursing in the broader sense.

The nurse under discussion here is the professional nurse. To be more precise, she is one of a group of professional persons within an occupation. This distinction is made because it is becoming fashionable nowadays to include everyone who drifts through a psychiatric ward as a part of the therapeutic team. Everyone who drifts through in uniform is, by popular definition, a member of the nursing team. A number of articles and books have appeared recently wherein the term "nurse" is footnoted to mean professional nurses, practical nurses, aides, attendants, technicians, and presumably the man who reads the hospital gas meter. (In this blanket approach, he cannot be omitted; he wears a uniform. Besides, he might be a transient father figure to someone.)

The point is that if there is not some immediate way to discern differences in function between the professional nurse and the brigade of "nursing others," then it is doubtful if professional nursing can be said to have a psychotherapeutic role of any notable dimension. Unless nurses can say "our reason for being here is because in this and that way we provide a unique service to patients," any claims they make to a therapeutic role are pretentious. The contribution of any profession, in any service setting, is valuable chiefly because of the distinctive service rendered to the client by that profession. In an interdisciplinary setting there will be areas of therapeutic overlap but the professional hard core of services within each discipline should stand out in bold relief. Eleanor Lambertsen is clear in this regard when she says:

> It is the prerogative of the practitioners of the profession to define this hard core of professional service. Related groups are concerned, but the final determination of the professional mission is the right and responsibility of the practitioner.[1]

The recent *entente cordiale* between psychiatric nursing, social scientists, and others makes it tempting to share this arduous task more fully than would be prudent. It might also be tempting, in an honest effort to be helpful to patients, to delegate the ancient prerogatives of nursing to other persons. This we almost did once before. We have been vacationing in administration, record keeping, and other more or less prestigeful resorts, while auxiliary workers fed, bathed, and cared directly for patients. Now, the cry is back to the bedside. Some outside observers feel it is too late to turn back, at least in more generalized hospitals.

Philosophy is the source from which all perceptions of past, present, and future role and function flow — an inner belief, a series of deeply held convictions. It would seem then that a professional nurse's philosophy of nursing, her professional value system, is the cornerstone on which her perception of psychotherapeutic function rests.

Perhaps the quickest way to determine a man's philosophy is to watch him live his life. Perhaps the quickest way to determining a nurse's concept of role and functioning is to note how and where she does her nursing. Setting influences the role and function of any psychiatric nurse. People generally select situations which suit their own philosophies. Unknowingly they may enter a setting essentially opposed to their beliefs. Then they generally sort themselves out or get sorted out, due to their anxieties or those of others.

A look at the psychiatric nursing scene reveals a spectrum of philosophies at work, ranging from a custodial view to a position verging on that of lay analyst. Each extreme, as well as more moderate versions in between, bespeaks commitment to some concept of role and function.

At one end of the line is the custodial concept. There are one or two custodial institutions left, despite a thunderous throwing open of doors and mass swallowing of tranquilizers. Nurses in such institutions demonstrate every day that they believe their role is primarily managerial. As it will be noted later, custodial management can well be a legitimate part of a psychotherapeutic role in nursing. It would seem that, like the grand old word "asylum" (originally meaning shelter from the storm), current usage has endowed "custodial" with an aura of disrepute. No matter what label is given to the routines of washing, feeding, bathing, or providing shelter from the storm, it is clear that somehow they must go on. It is the manner in which they go on that marks the difference for patients between detention on a psychiatric ward and creative psychotherapeutic nursing.

It would be well at this point to note that psychiatric nurses are not alone in attempting to conceptualize a psychotherapeutic role for nursing. Indeed it would appear that all nurses cannot lay any claims to being professional until this relationship between nurse and patient has taken definite form and shape, resting securely on a theoretical framework. Peplau has taken the lead in this endeavor, noting that the technical subrole is but one of several subroles flowing out of the counseling or psychotherapeutic role.[2]

Many writers have pointed out that professional workers tend to be guided by wide, generic directional systems, and are not bound by the structured minutiae of the technical worker. For this reason, the remaining comments concerning development of a psychotherapeutic role will be offered from a broad, generally accepted framework: the statement of functions and standards published in 1956 based on the work of Lesnik and Anderson. They say:

> Because professional nursing has been the subject of control for over 50 years, a study of legal decisions which have dealt with the identification of standards of conduct of specific functions in professional nursing may be relied upon to define and distinguish functions of professional nurses from those of other groups.[3]

They go on to establish six independent functions, the first of which is: the supervision of a patient involving the whole management of care, requiring the application of principles based upon the biologic, physical, and social sciences. This then could be the broad generic direction — related to the managerial subrole. Peplau notes that this role oversees the purposes of nursing care through the manipulation of the context or situation and speculates that, due to the physician's limited time, management of the patient's environment was inevitable.[4] So we can say that the nurse directs the play, manages the setting, and strongly influences the cast of characters.

All nurses know that a determined manager in white can rout a corps of physicians if she puts her mind to it, and she often does, it seems.[5] Maurice Greenhill has remarked that the nurse is the mistress of the ward situation. He also points out that, too often, she doesn't know it. The professional nurse is sensitively aware of what is going on; the others move about more or less blissfully ignorant of the fact that the patient's illness exists in a setting which may gravely influence the outcome of illness — particularly in any long-term illness and specifically mental illness.

The patient moves (we all move) in temperature, space, time, and light — a whole set of interdependent conditions that affect what he wears, where he sits, and what he does. The nurse then deals with the sights and sounds, the textures and the colors, the warp and woof of everyday life on the ward — with reality, in short — and with the task of defining and redefining the boundaries of reality to persons who are often none too sure of their own humanity, let alone the boundaries of the world in which they exist.

Consider one of these factors — space. Place anyone in a hospital for any length of time and some predictable things will happen. At first, the geographic constriction will be psychologically offset by continued and sustained interest in the outside world, unless the patient is very ill. In this regard note Lambertsen's comment, "the stage of health in which the nurse meets the client in a large measure determines the emphasis of the nursing functions."[6]

As time passes, more and more interest is turned to the new world in which the patient is immersed and proportionately less to the outside world. Hospitals are small worlds in themselves. Baziak and Denton note that it is possible for staff in hospitals to remain indoors for a week or two, eating, sleeping, moving about through tunnels, making purchases in the hospital gift shop and the like.[7] How much more the patient, who is not free to go, becomes involved in the culture of the sick, particularly in the mental hospital.

Eventually, the constricted artificial life of the hospital begins to assume undue proportions and begins to look more and more attractive. In the general hospital, this process is known as "hospital-itis;" of late, the word "colonization" has been applied to the same operation in a mental hospital.[8] The nurse is in a pivotal position to note the onset of this malady which in psychiatric hospitals has helped to create the dim, half world of the back wards. She is in a position to note it and take steps to prevent it or reverse it. The public health nurse is in a position to prevent a reverse operation within the patient's family, whereby they "close ranks" and gradually exclude the patient psychologically from their life.

Another illustration relates to the matter of touch and texture. The need to have physical contact with other people is a constant and universal phenomenon. French points out this culture is characterized by many taboos in regard to people's touching one another.[9] The seemingly simple matter of when to touch a patient or when to refrain is important, and requires precise professional judgment. Physical contact in caring for a child might be a crucial part of nursing care, while to touch some schizophrenic patients would distress them immeasurably at certain points in their illness. Conversely, some schizophrenics need to touch people and things frequently to assure themselves that others really exist, to try to establish boundaries between their bodies and the world, or perhaps to relieve anxiety through a ritualistic pattern of touching things to ward off some unformulated doom, by use of magic as it were.

A final example relates to what patients wear. In a crowded ward of one large public hospital there was much concern about keeping clothing on patients. Some of the concern came from our culture, which decrees that we cover ourselves appropriately, lest we be jailed or deemed a candidate for the mental hospital. But even in the mental hospital, it seems, one cannot be unclad in peace. The value system of this hospital indicated clothes under any and all circumstances. Blame would be placed if patients were not clothed; this was the real crux of the matter, the placing of blame.

Much of the concern was focused on one schizophrenic woman who went barefoot as much as she possibly could. A running battle went on between this patient and the nursing staff — a symbolic struggle, if you will. On the side of illness, and thus too frequently by definition on the side of wrong, was the lonely patient. Finally, after both sides were worn to a standstill, a perceptive nurse simply asked the patient about the matter. The patient stated with poignant dignity that touching the ward floor with her bare feet helped to maintain her contact with the real world. Her near terror at being cajoled into shoes became clear and opened the way for the nursing staff to plan other ways of helping her maintain contact with reality.

For the majority of the patients on this ward, wearing shoes would be desirable, inasmuch as in the well world, a precise definition of which is still to be developed, people wear shoes in most places. But for this one patient, at least for a time, it would be expert nursing judgment that she be allowed to doff her shoes when she needed to do so.

In summary, it is clear that much work is currently being done in regard to the formulation of a psychotherapeutic role of nursing in general, flowing in most instances (although by no means always) from psychiatric nursing literature. It would seem clear that the adequate definition of such a role will be one of the cornerstones for any rational claim to professionalization in nursing in the years ahead. Further, professional people are characterized by unique, independent functioning which is based not only on broad, general principles but on uniqueness of function as well. A series of independent functions have been identified, one of which has been developed as a possible broad base for identification of a psychotherapeutic role in nursing, one all nurses could consider, not psychiatric nurses alone.

It would appear that management and supervision of the patient's environment is an independent function of nursing. How it is done marks the difference between a therapeutic role and a mechanical, clerical approach to patient care. The limits here are boundless. Taking this one independent function alone, it is clear that by itself, it opens a view that is broad, a view that will have to be developed painstakingly before nursing is more than a few professionals submerged within an occupational group.

References

1. Lambertsen, Eleanor C. *Education for Nursing Leadership.* Philadelphia. J.B. Lippincott Co., 1958. p. 49.

2. Peplau, Hildegard. Therapeutic concepts. In National League for Nursing, *Aspects of Psychiatric Nursing.* New York,

The League, 1957, Section B. p. 9.
3. Lesnik, M.J. and Anderson, B.E. *Nursing Practice and the Law.* 2nd ed. Philadelphia. J.B. Lippincott Co., 1955, pp. 258-279.
4. Peplau, *op. cit.,* p. 12.
5. Burling, Temple and Others. *The Give and Take in Hospitals.* New York, G.P. Putnam's Sons, 1956, pp. 87-88.
6. Lambertsen, *op. cit.,* p. 81.
7. Baziak, Anna and Denton, R.K. The language of the hospital and its effects on the patient. *ETC* 17:261-268, Sept. 1960.
8. Goffman, Erving. *Asylums.* Garden City, N.Y., Doubleday and Co., 1961. p. 62.
9. French, T.M. *Basic Postulates.* (Integration of Behavior, Vol. 1) Chicago, University of Chicago Press, 1952.

Interpersonal Techniques: The Crux of Psychiatric Nursing

Hildegard E. Peplau

Miss Peplau (Pottstown, Pa., Hospital School of Nursing; B.A., Bennington; M.A., Ed.D., Teachers College, Columbia University) is professor of nursing at Rutgers University and chairman of the advanced program in psychiatric nursing in which graduate nurse students are trained for clinical specialization in psychiatric nursing.

Reprinted from *The American Journal of Nursing*, Vol. 62, June 1962.

The time is past when a nurse could become, in one lifetime, an expert in all clinical areas. Advances in all fields of knowledge and within nursing science itself point to the inevitability of clinical specialization.

When you begin to think about specialization, however, you think not only of a focus in a particular area but of considerable depth. As the scope of the specialists' work narrows, the depth intensifies at, I submit, the point of the uniqueness of the clinical area. The unique aspect of a clinical area is twofold: it is that which occurs in other clinical fields but is not emphasized to the same extent, and it is that which is almost entirely new — the uncommon, promising developments which result from thinking deeply about a particular facet of work in just one area.

Each of the areas of nursing practice has a particular clinical emphasis. This emphasis does not preclude attention to all the other aspects of the workrole of the nurse practitioner, but more time, effort, and thought are given to this particular facet. For example, nurses in public health programs emphasize health teaching, not to the exclusion of the technical aspects of nursing practice or of the supportive, reassuring, mother-surrogate type of nurse activities. But, by and large, nurses who visit patients in their homes spend a proportionately larger part of their time teaching. Medical-surgical nursing emphasizes technical care; pediatric nursing emphasizes the mother-surrogate role; in this paper I want to consider the particular emphasis of psychiatric nursing.

I have indicated various subroles of the workrole of nurses. Briefly, these include mother-surrogate, technician, manager, socializing agent, health teacher, and counselor or psychotherapist.[1]

Psychiatric nursing emphasizes the role of counselor or psychotherapist. It is true that this idea is not a universally accepted one in all psychiatric facilities. But note that I say "psychiatric nursing," not "nursing in psychiatric units."

There are two levels of professional nurse personnel practicing in psychiatric units — general practitioners (general duty nurses) and specialists (psychiatric nurses). Let me clarify the difference. A general practitioner is a nurse who has completed only her basic professional preparation. From my viewpoint, a "psychiatric nurse" is a specialist and, at this time, specialist status can be achieved by two routes — experience and education.

Before the passage of the Mental Health Act in 1946, experience was the route by which a nurse earned the title "psychiatric nurse;" since 1946, however, some 25 graduate-level, university-based programs in advanced psychiatric nursing have been established. There are stipends available for study in these programs. Any nurse who can qualify — because she has completed her full basic professional preparation and has the intellectual and personal qualifications for graduate study — can secure a stipend for graduate study toward becoming a clinical specialist in psychiatric nursing, that is, a "psychiatric nurse." From my point of view, then, the route of clinical specialization for any nurse who was graduated since 1946 is through a university-based graduate level program.

I realize this is a status problem but the profession of nursing will strengthen its position in relation to all other professional disciplines when it recognizes the culturally accepted fact that university education is the route for clinical specialization. There is good reason for this. Theoretically the university is free of the service commitment of the hospital — it can take objective distance, look dispassionately at the work of nurses, and dare to consider gross changes in the workrole.

When you are employed in a service agency, on the other hand, you become a participating member in its social system; ties of friendship and loyalty become binding as well as blinding, and dispassionate inquiry is greatly lessened. There is another reason why universities have culturally been charged with graduate education: the scope of established and newly formulated knowledge represented in a university faculty is ever so much wider than that represented in a professional staff group. It is access to this knowledge and its application to clinical observations that transform the student into an expert clinician.

There is clear distinction then between nursing in a psychiatric unit (what a general duty nurse does) and psychiatric nursing (what an expert clinical practitioner does). This distinction should be kept in the foreground, for in this paper I will refer to nurses and nursing when speaking of the common and basic elements, and to psychiatric nurses and psychiatric nursing when speaking of the more specialized clinical functions.

A psychiatric nurse is first of all an expert clinician. She may also be a teacher, supervisor, administrator, consultant, or researcher, but underlying all these functional positions there should be advanced clinical training. Such clinical expertness revolves around the field's unique aspect or emphasis — in this case, the role of counselor or psychotherapist. I want to develop the importance of this idea for the general practice of nursing in a psychiatric setting, but first, I wish to pinpoint why other aspects of the work in a psychiatric unit are not the central focus of psychiatric nursing.

The emphasis in psychiatric nursing is *not* on the mother-surrogate role. Some nurses believe that the unmet needs of a patient's infancy and early childhood can be met by the nurse taking on various mothering activities. This belief assumes that the corrective experience is largely an emotional one resulting from a relationship in which the nurse complements a need for mothering of the patient by supplying its counterpart — need-reducing mother-surrogate activities. This is analogous to the notion that when calcium deficiency produces tooth decay, supplying the calcium will fill up the cavities! A patient needs love, warmth, acceptance, support, and reassurance — not to supply the unmet needs of the past but for current reasons; having these emotional experiences makes it possible for the patient to come to grips with the earlier unmet needs on intellectual rather than on experiential grounds.

The notion that a made-up "good mother" experience will correct the patient's pathology is based on the assumption that the patient has not moved ahead in other areas compatible with chronological development — for example, language, vocabulary, and thought develop despite emotional deprivations.

To give mother-surrogate activities the central emphasis would be to de-emphasize these tools which have developed and can be utilized.

There is another inescapable fact; the small number of professional nurses in psychiatric facilities has for a long time required that the necessary mother-surrogate activities — the bathing, feeding, dressing, toileting, warning, disciplining, and approving the patient — be taken over largely by nonprofessional nursing personnel. I do not foresee that any great benefit would accrue even if the supply was such that professional nurses could take on fully these mothering activities. Note that I have not said that a nurse never bathes or feeds or dresses or warns a patient in a psychiatric unit; what I have said is that these mothering activities are not the central focus.

The emphasis in psychiatric nursing is *not* on the technical subrole. Some nurses believe that the cause of mental illness will ultimately prove to be some biochemical or otherwise organic problem, identifiable by the results of various laboratory test procedures and correctable by some technical manipulations analogous to the injection of insulin in the therapeutic management of a person diagnosed as diabetic. Other nurses in the past and present have believed that technical expertness in giving tubs, packs, coma insulin and care in the pre- and post-phases of electroconvulsive therapy or lobotomy would lead to solutions to mental illness. Technical expertness in giving medication or carrying out procedures associated with nursing is, in my opinion, not the desirable emphasis in psychiatric nursing.

Custodial Activities

The emphasis in psychiatric nursing is *not* on managerial activities. Historically, these have been aspects of custodial care with restraint, protection, cleanliness, and order the dominant themes. Many of the housekeeping activities associated with these themes have been shifted not only to nonprofessional personnel but to work details made up of working patients as well. The housekeeping activities have given way to a host of clerical and receptionist activities, which nurses have taken on, and which presumably have to do with the management of the patient's environment in the interest of his care. I submit that the time is near at hand when administrators will recognize that these clerical and receptionist activities can be performed far better and more cheaply by a high school graduate; that these are not "professional" activities but instead are largely busywork which keeps the nurse away from direct contact with patients.

The emphasis in psychiatric nursing is *not* on socializing-agent activities such as playing cards and games with patients, taking walks and watching TV with them and the like. In some basic schools of nursing, students are taught that these activities are central in the work of the nurse; I submit that the preparation of a nurse is not required for such activities; that the use of a nurse's social experience as an interesting diversionary activity in the patient's daily lie is not the best use of the time of a professional nurse. Nonprofessional nursing personnel, volunteers, and visitors can do this game-playing just as well as a nurse can. The professional education of the nurse is wasted; it is not needed to perform these activities which most laymen learn some time during their "teens."

Group activities along these lines might better be planned and carried out by the recreational department or some department other than nursing service (or nursing education since students are largely "used" for this purpose). I have not said that a professional nurse *never* plays cards with patients; however, these activities are not the central emphasis in psychiatric nursing and at most should take a bare minimum of the day's time of a professional nurse.

The emphasis in psychiatric nursing is *not* on health teaching although this subrole, in the workrole of the nurse, is an important one which needs to be developed further. I have pointed out that this is an important part of the work of nurses in public health. But the patients in the case load of these nurses are more often immediately able to use information than are patients in the psychiatric setting. Even so, teaching psychiatric patients about diet, nutrition, grooming, sex, and the like may be very helpful. There has also been one promising study reported in which psychiatric patients were taught a concept of anxiety to apply to their own experiences; several similar studies are now under way.[2]

The emphasis in psychiatric nursing is on the counseling or psychotherapeutic subrole. This generalization is based upon the assumption that the difficulties in living which lead up to mental illness in a particular patient are subject to investigation and control by the patient — with professional counseling assistance. It is also based on a second assumption: that formal knowledge of counseling procedure is absolutely essential for the more general type of approach which may be useful in very brief relationships with patients. Further, these general approaches are in the nature of "interpersonal techniques" useful in relation to specific problems — such as withdrawal, aggression, hallucinations, delusions, and the like — and these are the crux of psychiatric nursing.

There is being developed in psychiatric nursing a theory and procedure of nurse counseling. This development is proceeding along two lines:

1. A "surface type" of formal counseling procedure, such as a general nurse practitioner might use with patients in all clinical areas, is being described. Many schools of nursing already are beginning to teach interviewing — of a therapeutic in contrast to a biographical type — as a basis for counseling. A companion result of this development will surely be the identification and description of a variety of general approaches to specific problems — interpersonal techniques — which nurses can use in everday brief contacts with all types of patients.

2. Depth counseling, such as might be employed by a psychiatric nurse specialist who had completed two years of master's level clinical training, is also being described. Several nurses are now employed in situations in which they are doing long-term counseling of patients, utilizing the competencies secured through such clinical training. It is conceivable that in another decade or two nurses will share offices with psychiatrists and psychologists and social workers for the private practice of psychiatric nurse counseling, although now there are no publishable instances of such practices.

Teaching Students

In many basic schools of nursing, students are being taught counseling technique in connection with nurse-patient care studies, particularly in the psychiatric setting. I have talked with a number of teachers in these schools and their general conclusion seems to be that when the student has an opportunity to work directly with one patient — say in one-hour sessions twice a week over a period of ten weeks — a great deal of learning takes place.

The student gets more than a textbook picture of pathology; she gets a full view of the complexity of the difficulties of a psychiatric patient, of the variations which occur in particular patterns of behavior. Many students find out, for example, that there are infinite variations of the pattern of withdrawal and that observed changes in the behavior of a patient are more likely to be changes from one variant to another of a central pattern that persists. Thus, a patient who uses gross withdrawal — by muteness, for example — can, as a result of a nurse-patient relationship, eventually begin to speak; the verbalizations, however, are also classifiable as a variant of withdrawal, particularly when the patient talks but doesn't communicate anything descriptive of his difficulties.

In a carefully guided nurse-patient relationship, the nurse learns the art and science of counseling technique. She discovers that the art part of it is intuitively based — it is a clinical judgment which she herself makes, minute by minute, that this maneuver or that maneuver might conceivably be useful to the investigative effort. The student also learns the value of knowledge and procedures of their application to explain observations; this is the scientific part. The student gradually ceases to use such terms as anxiety, conflict, dissociation, and the like as mere labels for behavior; she begins to use these concepts as scientific tools to guide her in assessing the investigative effort under way and in getting more information. Both the nurse and patient need as much descriptive information about the patient's life experiences as can be obtained wihtout making the patient too uncomfortable. It is this information which will be worked over by the nurse and patient together so that the patient can understand and benefit from his previous experiences in living.

Another Benefit

Another important learning accrues from teaching counseling in the nurse-patient relationship. The student learns detachment; she learns — with the help of her teachers — how not to usurp the counseling time to meet her own needs; how to use the time, instead, to help the patient formulate and meet his needs. She learns to make clearer distinction between techniques that are useful to her socially, outside the professional work situation, and those specifically useful in a clinical situation.

Moreover, the student learns a lot about herself as she begins to understand her reactions to the patients' behavior and verbal content, her own need for approval, the points at which she is particularly vulnerable. Patients have a way of unwittingly locating the vulnerabilities of students — be it their need for approval, their sensitivity to their appearance, their embarrassment in discussion about sex, or any one of a host of similar problem areas.

Once a student nurse has had successive counseling interviews with a particular patient, and has responsibly reviewed her nurse-patient data with an expert psychiatric nurse teacher, she is able to transfer — or generalize — the learning products to much briefer relationships with patients. Students invariably report that learning about counseling of one patient helps them to use to better advantage the two-to-three-minute contacts they have with patients in the ward setting. Nor do I know of any other way for a student to achieve these understandings except as a result of talking with one patient about the patient's difficulties, in designated, time-limited sessions occurring over a period of time, and following each session by a substantial review of what went on with an expert psychiatric nurse. You can't tell students what to do along these lines and then expect them, magically, to be able to do it. The student must not only experience this day-to-day process but she must have interested and active help in examining, bit by bit, the interview data which she thus collects.

One result, then, of the nurse-patient inquiry is the ability to transfer a substantial amount of learning toward more generalized interpersonal techniques. I believe that such techniques are the crux of psychiatric nursing and it seems to me that it ought to be possible for psychiatric nurses to develop specific interpersonal techniques useful in intervening in specific patterns of pathological behavior of patients. And it is possible; several nurses I know are currently involved in developing and testing such techniques.

Steps to Abate Anxiety

One of the major difficulties of most, if not all, psychiatric patients is anxiety. We need a simple interpersonal technique which would be of value in the productive abatement of severe anxiety in patients. What might the steps of such a technique be? Could these steps be carried out by nonprofessional nursing personnel under the supervision of professional nurses who would have a deeper insight into the merits of the technique based upon the emotional experience of the nurse-patient investigation?

The steps are simple:

1. Encourage the patient to identify the anxiety as such. This is done by having all personnel help him recognize what he is experiencing at the point when he is actually anxious. Such anxiety is observable. In other words, the patient may well be unaware of his anxiety but another person — particularly a trained professional person — can observe the effects of anxiety and therefore infer its presence. So, a professional nurse would determine that a particular patient was anxious and unaware of it. Her behavior toward the patient and her supervision of the relationships which non-

professional personnel have with him would be guided by the aim: to help the patient identify the anxiety as such. This would be done by saying to the patient, for as long as it takes to achieve the recognition, "Are you uncomfortable," "Are you nervous," "Are you upset," Are you anxious?" With most psychiatric patients, it may take an amazingly long time to get a "Yes" answer, that is, to get him to recognize his anxiety. In many instances, the patient's responses will follow a sequence, beginning with "No" to "Sometimes I am," "Maybe," "A little," and finally "Yes, I am uncomfortable (or anxious)." When such "Yes" responses are obtained, the nurse can assume a modicum of awareness of anxiety; then, and not before then, the patient is ready for the second step in the interpersonal technique for utilizing anxiety constructively.

2. Encourage the patient to connect the relief-giving patterns that he uses to the anxiety which requires such relief. The nursing personnel focus their efforts on maintaining the patient's awareness of the anxiety and connecting it to his anxiety-relieving behavior. Thus, the nurse might observe that a patient was anxious. The nurse would ask, "Are you uncomfortable now?" If the patient replied, "Yes," the nurse would ask, "What do you do to get comfortable again when you are anxious?" This step would be repeated until it was clear to the professonal observer that the patient did, indeed, formulate the connection between his anxiety and the anxiety-relieving behavior he uses. Describing this behavior, he might say, "I cry," "I swing my foot," "I pace," "I talk to voices," "I worry about my family," and the like.

   Working in this manner with a particular patient, one graduate nurse student had the experience of hearing a patient say, "Yes, I am anxious right now; I am very anxious; I feel terrible, and I'm going over there and rock myself on that rocking chair good and hard and then I'll come back." A bit later, the patient did return to the nurse and commented, "Now I'm not so anxious; that rocking chair sure helps but I need to find out why I am anxious."

3. Encourage the patient to provide himself and the nurse with data descriptive of situations and interactions which go on immediately before an increase in anxiety is noticed. Once he has connected his anxiety-relieving behavior with his anxiety, the patient is ready for this third step: beginning the search for precipitating causes of the anxiety. Here the nursing personnel might ask, "What went on just before you got so uncomfortable?" The aim is to get the patient to describe the situations or interactions in which he was involved immediately preceding the developing increase in anxiety. Such description provides the nurse with a range of data about the patient so that she can begin to speculate (for herself) on probable causes of the anxiety.

   Here, the application of the concept of anxiety — which defines areas of causation — would be useful for the professional nurse. It cannot be over emphasized that in this step the patient is not searching for immediate, situational causes of the increase in his anxiety; he is merely providing a description of experience from which such causes can later be inferred.

4. Encourage the patient to formulate from the descriptive data the probable immediate, situational causes for the increase in his anxiety.

In Step 3 the professional nurse can begin to speculate as to causes; helping the patient to formulate his own view of the reasons for his anxiety is Step 4. Step 4 makes use of the descriptions which have accumulated out of several days of talks between the patient and the nursing personnel. The professional nurse might ask such questions as, "What have you noticed going on before you get anxious that might increase your discomfort?" Questions of this type encourage the patient to notice and to formulate cause-effect relations on his own.

Any patient who is able to utilize these four steps will show improvement in his ability to cope not only with living in the ward setting but with his pathology as well. Such a patient is most likely ready for a fifth step — referral for intensive counseling so that the causes of anxiety involving the connections between remote past experience and immediate situational experiences can be identified.

It is my premise that interpersonal techniques — such as the one I have indicated here — can be devised and utilized by nursing personnel in relation to problematic behavior patterns of psychiatric patients. I believe that these interpersonal techniques, rather than modifications of medical-surgical nursing techniques, are the crux of the practice of nursing in a psychiatric setting.

References

1. For a more complete discussion of subroles see Peplau's "Therapeutic Concepts" in *The League Exchange*, No. 26, pp. 1-30, published by the National League for Nursing, New York, 1957.

2. See "Teaching a Concept of Anxiety" by Dorothea Hays in *Nursing Research*, Vol. 10, pp. 108-113, Spring 1961 issue.

A Day Hospital for Psychiatric Patients

Anne Hargreaves, Patricia Warsaw, and Edith P. Lewis

Collaborating in the preparation of this article were Anne Hargreaves, (Boston City; B.S., M.S., Boston University) assistant professor of nursing at Boston University, who developed and directed the student program described in this paper; Patricia Warsaw, (Peter Bent Brigham), head nurse at Massachusetts Mental Health Center's Day Hospital; and Edith P. Lewis, contributing editor for the *Journal*.

Reprinted from *The American Journal of Nursing*, Vol. 62, No. 9, September 1962.

It is becoming less and less possible to speak of Boston's Massachusetts Mental Health Center as a hospital with a given "bed" capacity. As Dr. Milton Greenblatt, director of research and laboratories there, puts it: "We have facilities to care for something like 200 patients — but, actually, we have only about 100 beds. The rest of our patients are cared for on a day basis and go home to their own beds at night."

At the Center, an average of about 40 to 50 patients are cared for in what might be called by Day Hospital proper: a separate but integral unit of this psychiatric hospital. And about an equal number of persons receive day care on the inpatient services: that is, they spend the day with the patients who are in the hospital on a 24-hour basis, but return to their own homes at night.

Again quoting Dr. Greenblatt: "We are looking forward to a relative numerical dominance of day patients over full-time hospitalized cases. How far this process can be extended depends on future developments, particularly the education and cooperation of staff, relatives, and the community. Whatever the ultimate success, the day hospital idea has struck a severe blow to the 'bricks and plaster' answer to mental illness problems — that is, the construction of ever more full-time custodial type institutions to care for mental cases."[1]

It could be added that the day hospital concept of care has also struck a severe blow to the traditional practice of psychiatric nursing and is creating a new and dynamic concept of the nurse's role in psychiatric care.

The idea for a day hospital at the Massachusetts Mental Health Center began to germinate about 10 years ago when it was noted that a number of discharged patients were returning to the hospital almost daily — apparently simply to pass the time or to take refuge from the difficulties of life at home or in the community. They would sit in the lounge chairs in the lobby, greeting old friends among patients and staff as they passed through, occasionally joining in available recreational activities. Some interaction took place among themselves but their attempts at socialization were for the most part feeble and fumbling.

Obviously, some step was missing in the discharge of these individuals; some needs were not being met. Consequently, exploration was started to find out what brought these former patients back to the hospital so often — sometimes just to visit, sometimes for readmission — and to ascertain what more helpful service could be provided to aid in the transition to community life.

A somewhat tentative day program was inaugurated for this group, with the investigating social worker serving as staff person. A small room near the lobby — originally a cloak room — became the official "center." There the patients could check in and out, hang up their coats and hats, meet for group or individual discussions with the social worker, or take refuge when they were overwhelmed in the course of the day. An activity program was also provided for the group, dovetailing with ongoing social and recreational activities in the hospital. Eventually, students from the Boston University School of Nursing were assigned to this rudimentary day care program as part of their educational experience in psychiatric nursing. Along with their psychiatric nursing instructor from the university, they helped develop a program of meaningful therapeutic activity for this "unattached" group.

In its early years at the Massachusetts Mental Health Center, the day care idea, although soon a living program, was nevertheless a rather diffuse and loosely organized one. Patients came not by referral but on their own initiative. There were no set criteria for admission to the program; in fact, there was no clear-cut program. Medical responsibility for the patients was not clearly defined and nurse participation was limited to the activities of the psychiatric nursing faculty member from Boston University and her students.

Even under these limited circumstances, however, the day care program continued to demonstrate its usefulness as one way of caring for psychiatric patients. By the end of 1956, the Day Hospital was established as an official, functioning unit within the institution, with a large area equivalent to a ward setting given over to it. Psychiatrists were assigned to the unit and, in 1957, the first full-time professional nurse was added to the staff. Now, in 1962, the Day Hospital is a going concern, caring for 40 to 50 patients at any given time.

The Day Hospital in Action

The patient population runs the gamut from semi-acute, bordering on actue, to severely incapacitated chronic patients. The most common diagnoses are depression and schizophrenia. Within our present state of knowledge, drug addicts and patients with alcoholism or severe character disorders do not seem to benefit from this type of care.

At first, most of the Day Hospital patients were received from the inpatient services, the Day Hospital thus serving a primarily transitional function in returning these patients to full community living. Even in the beginning, however, from a quarter to a third of the patients were admitted to the Day Hospital without preceding inpatient services; too, practically all of the patients in the Day Hospital proper are admitted directly from the community on referral from physicians, community agencies, or outpatient and clinical services. On the whole, any patient who seems likely to benefit from therapy and who, along with his family, is willing to enter into a cooperative approach with the staff is considered suitable for admission.

The hospital day begins officially at 9:00 A.M. but the patients start arriving from 8:30 on. Occasionally, they drive their own cars to the hospital. Most often, they come by public transportation or are brought by a family member.

The Day Hospital operates from 9:00 to 4:00, Monday through Friday, but schedules are adjusted to the individual patient. Some arrive late or leave early, depending on transportation problems or family considerations. Some don't come every day. But each patient has his own schedule and is expected to adhere to it. If he doesn't put in an appearance at the given time and nothing has been heard from him, then the nurse phones his home — not to upbraid or discipline him, but to find out what the problem is and what can be done to help with it.

The Day Hospital is a self-contained unit within the larger hospital. A large living room is divided by halfway lattices into a number of smaller areas: a place to sit, read, or talk; a ping-pong and active games area; and a spot with a refrigerator and hot plate for coffee and snacks. Card tables, games, a piano, a sewing machine, and a radio are in frequent use. No television, though. This is considered too likely to foster withdrawal and isolation, but for special events — the World Series, for instance, a presidential inauguration, our first manned space flight — a television set is borrowed temporarily.

Adjacent to the large activity area are a number of smaller rooms: a sort of treatment or examining room with a small cot, which serves various purposes; a room with a record player for quiet listening or reading; offices for the psychiatrist, social worker, and other staff members; and a large, centrally located nursing office.

The latter bears little resemblance to the nursing office typical of the custodial type of institution: no locked doors, no shatterproof glass, no aspect whatsoever of an observation post in enemy territory. Instead it is a large, almost cluttered, somewhat shabby room, furnished with a desk, a few comfortable chairs, some straight ones, and plenty of "leaning" areas. A bulletin board on one wall contains not only official notices but also a random collection of cartoons culled from magazines and newspapers and poking fun at psychiatry. Patients as well as staff bring these in and they seem to be as much enjoyed by the one group as the other.

Aside from a medicine cabinet high on one wall, nothing is locked in this room and the door is rarely, if ever, closed. Patients, nurses, other staff members — in fact, anyone who has any business on the ward at all — wander freely in and out. At a given moment, a nurse may be giving a patient a medication in one corner; in another, an earnest conference is taking place between psychiatrist and social worker; and in still another, two patients are having a good-natured argument while waiting for the head nurse to hang up the phone and attend to them.

The atmosphere, not only in the nursing office, but throughout the entire Day Hospital, is definitely informal. Everyone wears street clothes and the visitor would be hard put to distinguish staff from patient, mostly because of the deceptively casual, give-and-take relationships that obtain between personnel and patients.

Neither the atmosphere nor the relationships, however, are as casual as they may seem. In almost every interaction between nurse and patient, for instance, the nurse's car is tuned for deeper implications, evidence of feelings and motivations, clues to problems and behavior.

In this calculatedly "open" environment, with no one arbitrarily dictating behavior or activities, the staff assumes — and makes clear in one way or another to the patients — that the latter are expected to act like responsible human beings. Realistic standards are set in matters of general behavior, dress, feeding, and toileting. When in the nursing office, patients are expected to respect the private conversations of others, to stay away from desk drawers, charts, and the like, and to make themselves scarce when requested. Rarely do they overstep their boundaries; they meet the expectations that are implicitly set before them.

The Therapeutic Goals

The philosophy of treatment in the Day Hospital, very generally stated, emphasizes four factors: psychotherapy, in individual or group settings or both; full use of the therapeutic milieu, with stress on meaningful staff-patient interrelationships; resocialization, as the patient is encouraged to take part in both the social and occupational activities of normal living; and a concerted effort to return the patient to full community living as soon as possible. Three months is the approximate period of hospitalization for Day Hospital patients.

Against the background of these general principles, the Day Hospital provides a place to which the patient can take his anxieties, people for him to relate to, and an opportunity for him to learn to understand his difficulties. The therapeutic plan is carefully modeled to meet each patient's individual needs, and is broad enough to include the family as well as the patient. Chemotherapy may also form part of the treatment and, in an occasional instance, convulsive shock therapy may be used.

Within the first few days of his admission, the patient's own doctor, nurse, and social worker meet with him and his family in an attempt to tailor a plan of care that will be most useful to all concerned. The same team — as well as other members of the staff who have become concerned with the patient — expedites this plan of care in cooperation with others, and reviews and re-evaluates it at frequent intervals in both formal and informal conferences.

The boundaries between the various disciplines represented on the Day Hospital staff tend to be fluid. Very roughly speaking, it might be said that the doctor is concerned with individual psychotherapy, the social worker with patient-family problems, and the nurse with maintaining a sociotherapeutic atmosphere and relationships. No one is yet prepared to spell out specifically, however, each one's "role" since the team approach is an integral part of the program.

Each staff member more or less works out his own relationship with the patient in line with the total therapeutic goal. There is free and frequent communication among all the personnel, a constant pooling and exchange of information, and cooperative planning as to approaches and attitudes.

The Patient's Day

The patient's day is not very formally structured. (Old line psychiatric nurses will remember the frequent calls: "Time for O.T., ladies" or "Time to go outdoors," and so on.) Each patient, however, is expected to spend at least two hours daily (this time increases as the patient improves) at some sort of work therapy: serving in the coffee or gift shop, typing in one of the offices, or lending a hand with the gardening in the greenhouse.

One of the most explicit objectives of this form of therapy is to build "work tolerance." The program is considered especially valuable, encouraging as it does a sense of responsibility, of participation in the normal workaday world of the well, of relationships with others, and of sharing in an activity of use to others.

In the course of the day, the patient will also have conferences, formal or informal, with doctor, social worker, or nurse. He will take part in the recreational activities on the ward or in other parts of the hospital. A small school with certified teachers is maintained for school-age patients, and they attend this regularly.

There may also be organized trips to a nearby bowling alley or to parks, museums, and other places of interest in the city. On occasion, the patient may prefer to sit quietly and read or listen to the radio. During the course of most days, too, he will spend some time with the nursing student who has been especially assigned to his case. Together they will explore feelings and attitudes as the student works on developing with the patient a relationship of true therapeutic significance.

Films are shown from time to time and there are also organized classes in such varied subjects as the modern dance, cooking, current events, or the Bible. Some of these classes are held in the Day Hospital itself. Others include patients from the other hospital services and may be conducted by occupational therapists, volunteers, or other hospital personnel, and may be held almost anywhere in the hospital. Generally speaking, however, it is the nurse who carries the major responsibility for group activities, although she brings in others — occupational therapists, theologians, volunteers — as needed.

Group meetings are held at scheduled times during the week, sometimes for the entire Day Hospital population, sometimes for a smaller segment of the group. Patients are expected to attend these sessions — one of the few structured elements in their day.

The group discussion leader may be the resident psychiatrist, a social worker, or one of the nurses. Each one of these, although drawing on the accepted principles of group dynamics, develops his own style of leadership and determines his own purpose. This means that both the content and form of the group sessions will depend to a considerable degree on the person leading the group.

The Nursing Staff

The nursing service of a 5-day-a-week day hospital has one great and unique advantage over conventional 24-hour nursing services: the same staff is there each day. For the nurses this means the elimination of one more problem in communication — passing on the day's information to the evening and then to the night staff. It means, too, that the nurses are on the scene during the patient's entire hospitalization, informed through their own presence of both problems and progress. A final and obvious advantage, of course, is that this system makes it possible to have more nurses available for day care.

For the patient, this setup not only cuts down on the number of people with whom he must establish relationships but, more importantly, assures him continuity of care, with a feeling of consistency in relationships. What may be important to him, for instance, is not just receiving a certain pill two or three times a day, but who gives it to him, her approach, and what the whole business of being medicated may signify to him. With the same nurse responsible for the same activities each day, a sense of stability and security is introduced into the patient's anxious world.

The professional nursing staff, which has grown steadily in numbers since the Day Hospital was first established, now numbers four: the head nurse, who has been with the unit since 1957, and three staff nurses. Stress for the staff in the early days was very great. Repeatedly they were asked to clarify the role of the nurse in the Day Hospital: how did it differ from social work? Was there a place for the nurse at all? The anxiety was great and often the nurses tended to fall back on traditional functions: ordering supplies, checking blood pressures, dispensing medications, and coordinating activities.

Today, however, there is no doubt that the nurse *is* a significant member of the staff of the day hospital, even though the nurses most intimately concerned are still exploring the full and exact potential of their contribution. As a social scientist who studied the day care program remarks, "The Day Hospital nurse engages in activities which are quite different from the traditional nurse's activities. Her work is much more oriented toward the patient's emotional life and toward his activity and participation in the unit."[2]

The head nurse, of course, in collaboration with the medical and social work staff, is the over-all administrator of the unit and coordinator of its activities. She is also a vital central link in the necessarily complex communication network. Finally, she is always available to talk with patients who may be having difficulties and to discuss with them problems arising from environmental stresses or intrapsychic conflicts.

Each of the three staff nurses has a specific area of responsibility. One is responsible for the social and recreational activities of the patients, both within and without the ward setting; another is in charge of medications and any physical treatments that may be indicated; and the third plans and supervises the patient's work program.

Each of these areas has its own special significance for the nurse-patient relationship that develops, as well as its own special problems. Take medications, for instance, which might seem to be the routine affair it usually is in a general hospital of checking cards, preparing medicines, and making a quick trip through the ward to dispense them. Not in the Day Hospital, however.

To begin with, the patients are expected to come to the nursing office at specified times to receive their medications: this is their responsibility. They may be consistently early or consistently late — or they may "forget" to come at all. They may watch carefully, almost suspiciously, to be sure they receive the "right" pills from the "right" bottle, or be completely indifferent to the process; they may report each possible side effect with anxiety, or ignore obvious ones completely; they may see medication time as an opportunity to socialize or discuss problems, or as something to be gotten over with as soon as possible.

Whatever their attitude or reaction, it is of concern to the medication nurse. It tells her something about their problems, and she recognizes that *her* reaction to *their* reactions may have as much significance as the medication itself. As soon as the nurse thinks it is feasible, incidentally, the patient is given a week's supply of his medication and expected to take care of it himself — this, to free him from dependence and to encourage self-reliance.

The fact that each nurse has her own special area of responsibility should not be interpreted as a return to the old "functional" approach to nursing. It means, rather, that each nurse has a specific contribution to make to the total therapeutic program, and a specific role to play in which she develops real expertness. This system also provides for consistency in nurse-patient relationships with the patient learning to whom he should turn and for what within this small community. Furthermore, each nurse, of course, develops relationships with all the patients — inside and outside her own particular area of responsibility — and she pools her observations and experiences with those of the rest of the staff.

Boston University School of Nursing undergraduate students have an eight-week clinical experience in psychiatric nursing in the Day Hospital during their senior year. In collaboration with the head nurse, their own instructor provides for a meaningful learning experience for them. Each nursing student is assigned to a doctor and social worker who join forces with her to make up a team which works with individual patients.

Often uneasy at first, the student soon grows in understanding of herself, the patient, and team interaction as she explores the developing relationship with "her" patients. Some patients she works with from admission through to discharge, participating in orientation, diagnostic and treatment plan formulation, and termination. In all, she contributes substantially to the total therapeutic plan.

Medical and social work students, in addition to nursing students, are also assigned to the Day Hospital. The entire student group brings to the unit youth, enthusiasm, and scientific curiosity which seem to have a wholesome and stimulating effect on the patients and staff. Through their presence, spontaneity, questions, and turnover, these students add even more flexibility and movement to an already dynamic environment.

Crisis Situations

Suicidal risk, of course, is always a concern of any institution or personnel caring for psychiatric patients. Its handling at the Day Hospital remains largely an area of judgment and of maintaining good communication with the patient and his family.

Occasionally, for this and other reasons, it becomes necessary to consider whether a particular patient at a particular time might not better be transferred to full-time hospitalization, at least for a while. Making the decision is again a matter of clinical judgment.

The patient or family may indicate, either verbally or in other ways, when this step seems indicated. The patient may seem overwhelmed in situations of daily living or may be temporarily "out of control." Sometimes his reactions or behavior constitute almost a direct request for someone to "take over," and the nurse's, doctor's, or social worker's ear soon becomes tuned to this unspoken plea.

What is important, when around-the-clock hospitalization for a period is decided upon, is that the situation be considered in the nature of a temporary upheaval, with a goal of returning the patient as rapidly as possible to the Day Hospital setting. In the meantime, while he is on full hospitalization, the Day Hospital staff still maintains contact with him so that ongoing medical and nursing relationships can be preserved.

Day Care on Inpatient Services

One of the outgrowths of the Day Hospital's demonstrated success in caring for patients who would once have been admitted for around-the-clock care has been the extension of day care to selected patients within the hospital's inservice population. Almost as soon as a patient is admitted to the Massachusetts Mental Health Center these days, consideration is given to the possibility of day care. Physician, nurse, and social worker discuss this with the patient and his family and, as soon as it seems therapeutically and socially feasible, day care is started.

This means that, on a given inpatient service, certain patients are in residence only during the day, returning to their own homes at night. (This situation is occasionally reversed. There have been instances where a patient holding a full-time job spends only his evenings and nights at the hospital, his therapeutic hours being arranged accordingly.) During his time at the hospital, the patient shares in all the activities — social, recreational, and therapeutic — of the full-time group.

Still another example of the flexibility of approach at the Massachusetts Mental Health Center is the fact that sometimes the family comes to the hospital instead of the patient returning to the family. One young mother on day care arrived at the hospital each day with her six-month-old baby. The sight of this baby placidly asleep in a playpen in an old-time seclusion room provides a sharp contrast between the old and the new in psychiatric care.

Implications for the Future

Until recently, hospitalization to most people has meant spending 24 hours a day under the direct care of the hospital staff when ill, and then being discharged home when well. With the rising costs of hospitalization, however, alternatives in care are developing — the system of progressive patient care in general hospitals, for instance, or the extension of home nursing care plans. Perhaps one of the most significant contributions to the present trend has been the increasing awareness of the fact that hospitalization, for both physical and mental illness, may create as many problems as it tries to resolve.

The traditional mental hospital system, with its borrowed medical-surgical orientation, fosters isolation, dependency, and a lack of self-direction. The mentally ill person's relationships with people, especially with his family, have broken down, and only in the setting of family and community relationships can effective therapy take place.

One of the most vexing problems in psychiatric therapy has been the loss of contact between patient and family; at first, this is unwittingly fostered by enforced separation, but eventually grows into lack of emotional investment as the months and years accumulate. It often becomes virtually impossible for the patient to return to the community after contact with home breaks down.

The advent of day care for psychiatric patients gets around many of these difficulties. It permits — in fact, almost insists — that the sick person continue his relationships with family and community. It provides an opportunity for psychiatric and nursing care to be truly therapeutic, integrated into a framework of more or less normal family and community living.

Also lending support to the day care idea is the fact that more and more individuals are seeking psychiatric help and at an earlier stage of illness than they once did. The public is becoming better informed about the importance of prevention and early recognition and treatment of mental illness, and the stigma once associated with psychiatric disorders is gradually disappearing.

Day hospitals — and, in some places, night hospitals — plus the development of psychiatric clinics and units in general hospitals make it more and more possible for these individuals to receive the help they need in a meaningful therapeutic setting and without too much disruption of their personal, family, and community relationships.

The patient in turmoil, needing full-time hospitalization during an acute phase, will probably be with us for some time to come. So, in all likelihood, will be the patient who needs temporary asylum from a very disturbed relationship with his family and community. The feeling at the Massachusetts Mental Health Center is, however, that as the medical and nursing staff become more comfortable with the trend toward noninstitutionalized care and more skilled in administering it, increasing numbers of patients can be cared for on a day care basis.

References

1. Kramer, B.M. *Day Hospital; A Study of Partial Hospitalization in Psychiatry.* Boston, Massachusetts Mental Health Center, 1960, Preface, pp. III-IV. (Mimeographed)

2. Ibid, Chap. 3, pp. 9-10.

The Joint Commission Report on Mental Illness and Health: Implications for Nursing Administration

Annie Laurie Crawford, R.N., M.Ed.

Ms. Crawford is with the Florida State Board of Health, Jacksonville, Florida.

Reprinted from *The American Journal of Psychiatry*, Vol. 119, No. 6, December 1962.

The report has identified three problem areas: *Manpower; Facilities;* and *Costs.* These are problems common to many programs, with some special dimensions for programs dealing with mental illness and health.

Recommendations providing a suggested blueprint for action are offered under three major headings: *Pursuit of New Knowledge; Better Use of Present Knowledge and Experience;* and *Cost.* The report is an impressive document with implications for nursing which usually challenge but sometimes dismay.

The problems identified by the Joint Commission are known to every nurse administrator. The extent to which the nurse administrator can meet the challenge of the recommendations by finding new and better ways of dealing with the problems will determine the effectiveness, to a significant degree, of the nursing profession in this as in other health programs.

The first task of the nurse administrator is to assure herself and her staff at least a potentially friendly climate for practice. The nature of the professional nurse's role and function in mental health and the care of mentally ill patients is not as clearly understood nor is it at all times as sharply defined as it is in many other health promoting and conserving programs. The direct or indirect effect of policies and decisions of numerous governmental agencies and units, such as the budget bureau, the Civil Service System, the institution or agency personnel officer, and others, on the climate for professional practice cannot be ignored. This is equally true in many instances for her professional organizations. She cannot assume, even when the evidence seems fairly conclusive, that people lack understanding (which they may) or wish to deliberately hamper her. While she may not, because of the administrative structure of the agency, have any face-to-face contact with the budget bureau director, her knowledge of the processes can help her clear shoals when dealing with her immediate supervisor. In her communications with her professional organizations she must be prepared to defend objectively and expertly her conviction that certain of the organization activities support while others hamper her administrative efforts to provide optimum nursing care for patients.

Next, it is necessary to consider the objectives of the nursing service. Are these clearly defined and available in a concise, realistic, understandable, and *stimulating statement,* and apparent in the *working environment* of every nursing unit in the hospital and in the community nursing agency? How competent in the nursing care of mentally ill patients, support to the family with mental health problems, and as a participant in preventive mental health programs is the nurse administrator? This is a vital question, particularly to directors of general hospital nursing services acquiring psychiatric inpatient units and to directors of public health and community nursing services, where an agency assumes family supportive and patient follow-up service.

The problem of *manpower,* of persons who seek out opportunities to nurse the mentally ill, has been with us since the first human being became mad. Since it is apparent that workers in the field of mental illness and mental health have been beset or immobilized by manpower shortages even when there was a surplus of people wanting jobs, the current widespread manpower shortage should do little to comfort us. It may be that national attention to the needs in our field will finally mobilize more creativity and industry in dealing with it. However, there would seem to be a serious question about whether we may not be required to shift gears hurriedly to more careful selection and more effective and realistic training because of a flood of young workers, and an increase of older women, in the labor market. (The Bureau of Labor Statistics reports that we will absorb 29 million additional workers by 1970 — most of them youths and older women.) There is already some evidence that some of these are nurses — and that others will be preparing for nursing in community colleges.

Large numbers of potential workers for this field were ignored in the 1930's. Nurses, most of whom had no training in psychiatric nursing, made the rounds of hospitals looking for work or sat by silent telephones awaiting calls for private duty, while thousands of mentally ill patients sat on dingy hospital wards, many of them tied into straight jackets, and from week to week did not even see a professional nurse. Even then some voices were raised, May Kennedy's, and your speaker often brought this question up at meetings. We believed then that it would have been possible to interest state hospital superintendents and the nurses in a cooperative effort to have hospitals offer housing and maintenance and plan educational programs useful to the nurses. If we reflect on the role of nursing in the development and expansion and in the excellence of general hospital patient care, we can reasonably speculate that the Commission Report might be telling a somewhat different story if nursing leadership could have been mobilized then. We know that public health nursing expanded and became a tremendous force for health during that period, often through installation of community nursing services under WPA. With this second opportunity to assume aggressive leadership in providing a decent standard of nursing care for the mentally ill, psychiatric nurses dare not fail to do so.

The manpower we need, and during the decade ahead will have a chance to get, will require the opportunity and tools to promote programs designed to prevent mental illness (with measurable results), to restore the mentally ill person to a healthy state, and to participate in rehabilitation which makes the person who has been sick a functioning member of society. The prestige and the remuneration which doing important work deserves will also be expected.

Nursing administration must recognize the enormous importance of volunteers, e.g., both the community worker and the summer college student for direct service to patients and for recruitment of workers. The patient's environmental climate is primarily the business of nursing. The psychiatric nurse in the mental health clinic, the public health nurse in the community, and the psychiatric nurse on the hospital ward, individually and collectively, have opportunity to promote immediate and long range goals for nursing service through productive contact with volunteers. These are the citizens of today and tomorrow whose knowledge of and tolerance for the ex-patient may mark the difference in whether he can survive at home during a crisis (for which the clinic is best equipped to help) or, following brief general hospital or extensive state hospital treatment, can return to a welcoming, not a rejecting, family and neighborhood.

In addition to regular orientation, instruction, and guidance for volunteers, nurses can conduct classes for other community groups (*Mental Hygiene* classes taught in the evening by the director of nursing were attended by stenographers, beauticians, saleswomen and others, in Idaho, early in the 1940's). Florida psychiatric and public health nurses, employed by county health departments, are meeting regularly with relatives of hospitalized mentally ill patients, with the focus on understanding, tolerating and setting limits when a relative returns from hospitalization.

The Commission has said that we must pursue *new knowledge*. The nurse administrator must prepare and support her staff so that they too, no matter how busy, *tolerate and encourage* thinkers in their ranks. One of the characteristics which sets the nurse apart, not only to the public, but to herself, is that of being a *doer*. The public health nurse has perhaps reached a higher level of achievement in allowing for thinking, but she too is sometimes shaken by the "be you a talking nurse or a doing nurse" question.

The report speaks of venture or risk capital; the nurse administrator will need to indulge in a good deal of venture or risk policy and procedure — even to make better use of present knowledge and experience. This will take courage, and the willingness to admit that the unworkable is, or for the time and place at least appears to be, unworkable. We have come a long way in recognizing the right and the *responsibility* of the physically ill person to participate freely in his own recovery process. We have not come even the first mile in many places toward allowing the mentally ill patient this right, nor preparing, even pushing him toward this responsibility. I do not believe that nurses should assume full credit for the *status quo* — we have distinguished friends and co-workers who share our failure to act. Let us be bold and imaginative now, and thus demonstrate that we have come of age professionally.

Nurse administrators will be expected in the *pursuit of new knowledge* and in the *better use of present knowledge and experience* to provide for more visible collaborative effort, in achieving and maintaining a healthy person and family, between the psychiatric nurse and the public health nurse, and among these nurses and others of the investigative and treatment groups (psychiatrists, public health physicians, behavioral scientists, and others).

The report suggests that we place more emphasis on the obvious that patients with major mental illnesses are different in significant ways from the physically ill. Almost everyone is aware that the mentally ill patient may at times behave impulsively and irresponsibly. This is not, I am sure, what the

Commission is referring to. I would endorse wholeheartedly the suggestion that we give more thoughtful attention to the significant difference and to the similarities, particularly in the orientation and training of students and new staff. Nursing administrators need to be sensitive to responses to staff members to, or even the stimulating of, bizarre behavior on the part of the patient. The manic is often charming — the paranoid patient a trouble maker, a convincing fabricator.

The diagnostic procedure and the planning of treatment for the mentally ill patient, in clinic or hospital (large state, small private, and to some extent in general hospital units) is one area where staff needs to understand certain differences clearly in order to participate appropriately in the "team or multidisciplinary approach."

Even as we emphasize differences we also need to be sure that the young staff nurse with traditional training is aware that there are some basic similarities between this and the approach which she daily experiences on the medical or surgical ward — the Lab report, the pathologist's findings, the result of x-ray reading, *etc.* This is a multidisciplinary approach but the emphasis for this "team" for whom the physician is undisputed captain is on presenting certain specifically confirmed information to the captain so that he can make a diagnosis and prescribe treatment.

In the case of the mentally ill patient, physicians, nurses, social workers, psychologists, occupational and recreational workers, aides and attendants sit around the table disclosing and discussing the most intimate aspects of the patient's life experience and relationships. Sometimes I have wondered a bit uncomfortably about how one could really distinguish a certain "staffing of a patient" from a general gossip session. I do not wish to imply that the staffing approach is inappropriate, but to emphasize the difference which I believe we must consciously prepare personnel to recognize and make use of in appropriate ways. We have at times emphasized the need for extensive information as a requisite for providing nursing to the point where nursing instructors and students feel frustrated and thwarted when the hospital's policy limits access to social and family history data and the psychiatrist refuses to sit down and discuss his patient with them. Until we have conclusive evidence that extensive information *gathered by others* about the patient facilitates nursing care success, we are on extremely tenuous ground when we demand this as an essential to demonstrate our nursing skills.

The nurse administrator might take the lead in planning staff conferences through which the nurse shares with her peers and co-workers what *she* has learned about a patient, and how she has used this information to facilitate a nursing care plan which is contributing to the promotion and restoration of health for the patient or is helping him and his family to learn more effective ways of dealing with crises.

Considering yet another dimension, members of the nursing staff need to consider the economic and social significance that confining all diabetics or heart disease victims in large barn-like institutions would have, and in so doing be challenged to find ways to help the mentally ill patient return to the community as a functioning member of society. Thus we avoid the immobilizing effect of professional preoccupation with "curing" which is sometimes more of an unrealistic attempt to make the patient into someone we like than a realistic plan to help him mobilize his resources to deal with his environment in an acceptable way. Humane treatment is not necessarily incompatible with coaxing, pushing (even shoving a little) a patient toward self responsibility.

One of the more obvious places where nursing can begin is in providing patients with an opportunity to behave and work responsibly while in hospital. As an example of this we might ask how much latent energy for nursing is sitting idly about the wards of many state hospitals. How many physically healthy schizophrenic women could and would profit by the assumption on the part of the nursing administration that they too, at some time in their lives, wanted to "nurse the sick." There are literally thousands of these women doing this work now — errand girls and aides on infirmary wards — and we can add a new approach for the already productive working patient by taking steps to help her see her work as an ingredient of her health potential. She needs to view her work as a step toward becoming a functioning member of society rather than as a pass to a few state hospital privileges.

Many can be trained by nurse supervisors and instructors, and made to feel that they are accepted and respected enough to be accorded status and trust. This does not imply *unsupervised responsibility* for the wellbeing of fellow patients. We might begin with lightly supervised or unsupervised responsibility for self by providing living quarters where the duty and the freedom to report for work is given. Let this be the base on which assignment to nurse's aide work is established. This would make sense to the patient and provide for her some sense of orderliness in progression to healthy activity.

The nursing aide is only one of many illustrations of steps toward responsible achievement the patient can and should take in the hospital. Of all personnel, nurses are in the most strategic position to assess the patient's readiness to and interest in going forth into a life of productivity. Nurses must assume more professional responsibility for bringing these observations to the psychiatrist.

The opportunity for innovation, for experimentation, and for creative action in planning for and providing nursing care available to the psychiatric nurse has always been its greatest appeal to me as a field of practice. To make credible this difference, and to provide the atmosphere for creative practice, is the ultimate in administration of nursing services to the mentally ill. I believe this is in keeping with the Commission Report implications in its recommendation that we make better use of existing knowledge and experience.

As an immediate and long range response to the Commission Report I believe that nursing administrators in state mental hospitals should immediately assume aggressive leadership in requiring an acceptable level of preparation of all workers through preservice, in-service and on-the-job training programs. The nursing administrator is the only person who can effectively demand and assume responsibility for requiring trained workers. This is only valid, however, if she has a plan. She will need to know what resources she can use, whether she can request assistance from vocational education, community colleges, and the extension service of the university. Many nurse administrators could begin by requiring that all schools of nursing sending students for instruction and clinical experience provide a faculty in this as in other clinical areas. Faculty members employed by the state hospital could then be released to instruct employed personnel, many of whom are at this time untrained workers assigned and paid to nurse the mentally ill.

The nurse administrator in the general hospital with a psychiatric unit or service often faces two inappropriate choices. If she can get a specialist she must often pay her a higher salary than she does other supervisors, adding to internal stresses, or she cannot find a specialist available and must therefore select from her staff the best equipped person. In this situation she needs easy ccess to consultation and an opportunity for some on-the-job training for the nurse selected. In Florida, nurse administrators have both resources available. Consultation is available in some areas through the county health department, if the mental health worker is a psychiatric nurse, in others through the State Board of Health training and research program. On-the-job training is available in the psychiatric unit of the university hospital. (If the director of nursing has had no prior preparation in psychiatric nursing, she should be the first to seek the on-the-job training.) It would seem that the specialist, when available, might best be used as a general nursing service supervisor, thus making her special skills available to all nursing service units.

In all types of facilities the nurse administrator should have specialist staff available to intensive care units so that the newly admitted patient can be continuously attended during the first days, or through crises. The modern general hospital considers an intensive care unit for medicine and surgery a necessity — expensively equipped and staffed with expert nurses. The psychiatric patient does not usually need the expensive equipment, but is in equally urgent need of the expert nursing care if recovery and rehabilitation are to be assured.

In the Commission's discussion of facilities many areas have direct and far reaching implications for nursing administration. The suggestion was made that large state mental hospitals be converted to multipurpose chronic disease hospitals with more nurses, occupational therapists and aides, and fewer psychiatrists. Is it to be expected that people, even chronically ill ones, will willingly submit to this type of isolation? What of the nurses and aides? There are hundreds of unfilled budgeted positions for professional nurses in isolated state mental hospitals now. There are few nurse positions unfilled in either general hospital or in mental health in public health. Outpatient departments and mental health clinics have too few psychiatric nurses, but this is because there are as yet few positions available to psychiatric nurses in these facilities.

I will only comment briefly on the *cost,* and not at all in terms of the cost of patient care as presently defined in all reports. Hospital insurance plans are constantly expanding, so today's figures are out-of-date tomorrow. I believe the nursing profession should put emphasis on the use of money where it seems most relevant — in recruiting, training and employing the nurses who will contribute significantly to abandonment of the need for large chronic disease institutions. We need particularly to expand our efforts in community nursing programs; we need to recruit talented youth and to strengthen preparation in psychiatric and public health nursing. In collaboration with psychiatric nurses, public health nurses can assume more responsibility in promotion of health, in prevention, in early case finding and referral, in support to individuals and families in time of crisis, and in support to the mentally ill patient who can manage at home on the job with this support. We need *enough* highly skilled psychiatric nurses to give direct care to patients when needed, and to instruct and supervise less skilled nursing personnel so that the patient is assured effective nursing care.

The Nurse as a Clinical Specialist

Mary M. Redmond

Ms. Redmond is Associate Professor, School of Nursing Education, Director of Psychiatric Mental Health Nursing, Catholic University of America.

Reprinted from *Military Medicine,* November 1957.

Nursing originated, spent its formative years, and is today being practiced in what you and I know as a clinical situation. This situation may be described as being concerned with a person who has a disease or condition for which he needs medical care. In the modern clinical setting, one finds many professional and non-professional people, technological and scientific tools, much general and special equipment, and frequently a particularly designed physical structure being useful in the medical care program.

The actual performance of nursing varies to some extent in every clinical setting and this poses a problem when one tries to describe the nurse as a clinical specialist. The components of a clinical setting are the patient, the personnel, and the environment. The person, who is commonly called the patient, is the heart of this setting. He is both the stimulus and the receptor of its action. The personnel become effective only to the degree that they recognize the significance of the patient. The environment, both in the physical and non-physical sense, becomes meaningful as it serves the purpose of the patient. We will not be concerned with the environment in this discussion only to the extent that we recognize the important contribution made to it by the people who live and work in it.

According to common usage, the term clinical nurse specialist implies that the nurse has a readiness to perform a superior quality of nursing. The clinical nurse specialist has educational preparation and/or experience in nursing which have given her an opportunity to increase her knowledge of medical and nursing science and to perfect her art and skill in the practice of nursing. The clinical specialties in nursing have developed largely in accordance with specialization in the field of medicine. Thus we have clinical nurse specialists in child and maternal health, cancer, tuberculosis, cardio-vascular disease, medical, surgical, neurological, and psychiatric nursing and many other areas. Nursing Education has organized nursing programs in graduate education to prepare clinical nurse specialists in some of these clinical areas. In other areas no educational program exists. The nursing profession as a whole differs from medicine in regard to specialization as it as not established standards for the practice of nursing in the various clinical fields. The medical profession has established qualifications, standards for practice and specialty board examinations to determine competence in many of the clinical areas of medicine. This may be a development in clinical specialization to which the nursing profession should give some attention.

As the science of nursing develops we recognize its significance and the various levels of performance in the nursing care of patients. Nursing in a general way is dependent upon physical, biological, and social science. It is also in a particular way dependent upon a knowledge of medicine, even of the special fields of medicine. For nurses to be equally prepared in all special areas of knowledge involved is both economically unsound and intellectually difficult at the same time. Therefore it seems to me to be potentially useful to examine preparation, qualifications and competencies desired in specialization in clinical nursing and to establish standards for practice of same. If we examine the practice of nursing in the various clinical areas we can identify the application of principles and concepts of the general and particular areas of science. Some sciences are more closely related to the practice of nursing in one clinical area than they are in another. For example, if we examine nursing activities or tasks in the care of patients with a cardiac illness, hemiplegia, psychiatric conditions or a child with cerebral palsy, we recognize the need for an applied knowledge of anatomy, physiology, pathology, psychology, epidemiology and other related sciences. The scientific ideas to which I refer are also used by all members of the health team, and the scientific knowledge which forms their basis makes it possible for the members of the health team to plan the patient's care, work together in his rehabilitation and aid families and the community in developing and understanding and assuming their responsibility in promotional, preventive and rehabilitation health programs.

Nursing in each of the highly specialized fields of medicine makes use of special skills, some of which are technical in nature but many of which are intellectual and judgmental. These skills are dependent upon human attitudes, understandings, and the personal characteristics of the nurse. The direct nursing care of patients in which the nurse gives care to the patients requires the artistic, often creative, use of skills so dependent upon scientific knowledge that when separated from it the actual nursing care becomes devoid of meaning and non-therapeutic. The indirect nursing care of patients in which the nurse performs tasks away from the patients, but related to his needs and welfare, likewise requires planning and implementation based on scientific knowledge. We have only to think of the recent treatment advances in the development of cardiology, surgery, psychiatry and tuberculosis to realize that the knowledge necessary to do therapeutic nursing is not static. Rather it requires new and dynamic concepts and is, therefore, based upon a continuous learning process which is both stimulating and challenging to the nurse who is a clinical specialist.

One may also think of the nurse as a clinical specialist, as being able to meet the nursing needs of patients regardless of their condition or disease entirely. Such a nurse has a high degree of actual or practical skill in nursing. This is identified in her work as she effectively accomplishes planning and administering nursing care, observation of patients, assisting physicians, creating and maintaining therapeutic environments, health teaching, socializing and other functions necessary in the rehabilitation of patients.

All clinical nursing is patient or family centered. To meet the nursing needs of patients is its goal. Some of the differences inherent in clinical nursing functions are due to the individual patients whose needs require different satisfactions. Patients' needs differ in many ways. His personality, self concept, future goal, family and cultural background, life's experience, occupational preparation and achievement always influence his needs. Likewise, his state of health, disease entity if sick, treatment reactions, and expectation of future dependencies or independency are determinants of his needs. They very often are grouped as physical, social, psychological, mental, spiritual and religious needs. However, it is well to think through these general terms in order to clarify their significance in the actual practice of nursing. It is also well to remember *no need* is found separately or alone but rather each depends and is entwined in another.

Each nurse is also an individual person and, therefore, brings to the practice of nursing characteristics unlike any other nurse. These characteristics influence the quality and effectiveness of the work done in nursing patients. They are so much a part of the person who is the nurse that it is difficult to see them, but they are reflected in the quality of nursing which she gives to patients.

The nurse-patient relationship is the enveloping structure in which all nursing activity occurs. The interaction which occurs in this relationship gives the patient the support, the nursing necessary for his comfort and promotion of sustained effort to meet with courage and realism the daily happenings in his period of stress. He develops from this experience strengths helpful in his future life.

Nursing has a goal of rehabilitation and recovery which it serves well. On the other hand realistic thinking makes us realize that recovery is not always possible. The nurse-patient relationship and the activities which it supports also brings comfort to the patient for whom recovery is impossible. In a measure this relationship stands its greatest test in the care of the dying patient whether he is young or old.

The nurse-patient relationship is predicated upon knowledge of oneself and the patient. This is brought about by physical and personal contact in a therapeutic social climate as the nurse ministers to the patient. She listens to him, communicates her respect, trust and love for him. She administers his medicine, diagnostic tests and treatments, observes his responses to treatment and other behavior, teaches and supports him in self care methods, guides and aids him in daily living activities and their modifications necessary for his rehabilitation. She assists him in planning for his self-development and healthy adjustment in his future life experiences. The communication going on between the nurse and the patient is both the cause and the means of their relationship. Communication is the means by which the nurse functions. In this way she knows the feelings of the patient and he realizes her feelings toward him. There is a supporting bond established which promotes his progress toward recovery or sustains and maintains his comfort in the event of the terminal illness.

The nurse has either the direction or the support of medical authority as she cares for patients. This gives her the responsibility of planning with the physician for the care of the patient and of reporting to him the patient's progress as she sees it. The nursing care that evolves in the nurse-patient relationship is both an integral part of this relationship and an extension of the overall comprehensive care of patients. Communications between nursing and allied professional workers is a pertinent means of insuring the effectiveness of the comprehensive care program.

Communications between allied workers are based upon knowledge and respect for each other's discipline as well as of each other. The morale, mutual understanding and co-operation of these allied workers in a comprehensive treatment program is reflected in the care of patients and in their rehabilitation. The nurse has a significant function in bringing about an effective communicating system to integrate and co-ordinate the excellent contributions of the many allied specialists that meet the needs of patients.

In summary my concept of the nurse as a clinical specialist may be briefly stated as follows:

Such a nurse will be specially qualified by educational preparation and/or experience to (1) competently develop the nurse-patient relationship, (2) give a fine quality of nursing care to meet the nursing needs of all patients, (3) perform expert nursing in a particular clinical setting in which medical specialization makes special demands on her knowledge and skill in giving care to individual patients who have particular disease conditions and (4) through her communications with patients and with allied professional and other workers, assists in an integration, co-ordination and extension of a comprehensive care which either influences the recovery of patients or sustains and comforts them in a terminal illness.

Bibliography

Anderson, Camilla: The Self-Image: A Theory of the Dynamics of Behavior, *Mental Hygiene*, 36:227-244, April, 1952.

Bird, Brian: Psychological Aspects of Pre-Operative and Post-Operative Care, *The American Journal of Nursing*, 55:685-687, June, 1955.

Brown, Esther Lucille: The Social Sciences and Improvement of Patient Care, *The American Journal of Nursing*, 1148-1151, September, 1956.

Caseley, Donald J.: Trends in Medical Practice — Their Implications for Nursing, *Nursing Outlook*, 57:300-302, May, 1957.

Greenhill, Maurice H: Interviewing with a Purpose, *The American Journal of Nursing*, 56:1259-1262, October, 1956.

Kreuter, Frances Reuter: What is Good Nursing Care, *Nursing Outlook*, 57:302-304, May, 1957.

Muller, Theresa: *Foundations of Human Behavior*, New York: G.P. Putnam's Sons, 1956.

Schwartz, Morris S. and Shockley, Emery: *The Nurse and the Mental Patient*, New York: Russell Sage Foundations, 1956.